Felice Eugenio Agrò

Editor

Body Fluid Management

From Physiology to Therapy

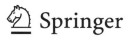 Springer

Editor
Felice Eugenio Agrò, MD
Commander to the Order of Merit of the Italian Republic
Full Professor of Anesthesia and Intensive Care
Chairman of Postgraduate School of Anesthesia and Intensive Care
Director of Anesthesia, Intensive Care and Pain Management Department
University School of Medicine Campus Bio-Medico of Rome
Rome, Italy

ISBN 978-88-470-2660-5   e-ISBN 978-88-470-2661-2

DOI 10.1007/978-88-470-2661-2

Springer Milan Dordrecht Heidelberg London New York

Library of Congress Control Number: 2012942793

© Springer-Verlag Italia 2013

9 8 7 6 5 4 3 2 1   2013 2014 2015 2016

Cover design: Ikona S.r.l., Milan, Italy
Typesetting: Graphostudio, Milan, Italy
Printing and binding: Esperia S.r.l., Lavis (TN), Italy

Printed in Italy

Springer-Verlag Italia S.r.l. – Via Decembrio 28 – I-20137 Milan
Springer is a part of Springer Science+Business Media (www.springer.com)

Body Fluid Management

This book is due for return on or before the last date shown below.

Preface

The present monograph is a useful guide to fluid management. It describes the physiological role of fluids and electrolytes in maintaining body homeostasis, underling the essential fundamentals needed for clinical practice.

It is addressed mainly to practitioners and post-graduates, but is clearly accessible to graduate students and undergraduates as well. It reviews, refreshes, and intensifies the basic concepts of fluid management while also providing a new perspective on its role in daily practice.

The book begins with a discussion of the core physiology of body water, specifically, the various compartments, as well as electrolytes, and acid-base balance. Subsequent chapters provide a detailed description of the main intravenous solutions currently available on the market and explain their role in the different clinical settings, presenting suggestions and guidelines but also noting the controversies concerning their use. At the end of each chapter the boxes "Key Concepts" and "Key Words" help the reader retaining the most relevant concepts of the chapter, while the box "Focus on..." suggests literature and other links that expand on the material discussed in the chapter, satisfy the reader's curiosity, and offer novel ideas.

The chapter on the economic issues associated with fluid management in clinical practice reflects the Editor's intent to include in this volume one of the most important issues in the daily routine of all practitioners.

Finally, the chapter "Questions and Answers" summarizes the main concepts presented in the volume. It offers a useful, rapid consultation as an overview at the end of the volume.

The contributions of different authors with expertise in specific clinical areas assure the completeness of the monograph and serve to offer a variety of perspectives that will broaden the reader's professional horizons and stimulate new research.

Rome, August 2012   Felice Eugenio Agrò

Acknowledgements

This monograph would not have been possible without the efforts of many people who, in one way or another, contributed and extended their assistance throughout its preparation and who have been instrumental in its successful completion.

First and foremost, I gratefully acknowledge my contributors, Marialuisa Vennari, Maria Benedetto, Chiara Candela, and Annalaura Di Pumpo, for their constant and steadfast support. Thank you for your patience and the care that you lavished in carrying out this project.

It is with great pleasure that I offer my deep and sincere gratitude to my friend, the engineer Gianluca De Novi, for his efforts and approach to creating the illustrations contained in this monograph.

I would also like to express my special and deep appreciation to Romina Lavia, Visiting Researcher in my department, who was responsible for the linguistic aspects of the book. She carried out her work with great enthusiasm, commitment and cheerfulness, and her contributions were both accurate and punctual. Throughout the preparation of this monograph, she provided several useful additions and suggestions, improving the stylistic aspects of the sentences and paragraphs in order to better emphasize the main focal points of each section. I am truly grateful for the generosity of her efforts and wish her great success in her chosen career.

I would also like to thank the Anesthesia, Intensive Care and Pain Management Department of the University School of Medicine Campus Bio-Medico of Rome for providing us with the environment and facilities conducive to completing this project. Special mention goes in particular to Carmela Del Tufo, Valeria Iorno, Claudia Grasselli, Chiara Laurenza, Francesco Polisca, Lorenzo Schiavoni, and Eleonora Tomaselli.

I take immense pleasure in thanking Gabriele Ceratti, Kerstin Faude, and Sayan Roy for the friendly encouragement they showed throughout the preparation of this book and the valuable insights they shared.

Finally, I thank Marco Pappagallo and Michelle do Vale for their unselfish and unfailing support as my advisers.

The evolution of this book also owes a personal and beloved note of appreciation to my wife, Antonella, and my children, Luigi, Giuseppe, Francesco, Tania, Matteo Josemaria, and Rosamaria. They have been a source of constant support during the writing of this book. Thank you for your understanding and endless love.

Felice Eugenio Agrò

Contents

Contributors

Hans Anton Adams MD, Head, Staff Unit Interdisciplinary Emergency- and Disaster-Medicine Hannover Medical School - INKM OE 9050, Hannover, Germany

Maria Benedetto MD, Postgraduate School of Anesthesia and Intensive Care, Anesthesia, Intensive Care and Pain Management Department, University School of Medicine Campus Bio-Medico of Rome, Italy

Umberto Benedetto MD, PhD, Visiting Researcher Postgraduate School of Anesthesia and Intensive Care, University School of Medicine Campus Bio-Medico of Rome, Italy

Laura Bertini MD, Chief Pain Management and Anesthesia Unit, S. Caterina della Rosa Hospital, Rome, Italy

Chiara Candela MD, Postgraduate School of Anesthesia and Intensive Care, Anesthesia, Intensive Care and Pain Management Department, University School of Medicine Campus Bio-Medico of Rome, Italy

Massimiliano Carassiti MD, PhD, Director of Intensive Care and Pain Medicine Unit, University School of Medicine, Campus Bio-Medico of Rome, Italy

Rita Cataldo MD, Director of Anesthesia Department, University School of Medicine Campus Bio-Medico of Rome, Italy

Edmond Cohen MD, Professor of Anesthesiology, Director of Thoracic Anesthesia, Mount Sinai Medical Center, New York, USA

Roberta Colonna MD, Postgraduate School of Anesthesia and Intensive Care, Emergency Department, Politechnical University-School of Medicine, Ancona, Italy

Gianluca De Novi PhD, Harvard University, Harvard Medical School, Imaging Department, Massachusetts General Hospital, Boston, MA, USA; Visiting Professor Postgraduate School of Anesthesia and Intensive Care, University School of Medicine Campus Bio-Medico of Rome, Italy

Annalaura Di Pumpo MD, Postgraduate School of Anesthesia and Intensive Care, Anesthesia, Intensive Care and Pain Management Department, University School of Medicine Campus Bio-Medico of Rome, Italy

Dietmar Fries MD, PhD, Department for General and Surgical Critical Care Medicine, Medical University Innsbruck, Austria

Maria Grazia Frigo MD, Chief Department Obstetric Anesthesia, Fatebenefratelli General Hospital, Isola Tiberina, Rome, Italy

Boleslav Korsharskyy MD, Department of Anesthesiology and Pain Medicine, Montefiore Medical Center, Albert Einstein College of Medicine, New York, USA

Romina Lavia PhD, International Doctoral School of Humanities, Department of Linguistics, University of Calabria; Visiting Researcher Postgraduate School of Anesthesia and Intensive Care, University School of Medicine Campus Bio-Medico of Rome, Italy

Pietro Martorano MD, Head of Neuroanesthesia and Post Neurosurgical Intensive Care Unit, AO "Ospedali Riuniti" Ancona, Italy

Florian R. Nuevo MD, Consultant Anesthesiologist, University of Santo Tomas Hospital, City of Manila, Philippines; Philippine Heart Center, Quezon City, Philippines

Robert Sümpelmann MD, PhD, Medizinische Hochschule Hannover, Klinik für Anästhesiologie und Intensivmedizin, Hannover, Germany

Peter Slinger MD, Department of Anesthesia, Toronto General Hospital, Toronto, On, Canada

Marialuisa Vennari MD, Postgraduate School of Anesthesia and Intensive Care, Anesthesia, Intensive Care and Pain Management Department, University School of Medicine Campus Bio-Medico of Rome, Italy

Carlo Alberto Volta MD, Anesthesia and Intensive Care Medicine, Section of Anesthesia and Intensive Care Medicine, University of Ferrara, S. Anna Hospital, Ferrara, Italy

Physiology of Body Fluid Compartments and Body Fluid Movements

Felice Eugenio Agrò and Marialuisa Vennari

1.1   Body Water Distribution

The human body is divided into two main compartments: intracellular space (ICS) and extracellular space (ECS). The ECS is divided into three additional compartments: intravascular space (IVS, plasma), interstitial space (ISS), and transcellular space (TCS) (Fig. 1.1). These compartments contain the body water and are surrounded by a semi-permeable membrane through which fluids pass from one space to another and which separates them.

The water within the body accounts for approximately 60% of body weight; it is mainly distributed in the ECS and ICS. The ICS contains nearly 55% of total body water, and the ECS approximately 45% (about 15 L in a normal adult). Among the three compartments the IVS accounts for about 15% of ECS water, the ISS for nearly 45%, and the TCS for about 40% (Fig. 1.1).

The TCS is a functional compartment represented by the amount of fluid and electrolytes continually exchanged (in and out) by cells with the ISS and by the IVS with the ISS (Fig. 1.2). Other fluids composing the ECS are secretions, ocular fluid, and cerebrospinal fluid [1].

1.2   Main Properties of Body Fluids and Semi-Permeable Membranes

Fluid and electrolyte balance is both an external balance between the body and its environment and an internal balance between the ECS and ICS, and between the IVS and ISS. This balance is based on the specific chemical and

M.Vennari (✉)
Postgraduate School of Anesthesia and Intensive Care, Anesthesia, Intensive Care and Pain Management Department, University School of Medicine Campus Bio-Medico of Rome, Rome, Italy
e-mail: m.vennari@unicampus.it

F. E. Agrò (ed.), *Body Fluid Management*,
DOI: 10.1007/978-88-470-2661-2_1, © Springer-Verlag Italia 2013

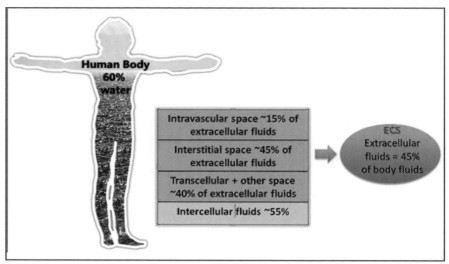

Fig. 1.1 Body water distribution representation

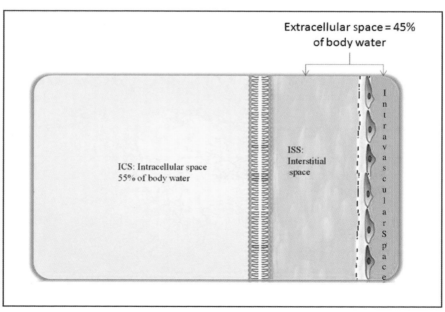

Fig. 1.2 The body's fluid compartments

Table 1.1 Main properties of body fluids

Properties	Plasma	Interstitial fluid	Intracellular fluid
Colloid-osmotic pressure (mmHg)	25	4	-
Osmolality (mOsmol/kg)	280	280	280
pH	7.4	7.4	7.2
Na^+ (mmol/L)	142	143	10
K^+ (mmol/L)	4	4	155
Cl^- (mmol/L)	103	115	8
Ca^{2+} (mmol/L)	2.5	1.3	< 0.001

physical properties of body fluids, such as ionic composition, pH, and protein content. It is also based on the properties of semi-permeable membranes, such as osmolarity, osmolality, tonicity, osmotic pressure, and colloid-osmotic pressure (Table 1.1).

1.3 Ionic Composition of Body Fluids

1.3.1 Sodium

1.3.1.1 Physiological Role
Sodium is the main determinant of ECS volume, being the most highly represented cation in the ECS. It plays a critical role in determining osmolarity and the volumes of the ICS and ECS. It contributes to renin-angiotensin-aldosterone system activation and regulates ADH secretion [2].

1.3.1.2 Daily Requirement
Sodium requirements depend on age: adults need about 1.5 mEq/kg/d, while newborns require a higher daily intake (2–3 mEq/kg/d), and neonates a lower one (0.5 mEq/kg/d) [2].

1.3.1.3 Normal Concentration
The normal sodium concentration in plasma and the ISS is about 142 mmol/L and it is higher than the ICS concentration (10 mmol/L) [2].

1.3.1.4 Metabolism
Sodium balance is determined by the balance among daily losses and daily intakes. Intakes are mainly due to alimentation, and losses to urinary excretion. Other losses may be due to vomiting, diarrhea, sweating, and burns. The kidneys are the central regulators of sodium homeostasis: they increase natriuresis after a sodium load and trigger antinatriuresis when sodium intake is reduced [2].

Sodium (Na+)
Sodium is one of the central ions in the human body. It is necessary for reg-
ulation of the blood and body-fluids volume, for the transmission of nerve
impulses, for cardiac activity, and for certain metabolic functions. It plays
an indirect hemodynamic role.

1.3.1.5 Hyponatremia

Definition
Hyponatremia is a condition of reduced plasma sodium concentration (< 135 mEq/L). Since sodium is closely related to water body balance, hyponatremia is associated with alterations of this balance. In particular, it may cause a reduction of ECS water.

Causes
The most common causes of hyponatremia are
- vomiting;
- sweating;
- diarrhea;
- burns;
- excessive administration of diuretics.

Hyperproteinemia or chylomicronemia may lead to a factitious (normotonic) hyponatremia. Hyperosmolality due to conditions such as hyperglycemia or mannitol overdose dilutes the ECS sodium concentration by drawing water from the ICS to the ECS. The syndrome of inappropriate antidiuretic hormone secretion (SIADH) is another cause of diluting hyponatremia. It can arise as a paraneoplastic syndrome or in association with pulmonary (sarcoidosis) or cranial disorders. In advanced heart failure, severe hypovolemia, and cirrhosis with ascites, ADH release is altered and the kidneys' capacity to dilute urine is reduced, leading to hyponatremia [2].

Signs and symptoms
Hyponatremia symptoms depend on the severity of the sodium deficit. Clinical features are:
- weakness;
- nausea;
- vomiting;
- modification of consciousness (agitation, confusion, coma, seizures);
- visual alteration;
- cramps;
- myoclonus.

When the sodium level falls below 123 mEq/L, cerebral edema occurs; at a sodium concentration of 100 mEq/L, cardiac symptoms develop.

In diluting hyponatremia, an increase in IVS volume can lead to pulmonary edema, hypertension, and heart failure [2].

Treatment

The first-line treatment of hyponatremia is elimination of the underlying cause. The second line is correction of the sodium deficit, generally through intravenous sodium administration.

The dose of sodium required to correct hyponatremia may be calculated using the following formula:

Sodium deficit (mEq) = (130 mEq - measured serum Na mEq) × Total body water

where Total body water = (body weight in kg) × (0.6 in men and 0.5 in women).

Thus, a 70 kg man with a plasma sodium of 120 mEq/L requires the administration of 1167 mEq of sodium:

Sodium deficit (mEq) = (130 mEq - 120 mEq) × (70 kg) × 0.6= 1167 mEq

A slow rate (maximum rate = 0.5 mEq/L/h) of correction is always indicated, because rapid correction can cause central pontine myelinolysis [3].

In case of hypervolemia, it may be preferable to utilize water restriction and a diuretic, such as furosemide.

1.3.1.6 Hypernatremia

Definition

Hypernatremia is a condition characterized by an ECS sodium concentration > 145 mEq/L. The total body sodium content, however, may be low, normal, or high.

Causes

The major causes of hypernatremia are:
- excessive loss of water;
- inadequate intake of water;
- lack or resistance to ADH (diabetes insipidus);
- excessive intake of sodium.

Signs and Symptoms

Generally, a slight increase in sodium concentration (e.g., 3–4 mmol/L) elicits intense thirst. Consequently, thirst is one of the first symptoms of hypernatremia. Other symptoms are:
- lethargy;
- reduction of consciousness, up to coma and convulsions;
- peripheral edema;

- myoclonus;
- ascites and/or pleural effusion;
- tremor and/or rigidity;
- increased reflexes.

If hypernatremia develops slowly, it is well tolerated because the brain is able to regulate its own volume in response to ECS volume and osmolarity changes. Acute and severe hypernatremia may lead to a shift of water from the ICS, causing brain shrinkage and tearing of the meningeal vessels, with the risk of intracranial hemorrhage [2].

Treatment

Hypernatremia management is based on normal osmolarity and volume restoration. It includes diuretics and the administration of hypotonic crystalloids or dextrose solutions. The rate of correction depends on the symptoms and the development of hypernatremia (acute, subacute, or chronic). Regardless, a more rapid correction may lead to brain edema [3].

1.3.2 Potassium

1.3.2.1 Physiological Role

Potassium is the main cation of the ICS (155 mEq/L). It plays a central role in determining the resting cell membrane potential, especially for excitable cells (neurons, myocytes), and it is crucial for renal function. It influences the transmission of nerve impulses and the contraction of muscle cells (included myocardial cells). It is also involved in a variety of metabolic processes, including energy production and the synthesis of nucleic acids and proteins [2].

1.3.2.2 Daily Requirement

Potassium needs depend on age. Newborns require 2–3 mEq/kg/d, while adults require a lower daily intake (1.0–1.5 mEq/kg/d). Metabolic status also influence potassium requirement (2.0 mEq/100 kcal).

1.3.2.3 Normal Concentration

The normal potassium concentration in plasma is about 4.5 mmol/L. Extreme hyperkalemia (>5.5 mEq/L) or hypokalemia (<3.5 mEq/L) can be life-threatening: either one may cause alterations in electrical impulse conduction, leading to the dysfunction of excitable cells. In particular, hyper- and hypokalemia may induce alterations in cardiac pacemaker activity, predisposing the patient to the onset of serious arrhythmias [2].

1.3.2.4 Metabolism

Potassium metabolism has two different regulatory mechanisms in relation to time. In the long term, the kidneys regulate serum potassium concentrations through the actions of aldosterone. An augmented ECS potassium concentration stimulates aldosterone production by the adrenal glands. Aldosterone acts on cortical collecting ducts, increasing potassium tubular secretion and reducing potassium reabsorption. Thus, renal potassium excretion increases when intake increases.

In the short term, many factors regulate potassium homeostasis: pH and bicarbonate concentration (acidosis causes hyperkalemia, while alkalosis causes hypokalemia); insulin secreted by the β-cells of the pancreas (the glucose pump uses potassium ions for cellular glucose transport); and β-adrenergic system activation (which reduces potassium plasma levels) [2].

> *Potassium (K⁺)*
> *Potassium is the major cation in the intracellular space. It is important in allowing cardiac muscle contraction and conduction and in sending nerve impulses. It plays a major role in kidney function.*

1.3.2.5 Hypokalemia

Definition
Hypokalemia occurs when the potassium plasma concentration is < 3.5 mEq/L. It may be caused by:
- an absolute deficiency of total body potassium stores;
- an abnormal shift of potassium from the ECS to the ICS (despite a normal total potassium).

Causes
Common causes of hypokalemia are:
- gastrointestinal losses;
- excessive renal excretion;
- reduced intake
with an absolute potassium deficit; and
- alkalosis;
- insulin therapy;
- catecholamine release;
- hypokalemic periodic paralysis
with a potassium shift from the ECS to the ICS.

Signs and Symptoms
In a normal adult, a net loss of 100–200 mEq of total body potassium corresponds to a reduction of 1 mEq/L of serum potassium. Accompanying signs and symptoms depend on the potassium level. Arrhythmias (frequently, atrial fibrillation and premature ventricular beat) and other electrocardiographic abnormalities (sagging of the ST segment, T wave depression, and U-wave elevation) may appear at potassium concentrations < 2.5 mEq/L [2].

Treatment

The rate of potassium administration must be adjusted considering the distribution within the ECS. The administration rate is limited to 0.5–1.0 mEq/kg/h. For potassium correction, intravenous potassium chloride is most commonly used [2].

1.3.2.6 Hyperkalemia

Definition

Hyperkalemia occurs when the potassium plasma concentration is > 5.5 mEq/L. It may be the consequence of an increase in total potassium body stores or of a shift of potassium from the ICS to the ECS (cellular lysis, acidosis).

Causes

Hyperkalemia may be due to:
- various renal and non-renal diseases;
- drugs;
- potassium shifts from the ICS to the ECS.

In most cases, hyperkalemia reflects a reduced renal excretion of potassium. Since potassium excretion is largely due to tubular secretion rather than glomerular filtration, hyperkalemia usually does not occur in patients with kidney diseases until a marked reduction of glomerular filtrate has developed, causing uremia.

Adrenal dysfunction (due to disease or drugs), with reduced aldosterone production, can lead to potassium retention. Cellular lysis (i.e., hemolysis or tumoral lysis after treatment) may cause hyperkalemia through a shift of potassium from the ICS to the ECS and should therefore be considered in the differential diagnosis [2].

Signs and Symptoms

Muscular weakness, up to paralysis, is one of the main manifestation of hyperkalemia. Cardiac signs are increased automaticity and repolarization of the myocardium, leading to ECG alterations and arrhythmias. Mild hyperkalemia (6–7 mEq/L) may appear with T waves and a prolonged P-R interval; severe hyperkalemia (10–12 mEq/L) may cause a wide QRS complex, asystole, or ventricular fibrillation [2].

Treatment

The management of hyperkalemia includes cardiac protection and treatments favoring the ICS redistribution of potassium. Rapid-effect therapies are the administration of calcium gluconate, insulin with glucose (considering the patient's glycemia), bicarbonate, and hyperventilation (to correct acidosis). They are used in acute as well as severe conditions. Additional therapies are resin exchange, dialysis, diuretics, aldosterone agonists, and β-adrenergic agonists. All of these approaches are effective in the long term [2].

1.3.3 Calcium

1.3.3.1 Physiological Role

Several extra- and intracellular activities are regulated by calcium action. Calcium is involved in: endocrine, exocrine, and neurocrine secretion; coagulation activation; muscle contraction; cell growth, enzymatic regulation; and in the metabolism of other electrolytes.

1.3.3.2 Normal Concentration

The normal plasma calcium concentration is 2–2.6 mEq/L. In an adult, 99% of total body calcium (generally 1.3 g) is contained in the teeth and bones. Only 1% of bone calcium is exchangeable with other body compartments to make up for any lack. Calcium may circulate in the plasma bound to albumin (40% of total plasma calcium) and free from proteins. Free calcium may be ionized and physiologically active (50% of total plasma calcium) or non-ionized and chelated with inorganic anions such as sulfate, citrate, and phosphate (10% of total plasma calcium). Free calcium is filtered by the kidneys, while the bound form is not. The amounts of the three forms may change and are altered by many factors, such as total plasma protein levels, percentage of anions associated with ionized calcium, and pH. In particular, pH modifies the bound fraction, while plasma proteins alter ionized and bound fractions. Generally, we measure total plasma calcium, which may be adjusted for protein plasma levels [2].

1.3.3.3 Metabolism

The correct balance of calcium reflects daily intake, intestinal absorption, and renal excretion. The kidneys are the main organ responsible for regulating calcium levels. The amount of filtered calcium is quite completely reabsorbed by the tubules.

The stability of serum calcium concentrations is the result of a complex interaction between three hormones: parathyroid hormone (PTH), 1,25-dihydroxycholecalciferol (vitamin D), and calcitonin.

PTH, released by the parathyroid glands, is probably the most important protection against hypocalcemia. After calcium depletion, PTH stimulates renal reabsorption and reduces excretion. It also induces a rapid mobilization of bone calcium and phosphate. Furthermore, PTH influences the metabolism of vitamin D, which increases the proportion of dietary calcium that is absorbed by the intestine.

Calcitonin is secreted by thyroid C cells. It tends to reduce the plasma calcium concentration by increasing cellular uptake, renal excretion, and bone synthesis. The effects of calcitonin on bone metabolism are much weaker than those of PTH [2].

Calcium (Ca⁺⁺)
Calcium is the most abundant mineral in the human body. It plays a vital
role in the coagulation cascade, in signal transduction pathways, and in
muscle contraction.

1.3.3.4 Hypocalcemia

Definition
Hypocalcemia is a calcium plasma concentration lower than 2 mEq/L. It refers
to ionized calcium levels in the plasma and develops when calcium concentrations are low but plasma protein levels are normal. It can be better recognized
by measuring only the ionized fraction.

Causes
Hypoalbuminemia is the most common cause of hypocalcemia.
Other causes are:
*   PTH deficiency (primary and secondary);
*   renal failure (reduced activation of vitamin D);
*   renal tubular diseases (increased calcium losses);
*   reduced calcium intake;
*   malabsorption;
*   vitamin D3 deficit;
*   cholestasis (deficit in vitamin D absorption).
    A deficiency of vitamin D may be due to reduced cutaneous activation (in
the elderly, reduced exposure to UV rays) and to a reduced intake (malabsorption, malnutrition).
    Hypocalcemia may also be due to acute hyperventilation or to excessive
blood cell transfusions that contain citrate. It is common also during sepsis but
the pathogenetic mechanisms are not fully understood.

Signs and Symptoms
The main clinical manifestations of hypocalcemia are due to the increased cardiac and neuromuscular excitability, and to the reduced contractile force of
cardiac and vascular smooth muscle.
    Tetanic syndrome, a result of increased neuromuscular excitability, is char-
acterized by numbness (especially around the mouth, lips, and tongue) and
muscle spasms, particularly in the hands, feet, and face (characteristic are
Chvostek and Trousseau signs).
    Regarding the cardiovascular alterations, hypocalcemia causes prolonga-
tion of the PQ interval, which predisposes patients to the onset of severe ventricular arrhythmias. Hypocalcemia may also lead to hypotension.
    Nervous symptoms are due to the impaired mental status [2].

Treatment
Hypocalcemia treatment should be causal, but should also be aimed at quickly increasing the serum calcium concentration. It may be corrected by administering 10% calcium chloride (1.36 mEq/mL) or calcium gluconate (0.45 mEq/mL) [2].

1.3.3.5 Hypercalcemia

Definition
Hypercalcemia is a plasma calcium concentration > 2.6 mEq/L.

Causes
Hypercalcemia may be caused by:
- increased intestinal calcium absorption;
- excessive skeletal calcium release;
- decreased renal calcium excretion.

Other causes are renal failure, hyperparathyroidism, tumors, and alteration of vitamin D production.

Signs and Symptoms
Main symptoms of hypercalcemia may be remembered using the rhyme: "groans (constipation), moans (psychic moans, e.g., fatigue, lethargy, depression), bones (bone pain, especially in hyperparathyroidism), stones (kidney stones), and psychiatric overtones (including depression and confusion)." Other symptoms are anorexia, fatigue, vomiting, and nausea. ECG alteration such as a short QT interval or widened T wave are suggestive of hypocalcemia. Symptoms are common at high calcium concentration (> 3 mEq/L). Severe hypocalcemia (> 3.75–4 mEql/L) is a medical emergency. It may lead to coma and cardiac arrest [2].

Treatment
Hypercalcemia management involves increased diuresis and plasma dilution. Accordingly, diuretics and saline solutions are used, because sodium reduces calcium re-absorption by the kidneys. Other treatments are calcitonin, bisphosphonate, glucocorticoids, and ambulation. It is always important to identify and cure the underlying cause.

1.3.4 Magnesium

1.3.4.1 Physiological Role
Magnesium is the physiological antagonist of calcium. It plays a crucial role in neuromuscular stimulation; it also acts as a cofactor of several enzymes involved in the metabolism of three major categories of nutrients: carbohydrates, lipids, and proteins.

1.3.5   Chloride

1.3.5.1 Physiological Role
Chloride is the most important anion of the ECS. Together with sodium, it determines the ECS volume. It is also responsible for the resting potential of the membrane, acid-base balance, and plasma osmotic pressure [2].

1.3.5.2 Normal Concentration and Metabolism
In the body, chloride is mainly present as sodium and potassium chloride. The normal plasma chloride concentration is 97–107 mEq/L. Blood levels are related to both the chloride present in red blood cells and the chloride free in the blood. Chloride absorption occurs in the first section of the small intestine, through an exchange with bicarbonate; elimination occurs primarily via the urine and feces, but also through sweat. Thus, chloride metabolism is strongly associated with that of sodium and bicarbonate and with systems regulating acid-base balance.

Chloride (Cl⁻)
Chloride is responsible for the extracellular fluid volume, together with sodium. It is particularly involved in acid-base balance and in signal transduction by nerve cells.

1.3.5.3 Hypochloremia

Definition
Hypochloremia is characterized by plasma chloride concentrations < 97 mEq/L.

Causes
Hypochloremia is always associated with other electrolytic and acid-base imbalances. The most common causes are increased renal or gastric losses (vomiting or gastric aspiration). Hypochloremia also appears with metabolic or respiratory alkalosis, subsequent to blood bicarbonate variation and acid-base equilibrium compensation.

The reduction in blood chloride levels leads to reduced bicarbonate excretion by the kidneys and increased sodium reabsorption [2].

Signs and Symptoms
Hypochloremia is often asymptomatic. Symptoms are generally linked to the other alterations that accompany hypochloremia.

Treatment
Hypochloremia must be treated by restoring plasma volume and acid-base balance. The underlying cause must be identified and cured.

1.3.5.4 Hyperchloremia

Definition
Hyperchloremia is as a condition characterized by plasma chloride concentrations > 110 mEq/L.

Causes
Hyperchloremia may be caused by:
- hyperparathyroidism (primary and secondary):
- excess intake;
- inadequate excretion due to renal failure and renal disease, such as renal tubular acidosis type I and type II.
    Other causes are diarrhea and drugs (diuretic, hormonal therapies).
    Predisposing conditions are hyponatremia and diabetes mellitus. Hyperchloremia can be also due to increased chloride intake (especially with intravenous fluid administration), with metabolic acidosis. In fact, hyperchloremia is always linked to this alteration of acid-base balance. One of the most common iatrogenic causes of metabolic acidosis is diuretics.

Signs and Symptoms
Hyperchloremia is often asymptomatic. It may be associated with inadequate control of glycemia in diabetic patients, with diarrhea, and with vomiting. When symptomatic, its manifestation may be weakness, thirst, and Kussmaul's breathing because of metabolic acidosis [1, 3].

Treatment
The basis of hyperchloremia management is treatment of the underlying condition. The goals of treatment are: (a) to restore an adequate plasma volume, (b) to interrupt the action of any drug potentially aggravating the hyperchloremia, and (c) to assess renal function [3].

1.3.6   Bicarbonate

1.3.6.1 Physiological Role
Bicarbonate is the main buffer system of the blood. It plays a crucial role in maintaining acid-base balance. Two-thirds of the CO_2 in the human body is metabolized as bicarbonate, through the action of carbonic anhydrase. The equilibrium between CO_2 and bicarbonate leads to the elimination of volatile acid. The bicarbonate buffer system is described by the following equilibrium reaction:

$$CO_2 + H_2O \leftrightarrow H_2CO_3 \leftrightarrow HCO_3^- + H^+$$

When there is an increased concentration of H+, the system reacts by shifting the reaction equilibrium to the left (towards the production of CO_2); if the concentration of H^+ is reduced, the system moves to the right, resulting in the production of H^+. The bicarbonate buffer system works "in concert" with several organs. In particular, if the reaction is shifted to the right, the kidneys eliminate the excess H^+. When the reaction moves to the left, producing more CO_2, the lungs increase the respiratory rate in order to eliminate the excess. This compensation is rapid and is regulated by chemoreceptors that record the change in pH and the increase in the partial pressure of CO_2 (pCO_2), and thus stimulate the respiratory center. Bicarbonate has a normal plasma concentration of about 24 mmol/L [3].

> **Bicarbonate (HCO_3^-)**
> Bicarbonate is the main buffer system of the blood. It cannot be incorporated into electrolyte solutions as this causes the precipitation of carbonates. Thus, anions metabolizable as bicarbonate are used, most commonly: lactate, malate, and acetate.

1.4 Acid-Base Balance

Acid-base balance represents a complex mechanism through which the body maintains a neutral pH, in order to prevent protein degradation and alterations in biochemical reactions. This mechanism includes an inorganic buffer system, i.e., bicarbonate, and an organic buffer, i.e., hemoglobin and plasma protein. The kidneys and lungs, as described in the previous section, are involved in the elimination of acids or bases that are overproduced or that have accumulated [4].

1.4.1 Interpretation of the Physiology of Acid-Base Balance

Acid-base balance interpretation has been traditionally approached in a qualitative manner, which explains the potential for misunderstanding and disagreement. Recently, the literature has redefined the role of acid-base alterations in the clinical setting, especially in critically ill patients. Consequently, a quantitative perspective has revised our knowledge of the main control mechanisms of acid-base balance and therefore of acid-base physiology in general [5].

1.4.1.1 The Three Approaches
There are three approaches to interpreting acid-base balance physiology (Fig.1.3).

They use distinct variables derived from a set of master equations that can be transferred from one approach to the other two [6].

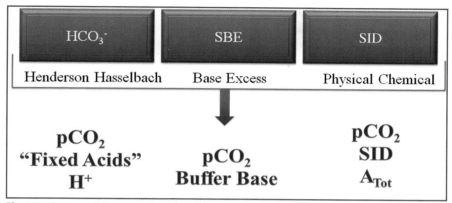

Fig. 1.3 Three possible approaches describing acid-base balance. Some factors (e.g., pCO_2) are considered by all approaches. *SBE,* Standard base excess; *SID,* strong ion difference; A_{tot}, total weak acid concentration

The Descriptive Approach

The traditional descriptive approach is based on arterial pH, pCO_2, and bicarbonate measurements. This approach originated at the end of the nineteenth century, when Henderson revisited the Law of Mass Action from an acid-base equilibrium perspective [7]. The result was:

$$[H^+] = Ka \bullet [HA]/ [A^-]$$

where H^+ is the hydrogen ion concentration in solution, HA is a weak acid, A^- a strong base and Ka the dissociation constant of the acid. Henderson's equation revealed that when [HA] = [A^-], [H^+] does not change as a result of small variations in the amount of acid or base in the solution.

In 1917, K.A. Hasselbach applied Henderson's equation to the main physiological buffer system (CO_2/HCO_3^-) using logarithms [6], giving rise to the Henderson-Hasselbach equation:

$$pH = pKa + log ([HCO_3^-]/[CO_2]).$$

The pCO_2 value describes the respiratory contribution (CO_2 elimination) to acid-base imbalances, while the metabolic contribution (acid overproduction, accumulation, reduced metabolism) is described by the bicarbonate concentration in the blood.

Since the 1940s, researchers have recognized the limitations of this approach to acid-base physiology: blood bicarbonate concentration is useful in determining the type of acid-base abnormality, but it is not able to quantify the amount of acid or base excess in the plasma unless pCO_2 is held constant [7]. This observation promoted research into a quantitative approach to acid-base balance, in order to quantify the metabolic component [7].

The Semi-quantitative Approach

In 1957, K.E. Jörgensen and P. Astrup developed a tool to calculate bicarbonate concentration, in which fully oxygenated whole blood was equilibrated with a pCO_2 of 40 mmHg at 37°C. This was called *standard bicarbonate*. However, subsequent studies determined the role of the body's other buffer systems (albumin, hemoglobin, and phosphates), which were not considered as either the bicarbonate concentration or the standard bicarbonate method.

In 1948, Singer and Hastings defined the sum of the non-volatile weak-acid buffers and bicarbonates as the "buffer base" [6] This led to several revisions of the method to calculate changes in the buffer base, including the base excess (BE) methodology [7-11]. BE is the quantity of metabolic acidosis or alkalosis, defined as how much base or acid should be added to an in vitro whole blood sample to reach a pH of 7.40, while the pCO_2 is maintained at 40 mmHg. The most widely used formula for calculating BE is the equation of Van Slyke [7, 13-15]:

$$BE = (HCO_3^- - 24.4 + [2.3 \times Hb + 7.7] \times [pH - 7.4]) \times (1 - 0.023 \times Hb)$$

where HCO_3^- and hemoglobin (Hb) are expressed in mmol/L. The standard base excess (SBE) is the BE when corrected for the buffer effect of hemoglobin; it better quantifies the acid-base status in vivo [15,16]. Nonetheless, when applied in vivo BE is still inadequate, since it changes slightly with fluctuations in pCO_2.

The Quantitative Approach

Another approach to acid-base pathophysiology is the calculation of the anion gap (AG) [8], which is the difference in the main measured plasma anion and cation concentrations $[(Na^+ + K^+) - (Cl^- + HCO_3^-)]$, expressed in mEq/L. The AG corresponds to the difference between non-measured anions and cations $[(Ca^{2+} + Mg2^+) - (PO_4^{3-} + SO_4^{2-} + organic\ anions + proteins)]$. Generally, AG values indicate a variation in the concentration of organic anions (lactic acidosis, ketoacidosis). A possible limit of the AG is the wide variability in both plasma albumin concentrations and renal function with respect to phosphate storage, especially in critically ill patients [7].

In the 1980s, P. Stewart introduced a new approach based on the Law of Mass Conservation, the electroneutrality of water, and three independent variables [7]:

- the *strong ion difference* (SID), which is the difference in the total amount of strong anions and cations
$SID = ([Na^+] + [K^+] + [Ca^{2+}] + [Mg^{2+}]) - ([Cl^-] + [A^-] + [SO_4^{2-}])$ (Fig. 1.4).
- PCO_2.
- Total weak acid concentration (A tot).

Stewart's approach considers the pH and the bicarbonate concentration as dependent variables.

The undissociated form of weak acids (HA) is neutral; the dissociated form (A^-) is negative. Their concentrations reflect the Law of Mass Conservation

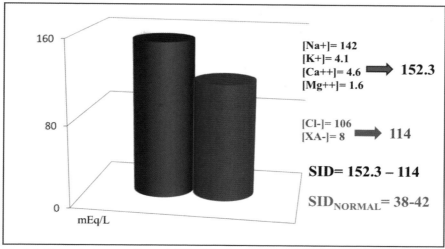

Fig. 1.4 Water electroneutrality and SID. *SID,* Strong ion difference; *XA-,* dissociated organic acids

$([Atot] = [A^-] + [HA])$ and the dissociation equilibrium $([H^+]*[A^-] = Ka * [HA])$.

In order to respect electroneutrality, SID determines the dissociation equilibrium of weak acids:

$$[SID] + [H^+] = [HCO_3^-] + [A^-] + [CO_3^{2-}] + [OH].$$

Consequently, it is physiologically positive and must be balanced by a corresponding excess of negative charges, between 38 and 42 mEq/L [7, 17].

When the concentration of non-volatile organic anions (e.g., lactate) increases, SID decreases [6, 16]. For example, if lactate increase to 20 mEq/L, the SID will decrease by the same value.

When CO_2 increases, bicarbonate increases to compensate for the respiratory acidosis and SID remains unmodified. For each 1 mEq/L increase in bicarbonate due to an increase in CO_2, A^- will necessarily decrease by 1 mEq/L, maintaining SID value.

SID decreases in metabolic acidosis and increases in metabolic alkalosis [7, 17].

1.4.1.2 Conclusions

The quantitative and qualitative approaches described above are easily interchangeable through simple mathematical manipulations [7].

Quantitative indices, such as the SID, may be used to understand the pathophysiological mechanisms underlying acid-base alterations, while descriptive indices, such as standard base excess (SBE) and the Henderson-Hasselbalch equation, can be applied to classify acid–base imbalances. The chemical behavior of the main plasma ions is also relevant for the behavior of infused fluids and their effects on the whole body [7].

1.5   Osmolarity and Osmolality

Osmolarity and osmolality are two of the main colligative properties of a solution. In fact, they are related to the number of dissolved particles. An understanding of the concepts described in the following sections requires a definition of the term "osmole": the number of particles dissolved in a solution.

1.5.1   Osmolarity

Osmolarity measure the concentration of a solution, expressed as the number of particles of solute per 1 L solution. Osmolarity is measured in milliosmoles per liter of solution (mOsm/L). It is calculated as the product of the molarity and the Van't Hoff coefficient, which considers the degree of dissociation of the solute present in the solution. For example, if a solution contains 1 mole of glucose or 1 mole of NaCl it will be 1 osmolar with respect to glucose (which does not dissociate in solution), while it will be 2 osmolar with respect to NaCl (which dissociates in solution into sodium ions and chloride ions) [18, 19].

1.5.2   Osmolality

Osmolality is another measure of the concentration of a solution, expressed as the number of particles per 1 kg water of solution. Osmolality is measured in milliosmoles per kilogram of water (mOsm/kg). Even if the concepts of osmolality and osmolarity are often associated, their meaning is indeed slightly different; in fact, osmolarity is an expression of solute osmotic concentration per volume of solution, whereas osmolality is per mass of solvent. Plasma osmolality is primarily regulated by ADH, a hormone produced by the pituitary gland in response to any increase in plasma osmolality (closely determined by the plasma sodium concentration). ADH determines an increase in water reabsorption by the kidney and thus correction of the increased osmolality [20, 21].

1.6   Osmotic Pressure, Tonicity, and Oncotic Pressure

1.6.1   Osmotic Pressure

Osmotic pressure (μ) is a property of solutions with different osmolarities and separated by a semi-permeable membrane. It is the force exerted by the sum of

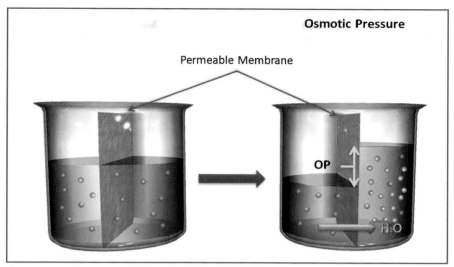

Fig. 1.5 In biological membranes, the movements of water in or out of the cells depends on the electrolyte concentration. According to the osmotic pressure, water diffuses from areas of low to those of high electrolyte concentration

osmotically active particles (electrolytes) that do not freely pass through semi-permeable biological membranes (which allow the passage of water but not of all solutes). When two solutions consist of the same solvent, but different concentrations of solute and are separated by a semi-permeable membrane, the solvent moves from the solution with a lower solute concentration to the solution with a higher one, to equilibrate the electrolyte concentration at the two sides of the membrane. This movement can be thwarted, arrested, or even reversed by applying pressure to the high-concentration compartment in order to oppose the passage of solvent through the semi-permeable membranes. This pressure is called the *osmotic pressure* [21-22].

1.6.1.1 Osmotic Pressure and Fluid Movement Across Biological Membranes

Osmotic pressure is one of the forces that regulate fluid movement across biological membranes. Thus, water will pass from low- to high-electrolyte concentration compartments to re-equilibrate the concentration on either side of the membrane [21, 22] (Fig. 1.5).

1.6.2 Tonicity

Tonicity is a comparative measure of the osmotic pressure of two solutions separated by a semi-permeable membrane. Under this condition, water shifts from the solution with lower osmotic activity (hypotonic solution with lower number of solute particles) to the solution with increased osmotic activity (hypertonic solution with higher number of solute particles). The osmotic pressure gradient between the two solutions is described as the tonicity [20].

1.6.2.1 Blood Tonicity

The tonicity of the blood is 288 ± 5 mOsm/kg H_2O. Plasma tonicity can be calculated by measuring the plasma concentrations of Na, Cl, glucose, and urea but the main determinant of plasma tonicity is the Na concentration. In addition, since plasma tonicity determines water's tendency to move in and out of the cell, the Na concentration is the main determinant of the relative volumes of the intra- and extracellular fluids [21].

1.6.2.2 Tonicity of Infused Solutions

In terms of blood tonicity, three different groups of infusible solutions can be distinguished:
*   hypotonic solutions, with lower tonicity than blood;
*   isotonic solutions, with similar tonicity to blood;
*   hypertonic solutions, with higher tonicity than blood.

The infusion of a hypotonic solution reduces the plasma osmotic pressure and causes water to move from the ECS to the ICS. An isotonic solution has the same tonicity as blood, such that the plasma osmotic pressure is maintained, without causing electrolyte imbalances. Finally, hypertonic solutions increase the plasma osmotic pressure, causing water movement from the ICS to the ECS.

1.6.3   Oncotic Pressure

Oncotic pressure, or colloid-osmotic pressure (π), is a form of osmotic pressure exerted by macro-molecules (proteins, particularly albumin) that cannot easily cross the semi-permeable membrane [21].

1.6.3.1 Oncotic Pressure and Fluid Movement Across Biological Membranes

Colloid-osmotic pressure is another force that regulates fluid movement across biological membranes. Thus, water will pass from low- to high-protein concentration solutions [21, 22] (Fig. 1.6).

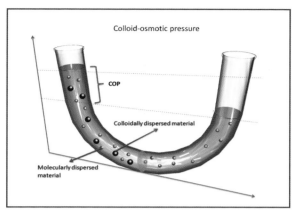

Colloid-osmotic pressure

COP

Colloidally dispersed material

Molecularly dispersed material

Fig. 1.6 According to the colloid-osmotic pressure, water diffuses from areas of low to those of high macromolecular concentration. Since biological membranes are impermeable to macromolecules, water migrates towards the latter

1.7 Fluid Movement Through Capillary Membranes

Fluids movements across capillary membrane are regulated by physical forces and the specific properties of both the semi-permeable membrane and the different compartments separated by it. Accordingly, electrolyte and protein concentrations as well as osmotic properties play a crucial role, as expressed in the Starling Equation.

1.7.1 Starling Equation

The Starling equation describes fluid movement through capillary membranes (Fig. 1.7):

$$J_v = K_f ([P_c-P_i] - \sigma [\pi_c-\pi_i]).$$

According to this equation, water flow depends on six variables:
1. Capillary hydrostatic pressure (P_c).
2. Interstitial hydrostatic pressure (P_i).
3. Capillary oncotic pressure (π_c).
4. Interstitial oncotic pressure (π_i).
5. Filtration coefficient (Kf).
6. Reflection coefficient (σ).

The equation states that the net filtration (J_v) is proportional to the net driving force ($[P_c - P_i] - \sigma [\pi_c - \pi_i]$). If this value is positive, water leaves the IVS (filtration). If it is negative, water enters the IVS (absorption) (Fig. 1.7).

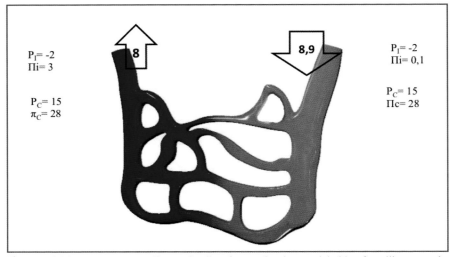

$P_I = -2$
$\Pi_i = 3$

$P_C = 15$
$\pi_C = 28$

$P_I = -2$
$\Pi_i = 0,1$

$P_C = 15$
$\Pi_C = 28$

Fig. 1.7 Fluid movement according to Starling forces. On the arterial side of capillary vessels, forces displacing water overcome those drawing it in. The opposite occurs on the venous side

Key Concepts
- Definition of body-water compartments and their composition
- Properties of semi-permeable membranes

Key Words
- Body water compartments (ECS, ISS, IVS, ICS)
- Electrolytic composition
- Acide-base balance
- Strong ion difference
- Semi-permeable membranes
- Osmolarity
- Osmolalitity
- Tonicity; blood tonicity
- Fluids movements
- Starling equation

Focus on...
- Venkatesh B, Morgan TJ, Cohen J (2010) Interstitium: the next diagnostic and therapeutic platform in critical illness. Crit Care Med (10 Suppl):S630-636

References

1. Chappell D, Jacob M, Hofmann-Kiefer K, Conzen P, Rehm M (2008) A rational approach to perioperative fluid management Anesthesiology 109:723-40
2. Miller RD (2009) Miller's anesthesia, 7 edn. Churchill Livingstone, UK
3. Bernsen HJ, Prick MJ (1999) Improvement of central pontine myelinolysis as demonstrated by repeated magnetic resonance imaging in a patient without evidence of hyponatremia. Acta Neurol Belg 99:189–93
4. Kellum JA, Weber PAW (2009) Stewart's textbook of acid-base, 2 edn. Lulu.Enterprises, UK
5. Kellum JA (2000) Determinants of blood pH in health and disease. Critical Care 4:6-14
6. Kellum JA (2005) Making strong ion difference the euro for bedside acid-base analysis. Intens Car and Emerg Medicine14:675-685
7. Kellum JA (2005) Clinical review: Reunification of acid–base physiology. Critical Care 9:500-507
8. Astrup P, Jorgensen K, Siggaard-Andersen O (1960) Acid-base metabolism: new approach. Lancet 1:1035-1039
9. Siggaard-Andersen O (1962) The pH-log PCO2 blood acid-base nomogram revised. Scand J Clin Lab Invest 14:598-604
10. Grogono AW, Byles PH, Hawke W (1976) An in vivo representation of acid-base balance. Lancet 1:499-500
11. Severinghaus JW (1976) Acid-base balance nomogram–a Boston-Copenhagen détente. Anesthesiology 45:539-541
12. Siggaard-Andersen O (1974) The acid-base status of the blood, 4 edn. William and Wilkins, Baltimore
13. Siggaard-Andersen O (1977) The Van Slyke equation. Scand J Clin Lab Invest 146:15-20
14. Wooten EW (1999) Analytic claculation of physiological acid-base parameters in plasma. J Appl Physiol 86:326-334
15. Brackett NC, Cohen JJ, Schwartz WB (1965) Carbon dioxide titration curve of normal man. N Engl J Med 272:6-12
16. Prys-Roberts C, Kelman GR, Nunn JF (1966) Determinants of the in vivo carbon dioxide titration curve in anesthetized man. Br JAnesth 38:500-550
17. Kellum JA, Kramer DJ, Pinsky MR (1995) Strong ion gap: a methodology for exploring unexplained anions. J Crit Care 10:51-55
18. Hendry EB (1961) Osmolarity of human serum and of chemical solutions of biological importance. Clin Chem 7:156-164
19. Olmstead EG, Roth DA (1957) The relationship of serum sodium to total serum osmolarity: a method of distinguishing hyponatremic states. Am J Med Sci 233:392-399
20. Glasser L, Sternglanz, PD, Combie J et al (1973) Serum osmolality and its applicability to drug overdose. Am J Clin Path 60:695-699
21. Voet D, Voet JG, Pratt CW (2001) Fundamentals of biochemistry. Wiley, New York
22. Mansoor MA, Sandmann BJ (2002) Applied physical pharmacy. McGraw-Hill Professional

Properties and Composition of Plasma Substitutes

2

Felice Eugenio Agrò and Maria Benedetto

2.1 Isotonicity

The choice of a non-blood plasma substitute should be guided by the properties of the targeted fluid space. Ideal IV fluids should be isotonic, should not cause electrolyte imbalance, and should contain metabolizable anions [1]. According to blood tonicity, the infusion of hypotonic or hypertonic solutions will change plasma osmotic pressure, resulting in an abnormal water flow.

2.1.1 Hypotonic Solutions

A hypotonic solution reduces plasma osmotic pressure, leading to the movement of water from the ECS to the ICS [2]. Cellular edema and lysis (i.e., hemolysis) may occur (Fig. 2.1). Larger volumes of hypotonic solutions have been known to produce a transient increase in intracranial pressure (ICP) [3], because of cerebral edema. The magnitude of this increase can be predicted by the reduction of plasma osmolarity [4]. Patients with an osmolality below 240 mOsmol/kg will fall into a coma, with a mortality rate of 50% [5]. Consequently, the infusion of large amounts of hypotonic solutions should be avoided, especially in cases of intracranial lesions such as cerebral hemorrhage and edema, cancer, or subdural hematoma.

M. Benedetto (✉)
Postgraduate School of Anesthesia and Intensive Care, Anesthesia, Intensive Care and Pain Management Department, University School of Medicine Campus Bio-Medico of Rome, Rome, Italy
e-mail: m.benedetto@unicampus.it

F. E. Agrò (ed.), *Body Fluid Management*,
DOI: 10.1007/978-88-470-2661-2_2, © Springer-Verlag Italia 2013

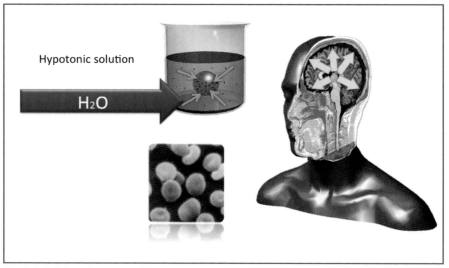

Fig. 2.1 Cellular edema caused by hypotonic solutions

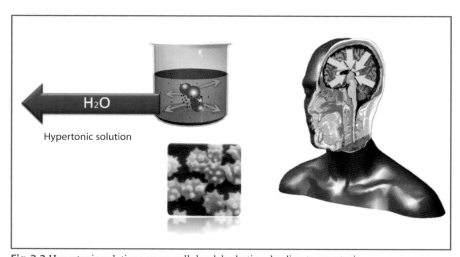

Fig. 2.2 Hypertonic solutions cause cellular dehydration, leading to apoptosis

2.1.2 Hypertonic Solutions

Hypertonic solutions increase plasma osmotic pressure, leading to water movement from the ICS to the ECS and cellular dehydration and, eventually, apoptosis (Fig. 2.2).

Many clinical settings may increase plasma osmotic pressure, with a very high mortality. In both hyperosmolar hyperglycemic non-ketotic syndrome and diabetic ketoacidosis, mortality is clearly correlated with plasma osmolality [6]. Hypovolemic shock also triggers hyperglycemia with hyperosmolarity [7], through the release of epinephrine [8] or through an increase in lactate blood levels [9]. In patients with multiple injuries, a hyperosmolar state correlates with increased mortality [9, 10]. It has been shown that in acute stroke patients, [11] multiple trauma patients [12], and ICU patients [13], non-survivors had a higher plasma osmolarity than survivors.

2.2 Electrolytic and Acid-Base Balances

When establishing fluid therapy, both acid-base and electrolyte iatrogenic disorders must be avoided [15, 16]. Generally, metabolic acidosis with hyperchloremia and hyperkalemia is the most frequent alteration [17, 18].

2.2.1 Balanced Plasma-Adapted Solutions

Depending on the electrolytic composition, IV solutions may be classified as balanced or unbalanced and plasma-adapted or not plasma-adapted. A balanced plasma-adapted solution is qualitatively and quantitatively similar to plasma. It contains sodium, chloride, potassium, magnesium, and calcium in the same concentrations as plasma and has metabolizable anions [1]. Except for the risk of fluid overload, the infusion of this solution reduces the incidence of side effects related to fluid management.

2.2.1.1 Balanced Plasma-Adapted Solutions and Hyperchloremia

Compared to other solutions, a balanced plasma-adapted solution has a lower chloride content. Clinical studies have revealed that chloride excess causes a specific splanchnic and renal vasoconstriction, interferes with cellular exchanges, and reduces the glomerular filtration rate (GFR), leading to sodium and water retention [19, 20]. Hyperchloremia is often associated with metabolic acidosis and may cause a further reduction in GFR [20]. It has been shown that balanced and plasma-adapted solutions help to avoid hyperchloremic acidosis, while assuring the same volume effect as unbalanced solutions but potentially reducing morbidity and mortality [1].

2.2.1.2 Balanced Plasma-Adapted Solutions and Physiological Buffer System

Currently available solutions used throughout the world do not contain the physiological buffer base bicarbonate because it cannot be incorporated into polyelectrolyte solutions, since carbonate precipitation would occur. For this reason, any fluid infusion may cause "dilutional" acidosis, i.e., a dilution of the HCO_3 concentration, while the CO_2 partial pressure (buffer acid) remains constant [21, 22]. This alteration may have catastrophic consequences, especially in critically ill patients with pre-existing acidosis. Replacing HCO_3- with metabolizable anions reduces the risk of dilutional acidosis. Metabolizable anions are organic anions that may be converted to HCO_3 by tissues. The main metabolizable anions are gluconate (gluconic acid), malate or hydrogen malate (malic acid), lactate (lactic acid), citrate (citric acid), and acetate (acetic acid). In IV fluid, the most frequently used metabolizable ions are acetate, malate, and lactate.

Acetate and malate are contained in plasma in very low concentrations. They may be metabolizable in all tissues, especially in muscles, liver, and heart [23]. Acetate is an early-onset (within 15 min) alkalizing anion [25-27], while malate has a slower action [26, 27].

2.2.1.3 Balanced Plasma-Adapted Solutions and Lactate

The most commonly used metabolizable anion is lactate, which is normally produced in the human body. In fact, lactate is the main product of anaerobic glycolysis. It is metabolizable only by the liver. However, the use of lactate has been matter of debate in clinical practice and in the literature, especially with respect to patients with pre-existing lactic acidosis. This condition is a manifestation of disproportionate tissue lactate formation due to impaired hepatic lactate metabolism [28, 29]. Lactate levels are a major criteria in the routine evaluation of critically ill patients [30-38]; indeed, changes in lactate concentration can provide an early and objective evaluation of patient responsiveness to therapy [38]. Furthermore, plasma lactate levels in the first 24–48 hours has a high predictive power for mortality in patients with various forms of shock, including cardiac, hemorrhagic, and septic shock [31, 33, 37-50]. In these situations, the administration of lactate-containing fluids may exacerbate the already existing lactic acidosis and interfere with lactate monitoring for diagnostic purposes [29, 50].

2.2.1.4 Balanced Plasma-Adapted Solutions and Base Excess

Another indicator of acidosis is base excess (BE). Since 1990, clinical trials have demonstrated that evaluating BE at the time of admission of critically ill patients is indeed the best prognostic indicator for mortality, complication rate, and transfusion needs, even in pediatric patients [51-59]. Persistent base disorders above or below 4 mmol/L differ with respect to mortality rate: 9% and 50%, respectively [60]. This is especially true for trauma patients, due to the risk of hemorrhagic shock [61-64]. Balanced, plasma-adapted solutions reduce the risk of acidosis and BE alterations. Common sense suggests that in critically ill patients any use of lactate-containing solutions should be avoided [65, 66] since the increase in lactate levels can precipitate pre-existing lactic acidosis or create diagnostic confusion regarding acid-base alterations (lactate and BE are independent indicators of mortality) [67, 68].

2.3   Conclusions

The use of isotonic, balanced and plasma-adapted solutions with metaboliz-able anions such as malate and acetate reduces the risk of iatrogenic acidosis, electrolytic imbalances and cerebral edema (Fig. 2.3).

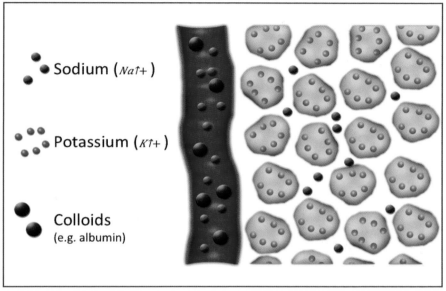

Fig. 2.3 Representation of sodium, potassium and albumin in the human body complements. Sodium is the main determinant of plasma tonicity and fluid distribution across body compartments. The sodium contained in an i.v. solution influences its pharmacokinetics

Key Concepts
- Influence of tonicity on the cell wall
- Definition of balanced and unbalanced solutions
- Definition of plasma-adapted and non-plasma-adapted solutions
- Comparison of the chemical composition and side effects of balanced and unbalanced solutions
- Comparison of the chemical composition and side effects of plasma-adapted and non-plasma-adapted solutions
- Dilutional and hyperchloremic acidosis: pathophysiology and prevention

Key Words
- Hypotonic, hypertonic, and isotonic solutions
- Balanced plasma-adapted solutions
- Metabolizable anions
- Base excess

Focus on...
- Wolf MB, Deland EC (2011) A mathematical model of blood-interstitial acid-base balance: Application to dilution acidosis and acid-base status. J Appl Physiol 110:988-1002
- Berend K (2010) Misconceptions about hyperchloremic acidosis. J Crit Care 25(3):532; author reply 532-3
- Use of the sodium-chloride difference and chloride-sodium ratio as surrogates for strong ion difference in the evaluation of metabolic acidosis in critically ill patients

References

1. Zander R (2006) Infusion fluids: why should they be balanced solutions? Eur Journ Hospital Pharmacy Practice 12:60-62
2. Williams EL, Hildebrand KL, McCormick SA et al (1999) The effect of intravenous lactated Ringer's solution versus 0.9 % sodium chloride solution on serum osmolality in human volunteers. Anesth Analg 88:999-1003
3. Tommasino C, Moore S, Todd MM (1988) Cerebral effects of isovolemic hemodilution with crystalloid or colloid solutions. Crit Care Med 16:862-868
4. Schell RM, Applegate RL, Cole DJ (1996) Salt, starch, and water on the brain. J Neurosurg Anesth 18:179-182
5. Arieff AI, Llach F, Massry SG (1976) Neurological manifestations and morbidity of hyponatremia: Correlation with brain water and electrolytes. Medicine 55:121-129

6. Jayashree M, Singhi S (2004) Diabetic ketoacidosis: Predictors of outcome in a pediatric intensive care unit of a developing country. Pediatr Crit Care Med 5:427-433
7. Boyd DR, Mansberger AR Jr (1968) Serum water and osmolal changes in hemorrhagic shock: An experimental and clinical study. Amer Surg 34:744-749
8. Järhult J (1973) Osmotic fluid transfer from tissue to blood during hemorrhagic hypotension. Acta Physiol Scand 89:213-226
9. Kenney PR, Allen-Rowlands CF, Gann DS (1983) Glucose and osmolality as predictors of injury severity. J Trauma 23:712-719
10. Kaukinen L, Pasanen M, Kaukinen S (1984) Outcome and risk factors in severely traumatized patients. Ann Chir Gynaecol 73:261-267
11. Bhalla A, Sankaralingam S, Dundas R et al (2000) Influence of raised plasma osmolality on clinical outcome after acute stroke. Stroke 31:2043-2048
12. Abel M, Vogel WM (1982) Osmolalitätsparameter und Nierenfunktion polytraumatisierter Intensivpatienten. Infusionsther 9:261-264
13. Holtfreter B, Bandt C, Kuhn SO et al (2006) Serum osmolality and outcome in intensive care unit patients. Acta Anaesthesiol Scand 50:970-977
14. Horn P, Münch E, Vajkoczy P et al (1999) Hypertonic saline solution for control of elevated intracranial pressure in patients with exhausted response to mannitol and barbiturates. Neurol Res 21:758-764
15. Dorje P, Adhikary G, Tempe DK (2000) Avoiding iatrogenic hyperchloremic acidosis: Call for a new crystalloid fluid. Anesthesiology 92:625-626
16. Mikhail J (1999) The trauma triad of death: Hypothermia, acidosis, and coagulopathy. AACN Clin Iss 10:85-94
17. Funk GC, Doberer D, Heinze G et al (2004) Changes of serum chloride and metabolic acid-base state in critical illness. Anaesth 59:1111-1115
18. Miller LR, Waters JH, Provost C (1996) Mechanism of hyperchloremic metabolic acidosis. Anesthesiology 84:482-483
19. Quilley CP, Lin YS, McGiff JC (1993) Chloride anion concentration as a determinant of renal vascular responsiveness to vasoconstrictor agents.. Br J Pharmacol 108:106-108
20. Wilcox CS (1983) Regulation of renal blood flow by plasma chloride. J Clin Invest 71:726-735
21. Shires GT, Holman J (1948) Dilution acidosis. Ann Intern Med 28:557-559
22. Asano S, Kato E, Yamauchi M et al (1966) The mechanism of the acidosis caused by infusion of saline solution. Lancet 1245-1246
23. Lundquist F (1962) Production and utilization of free acetate in man. Nature 193:579-580
24. Richards RH, Vreman HJ, Zager P et al (1982) Acetate metabolism in normal human subjects. Am J Kidney Dis 2:47-57
25. Mudge GH, Manning JA, Gilman A (1949) Sodium acetate as a source of fixed base. Proc Soc Exp Biol Med 71:136-138
26. Knowles SE, Jarrett IG, Filsell OH et (1974) Production and utilization of acetate in mammals. Biochem J 142:401-411
27. Akanji AO, Bruce MA, Frayn KN (1989) Effect of acetate infusion on energy expenditure and substrate oxidation rates in non-diabetic and diabetic subjects. Eur J Clin Nutr 43:107-115
28. Johnson V, Bielanski E, Eiseman B (1969) Lactate metabolism during marginal liver perfusion. Arch Surg 99:75-79
29. Levraut J, Ciebiera JP, Chave S et al (1998) Mild hyperlactatemia in stable septic patients is due to impaired lactate clearance rather than overproduction. Am J Respir Crit Carte Med 157:1021-1026
30. Abramson D, Scalea TM, Hitchcock R et al (1993) Lactate clearance and survival following injury. J Trauma 35:584-589
31. Bakker J, Gris P, Coffermils M et al (1996) Serial blood lactate levels can predict the development of multiple organ failure following septic shock. Am J Surg 224:97-102
32. Cowan BN, Burns HJ, Boyle P et al (1984) The relative prognostic value of lactate and haemodynamic measurements in early shock. Anaesthesia 39:750-755

33. Falk JL, Rachow EC, Leavy J et al (1985) Delayed lactate clearance in patients surviving cir-
     culatory shock. Acute Care 11:212-215
34. Friedman C, Berlot G, Kahn RJ et al (1995) Combined measurement of blood lactate con-
     centrations and gastric intramucosal pH in patients with severe sepsis. Crit Care Med 23:1184-
     1193
35. Henning RJ, Weil MH, Weiner F (1982) Blood lactate as a prognostic indicator of survival in
     patients with acute myocardial infarction. Circ Shock 9:307-315
36. McNelis J, Marini CP, Jurkiewicz A et al (2001) Prolonged lactate clearance is associated with
     increased mortality in the surgical intensive care unit. Am J Surg 182:481-485
37. Vincent JL, DuFaye P, Beré J et al (1983) Serial lactate determinations during circulatory shock.
     Crit Care Med 11:449-451
38. Rivers E, Nguyen B, Havstad S et al (2001) Early goal-directed therapy in the treatment of
     severe sepsis and septic shock. N Engl J Med 345:1368-1377
39. Levraut J, Ichai C, Petit I et al (2003) Low exogeneous lactate clearance as an early predic-
     tor of mortality in normolactemic critically ill septic patients. Crit Care Med 31:705-710
40. Weil MH, Michaels S, Rackow EC (1987) Comparison of blood lactate concentrations in cen-
     tral venous, pulmonary artery, and arterial blood. Crit Care Med 15:489-490
41. Marecaux G, Pinsky MR, Dupont E et al (1996) Blood lactate levels are better prognostic in-
     dicators than TNF and IL-6 levels in patients with septic shock. Intens Care Med 22:404-408
42. Holm C, Melcer B, Hörbrand F et al (2000) Haemodynamic and oxygen transport responses
     in survivors and non-survivors following thermal injury. Burns 26:25-33
43. Azimi G, Vincent JL (1986) Ultimate survival from septic shock. Resuscitation 14:245-253
44. Cady LD, Weil MH, Afifi AA et al (1973) Quantitation of severity of critical illness with spe-
     cial reference to blood lactate. Crit Care Med 1:75-80
45. Callaway D, Shapiro N, Donnino M et al (2007) Admission lactate and base excess predict
     mortality in normotensive elder blunt trauma patients. Acad Emerg Med 14:5(Suppl 1) S152
46. Milzmann D, Boulanger B, Wiles C et al (1992) Admission lactate predicts injury severity
     and outcome in trauma patients. Crit Care Med 20:S94
47. Peretz DI, Scott MH, Duff J et al (1965) The significance of lacticacidemia in the shock syn-
     drome. Ann NY Acad Sci 119:1133-1141
48. Rixen D, Raum M, Bouillon B et al (2001) Base deficit development and its prognostic sig-
     nificance in posttrauma critical illness. An analysis by the DGU Trauma Registry. Shock
     15:83-89
49. Vitek V, Cowley RA (1971) Blood lactate in the prognosis of various forms of shock. Ann
     Surg 173:308-313
50. Weil MH, Afifi AA (1970) Experimental and clinical studies on lactate and pyruvate as indi-
     cators of the severity of acute circulatory failure (shock). Circulation 41:989-1001
51. Davis JW, Parks SN, Kaups KL et al (1996) Admission base deficit predicts transfusion re-
     quirements and risk of complications. J Trauma 41:769-774
52. Rixen D, Raum M, Bouillon B et al (2001) Base deficit development and its prognostic signif-
     icance in posttrauma critical illness. An analysis by the DGU Trauma Registry. Shock 15:83-89
53. Rutherford EJ, Morris JA, Reed GW et al (1992) Base deficit stratifies mortality and derter-
     mines therapy. J Trauma 33:417-423
54. Siegel JH, Rivkind AI, Dalal S et al (1990) Early physiologic predictors of injury severity and
     death in blunt multiple trauma. Arch Surg 125:498-508
55. Davis J, Kaups KL, Parks SN (1998) Base deficit is superior to pH in evaluating clearance
     of acidosis after traumatic shock. J Trauma 44:114-118
56. Oestern H-J, Trentz O, Hempelmann G et al (1979) Cardiorespiratory and metabolic patterns
     in multiple trauma patients. Resuscitation 7:169-184
57. Randolph L, Takacs M, Davis K (2002) Resuscitation in the pediatric trauma population: Ad-
     mission base deficit remains an important prognostic indicator. J Trauma 53:838-842
58. Sander O, Reinhart K, Meier-Hellmann A (2003) Equivalence of hydroxyethyl starch HES
     130/0.4 and HES 200/0.5 for perioperative volume replacement in major gynaecological sur-
     gery. Acta Anaesthesiol Scand 47:1151-1158

59. Smith I, Kumar P, Molloy S et al (2001) Base excess and lactate as prognostic indicators for patients admitted to intensive care. Intensive Care Med 27:74-83
60. Kincaid, EH, Miller PR, Meredith JW et al (1998) Elevated arterial base deficit in trauma patients: A marker of impaired oxygen utilisation. J Am Coll Surg 187:384-392
61. Ruttmann TG, James MFM, Finlayson J (2002) Effects on coagulation of intravenous crystalloid or colloid in patients undergoing peripheral vascular surgery. Br J Anaesth 89:226-230
62. Jacob M, Chappell D, Hofmann-Kiefer K et al (2007) Determinanten des insensiblen Flüssigkeitsverlustes. Anaesthesist 56:747-76
63. Hahn RG, Drobin D (2003) Rapid water and slow sodium excretion of acetated Ringer's solution dehydrates cells. Anesth Analg 97:1590-1594
64. Lynn M, Jeroukhimov I, Klein Y et al (2002) Updates in the management of severe coagulopathy in trauma patients. Intensive Care Med 28:S241-S247
65. Ho AM, Karmakar MK, Contardi LH et al (2001) Excessive use of normal saline in managing traumatized patients in shock: A preventable contributor to acidosis. J Trauma 51:173-177
66. Lang W, Zander R (2005) Prediction of dilutional acidosis based on the revised classical dilution concept for bicarbonate. J Appl Physiol 98:62-71
67. Wilkes NJ, Woolf R, Mutch M et al (2001) The effect of balanced versus saline-based hetastarch and crystalloid solutions on acid-base and electrolyte status and gastric mucosal perfusion in elderly surgical patients. Anesth Analg 93:811-816
68. Waters JH, Gottlieb A, Schönwald P et al (2001) Normal saline versus lactated Ringer's solution for intraoperative fluid management in patients undergoing abdominal aortic aneurysm repair: An outcome study. Anesth Analg 93:817-822

How to Maintain and Restore Fluid Balance: Crystalloids

3

Florian R. Nuevo, Marialuisa Vennari and Felice Eugenio Agrò

3.1 Understanding Fluid Balance

In clinical practice, it is important to distinguish whether the fluid imbalance is due to an absolute volume deficit or to a relative volume deficit and/or whether this hypovolemia presents concurrent electrolyte imbalance problems. Absolute volume deficits can be due to massive blood loss or to severe dehydration issues. Relative volume deficits can be due to vasodilatation brought about by sepsis, anesthetic drug effects, or anaphylaxis.

Hypovolemia can also occur in the absence of evident fluid loss, secondary to generalized alterations of the endothelial barrier and resulting in diffuse capillary leak, with the passage of fluid and proteins from IVS (intravascular space) to ISS (interstitial space) (i.e., sepsis). The organism tries to compensate hypovolemia through the redistribution of blood flow to vital organs (heart and brain), at the expense of intestinal, renal, muscular, and skin perfusion. These alterations in the endothelial barrier together with the fluid shifts across fluid compartments can lead to osmotic and oncotic pressure changes, which bring about concurrent shifts in the electrolyte concentrations of the respective fluid compartments. Additional compensations include activation of both the sympathetic nervous system (SNS) and a hormonal response, namely, the renin-aldosterone-angiotensin system (RAAS). Initially, these compensatory systems are beneficial but eventually they become deleterious and may worsen outcome, especially in critically ill patients.

The Task Force of the American College of Critical Care Medicine reported that in approximately 50% of patients with sepsis adequate volume

M. Vennari (✉)
Postgraduate School of Anesthesia and Intensive Care, Anesthesia, Intensive Care and Pain Management Department, University School of Medicine Campus Bio-Medico of Rome, Rome, Italy
e-mail: m.vennari@unicampus.it

F. E. Agrò (ed.), *Body Fluid Management*,
DOI: 10.1007/978-88-470-2661-2_3, © Springer-Verlag Italia 2013

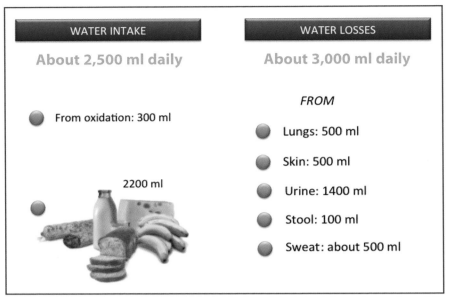

Fig. 3.1 Physiological water balance. Water intake is mainly derived from alimentation, while water losses are mainly due to diuresis

Table 3.1 Main commercially available plasma substitutes

Crystalloids	Colloids	Other fluids
NaCl 0.9%- 0.45%	Dextrans	Dextrose 5%
Ringer's solution	Albumin	Mannitol
Ringer Lactate/Acetate	Gelatins	Other electrolytic solutions
Sterofundin® ISO	Hydroxyethyl starches	…

restoration alone can achieve hemodynamic improvement by reversing hypotension [1].

In an adult, normal fluid intake is about 2500 ml/day, while water losses are about 3000 ml/day (Fig. 3.1). A gain or loss of water, influences both acid-base balance and electrolyte homeostasis in the body fluid compartments (see Chapter 1).

The problem at hand is then, how to restore fluid balance?

The solution to this problem is not the simple administration of any type of fluid.

Starting in 1913 [2], an extensive literature on fluid therapy has been published. Although there is consensus regarding the avoidance of blood transfusions (except in case of clear indications), debate remains about the ideal composition of IV fluids. Different solutions are available commercially; each one has its specific indications and side effects: crystalloids, colloids, and other fluids, such as dextrose solutions, mannitol solutions, and other concentrated solutions (Table 3.1).

3.2 Crystalloids

Low-molecular weight salts, dissolved in water, constitute crystalloids. The salts pass freely from the IVS to the ISS and vice versa [3].

3.2.1 Classification

Based on their tonicity, crystalloids can be classified as hypotonic, isotonic, or hypertonic. Four generations of crystalloids are available on the market (Fig. 3.2).

Many research studies have focused on producing more balanced and plasma-adapted crystalloids to replace those of the first generation. So far, the rational use of crystalloids remains a clinical problem. An improper choice of fluid and incorrect volume replacement cause disturbances in acid-base and electrolyte balances, such as hyperchloremic metabolic acidosis, and can interfere with lactate monitoring among critically ill patients and major surgery patients.

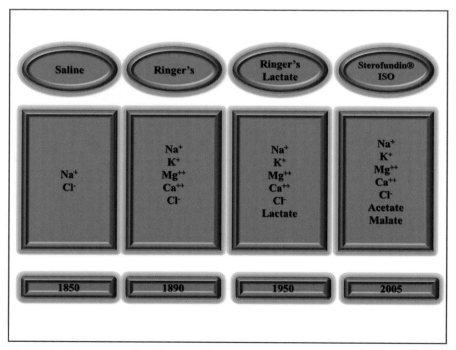

Fig. 3.2 Evolution of crystalloids' composition through the time. Comparison between the main crystalloids currently available on the market

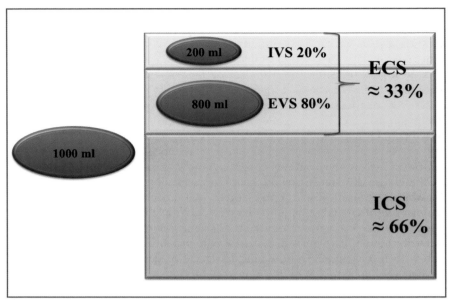

Fig. 3.3 Representation of isotonic crystalloid distribution. *ICS*, intracellular space; *IVS*, intravascular space; *ECS*, extracellular space; *EVS*, extravascular space

3.2.2   Pharmacokinetics: Distribution and Duration of Action

An isotonic crystalloid is distributed in the IVS (20%) but mostly in the EVS (80%) (Fig. 3.3). Accordingly, the efficiency of these solutions to expand the plasma volume is only 20%; the remainder is sequestered in the ISS [4-10].

Olsson et al. [11] found that approximately 30% of infused crystalloids remain within the vascular space for only 30 min. Thus, the use of crystalloids to replace severe volume deficits following massive blood or rapid fluid loss is not able to effectively restore fluid balance and blood pressure [12]. The volume expansion effect of crystalloids is short-term because of their rapid movement from the IVS into the ISS. Attaining the targeted goal of adequate blood pressure requires massive, repetitive infusions of crystalloids, which can lead to side effects such as interstitial edema and electrolyte imbalances.

3.2.3   Physiological Properties of the Main Crystalloids

The main properties of the most widely used crystalloids are described in Table 3.2.

Table 3.2 Properties of the main crystalloids

Electrolyte or parameter	Plasma	0.9% NaCl	Ringer lactate	Ringer acetate	Sterofundin®
Colloid-osmotic pressure (mmHg)	25	-	-	-	-
Osmolality (mOsm/Kg)	287	308	277	256	291
Sodium (mEq/L)	142	154	131	130	145
Potassium (mEq/L)	4.5	-	5.4	5	4
Magnesium (mEq/L)	1.25	-	-	1	1
Chloride (mEq/L)	103	154	112	112	127
Calcium (mEq/L)	2.5	-	1.8	1	2.5
Lactate (mEq/L)	1	-	28	-	-
Bicarbonate (mEq/L)	24	-	-	-	-
Acetate/Malate (mEq/L)	-	-	-	27/-	24-5

3.2.4 Normal Saline Solution

The standard 0.9% NaCl solution is also known as a normal or physiological saline solution. It contains only sodium and chloride, at high concentrations (154 mmol/L). Consequently, its administration may cause hyperchloremic acidosis and sodium overload, especially in patients with renal dysfunction or cardiac insufficiency. Moreover, it is a hypertonic fluid (osmolality 308 mosm/kg), implying the possibility of the consequences described in Chapter 2. As a result, normal saline solution is not actually normal, because it is neither isotonic, nor balanced, nor plasma-adapted.

3.2.5 Ringer Lactate and Ringer Acetate

Ringer solutions are second-generation crystalloids. Compared to saline solutions, they contain less sodium (130 mmol/L) and less chloride (112 mmol/L). They also contain potassium, calcium, magnesium (Ringer acetate), and metabolizable ions: lactate (Ringer lactate) and acetate (Ringer acetate). Ringer lactate may interfere with lactate monitoring and may precipitate or aggravate a lactic acidosis, especially in critical patients. Therefore, Ringer acetate is preferred. Both Ringer solutions are more plasma-adapted than normal saline, but are nonetheless unbalanced.

3.2.6   Latest-Generation Crystalloids

The ionic composition of the latest-generation crystalloids is very close to that of plasma: a lower chloride content than normal saline, together with two metabolizable ions (acetate and malate) rather than only one (acetate or lactate) as in Ringer solutions. As a result, these are isotonic, balanced, and plasma-adapted solutions that reduce the risk of chloride excess and dilutional acidosis, with a decreased influence on lactate monitoring, lactic acidosis, and base excess (BE). Furthermore, when these latest-generation crystalloids were administered to patients with sellar tumors, good correction of hypernatremia and metabolic alkalosis was achieved [13, 14].

3.2.7   Old and New Crystalloids: The Debate on Chloride Excess and Dilutional Acidosis

Over the past decades, clinicians have routinely restored fluid in the IVS with crystalloids. However, due to the rapid fluid shifts and large distribution volume of crystalloids, large volumes must be administered. This in turn causes fluid overload, particularly interstitial edema and potentially pulmonary edema, as well as dilutional acidosis [5, 6, 15]. Nevertheless, mortality due to dilutional acidosis is a lower than that associated with lactate acidosis [16, 17]. Sodium and chloride are excreted more slowly than free water, which is rapidly eliminated by the kidneys [18-22], an effect due to hyperchloremia. Fluid elimination is reduced through a suppression of the renin-angiotensin-aldosterone system [23]. The result is a weight gain that may increase mortality [24].

3.2.8   The Albumin Hemodilution Phenomenon

A major side effect of crystalloid volume replacement involves the plasma albumin concentration. Large-volume infusions of crystalloids can lead to albumin hemodilution effects [25] and cause a reduction in colloid oncotic pressure (COP). Moreover, the volume expansion may cause tissue edema [26], and thus albumin leakage. In critically ill patients, a reduction in COP is associated with a mortality rate of approximately 50% [27, 28]. Excessive use of crystalloids results in the development of "compartment syndrome" as well [29].

3.2.9 Clotting Disorders

It is common knowledge that crystalloids administration is an economical mean of volume replacement, with an apparently lower risk of clotting disorders. However, Ruttmann et al. [30, 31] and Ng et al. [32] have shown that dilution with crystalloids in vivo resulted in a significant potentiation of coagulation, due to a decreased concentration of antithrombin III [30]. The resultant hypercoagulability is unrelated to the type of crystalloid, but is related to the amount of crystalloid infused and consequently to the rate of hemodilution. It is also associated with an increased risk for peri-operative deep vein thrombosis.

3.2.10 Hypertonic Crystalloids

Hypertonic crystalloid solutions (HCS) contain higher sodium concentrations, ranging from 3% to 7.5%. HCS have a transient volume effect, but if used together with colloids, they demonstrated a prolonged efficacy of volume expansion [36].

By itself, HCS may improve the cardiovascular system, with only a small volume needed for fluid replacement (4 mL/kg). The effects can be due to the following mechanisms:
- direct myocardial, positive inotropic effect;
- direct vasodilator effect (both the systemic and the pulmonary circulation);
- reduced venous capacitance;
- improved volume effect due to fluid shifts into the vascular compartment from intravascular space.

Initially, there was enthusiasm for the use of HCS in patients with refractory hypovolemic shock states, but the practice faded because of the danger of side effects if HCS are not properly used. There is a rapid shift of water from EVS into IVS (plasma compartment), without a reduction in COP. However, to obtain this effect, an adequate volume status of both the intracellular and the interstitial spaces is necessary, so that the prolonged usage of HCS is contraindicated [37].

Both Wade et al. [38] and Bunn et al. [39] reported, in their meta-analyses, that there is no significant improvement in outcome in critical and trauma patients by using HCS alone. They hypothesized that the combined use of HCS and dextran would be superior to isotonic fluid resuscitation.

Key Concepts
- Definition of volume deficit and interstitial/intracellular water deficit
- Description of physiological compensatory mechanism in hypovolemia
- Description of isotonic crystalloid distribution
- Description of the electrolytic and physical properties of the most commonly used crystalloid solution
- Last generation crystalloids

Key Words
- Hypovolemia
- Dehydration
- Plasma substitutes
- Crystalloids solutions
- Normal saline solution
- Ringer lactate
- Ringer acetate
- Latest-generation crystalloids

Focus on...
- Liszkowski M, Nohria A (2010) Rubbing salt into wounds: hypertonic saline to assist with volume removal in heart failure. Curr Heart Fail Rep 7(3):134-9
- Patanwala AE, Amini A, Erstad BL (20101) Use of hypertonic saline injection in trautrauma. Am J Health Syst Pharm 67(22):1920-8

References

1. Task Force of the American College of Critical Care Medicine, Society of Critical Care Medicine (1999) Practice parameters for hemodynamic support of sepsis in adult patients in sepsis. Crit Care Med 27:639-6
2. Loeb J (1913) Avogadro's Law and the absorption of water by animal tissues in crystalloid and colloid solutions. Science:427-439
3. Voet D, Voet JG, Pratt CW (2001) Fundamentals of Biochemistry (Rev. ed.). New York, Wiley, p. 30
4. Lamke LO, Liljedahl SO (1976) Plasma volume changes after infusion of various plasma expanders. Resuscitation 5:93-102
5. Reid F, Lobo DN, Williams RN et al (2003) (Ab)normal saline and physiological Hartmann's solution: a randomized double-blind crossover study. Clin Sci 104:17-24
6. Grathwohl KW, Bruns BJ, LeBrun CJ et al (1996) Does haemodilution exist? Effects of saline infusion on hematologic parameters in euvolemic subjects. South Med 89:51-55

7. Greenfield RH, Bessen HA, Henneman PL (1989) Effect of crystalloid infusion on hematocrit and intravascular volume in healthy, no bleeding subjects. Ann Emerg Med 18:51-55
8. Hauser CJ; Shoemaker WC, Turpin I et al (1980) Oxygen transport responses to colloids and crystalloids in critically ill surgical patients. Surg Obstet 150:811-816
9. Hahn RG, Drobin D, Stähle L (1997) Volume kinetics of Ringer's solution in female volunteers. Br J Anaesth 78:144-148
10. Takil A, Eti Z, Irmak P et al (2002) Early postoperative respiratory acidosis after large intravascular volume infusion of lactated Ringer's solution during major spine surgery. Anesth Analg 95:294-298
11. Olsson J, Svense´n CH, Hahn RG (2004) The volume kinetics of acetated Ringer's solution during laparoscopic cholecystectomy. Anesth Analg 99:1854–60
12. Drummond JC, Petrovitch CT (2005) Intraoperative blood salvage: fluid replacement calculation. Anesth Analg 100:645-9
13. Ribeiro MA Jr, Epstein MG, Alves LD (2009) Volume replacement in trauma Ulus Trauma. Acil Cerrahi Derg 15:311-6
14. Popugaev KA, Savin IA, Kurdiumova NV, Luk'ianov VI (2009) Experience in using normofundin and sterofundin solutions for the correction of hypernatremia. Anesteziol Reanimatol 5:39-41
15. Waters JH, Gottlieb A, Schönwald P et al (2001) Normal saline versus lactated Ringer's solution for intraoperative fluid management in patients undergoing abdominal aortic aneurysm repair: An outcome study. Anesth Analg 93:817-822
16. Brill SA, Stewart TR, Brundage SI et al (2002) Base deficit does not predict mortality when secondary to hyperchloremic acidosis. Shock 17:459-462
17. Gunnerson, KJ, Saul M, He S et al (2006) Lactate versus non-lactate metabolic acidosis: a retrospective outcome evaluation of critically ill patients. Crit Care 10:R22
18. Hahn RG, Drobin D (2003) Rapid water and slow sodium excretion of acetated Ringer's solution dehydrates cells. Anesth Analg 97:1590-1594
19. Drobin D, Hahn RG (2002) Kinetics of isotonic and hypertonic plasma volume expanders. Anaesthesiology 96:1371-1380
20. Drobin D, Hahn RG (1999) Volume kinetics of Ringer's solution in hypovolemic volunteers. Anesthesiology 90:81-91
21. Holte K, Jensen P, Kehlet H (2003) Physiologic effects of intravenous fluid administration in healthy volunteers. Anesth Analg 96:1504-1509
22. Lobo DN, Stanga Z, Simpson JA et al (2001) Dilution and redistribution effects of rapid 2-litre infusions of 0.9% (w/v) saline and 5 % (w/v) dextrose on haematological parameters and serum biochemistry in normal subjects: A double-blind crossover study. Clin Sci 101:173-179
23. Drummer C, Gerzer R, Heer M et al (1992) Effects of an acute saline infusion in fluid and electrolyte metabolism in humans. Am J Physiol 262:F744-F754
24. Zander R (2009) Fluid Management. Bibliomed, Medizinische Verlagsgesellschaft mbH, Melsungen
25. Sitges-Serra A, Arcas G, Guirao X et al (1992) Extracellular fluid expansion during parenteral refeeding. Clin Nutr 11:63-68
26. Cervera AL, Moss G (1974) Crystalloid distribution following haemorrhage and haemodilution: mathematical model and prediction of optimum volumes for equilibration at normovolemia. J Trauma 14:506-520
27. Morissette M, Weil MH, Shubin H (1975) Reduction in colloid osmotic pressure associated with fatal progression of cardiopulmonary failure. Crit Care Med 3:115-117
28. Rackow E, Fein AI, Leppo J (1977) Colloid osmotic pressure as a prognostic indicator of pulmonary oedema and mortality in the critically ill. Chest 72:709-713
29. Cotton BA, Guy JS, Morris Jr JA et al (2006) The cellular, metabolic, and systemic consequences of aggressive fluid resuscitation strategies. Shock 26:115-121
30. Ruttmann TG, James MFM, Finlayson J et al (2002) Effects on coagulation of intravenous crystalloid or colloid in patients undergoing peripheral vascular surgery. Br J Anaesth 89:226-30

31. Ruttmann TG, James MFM, Lombard EM et al (2001) Haemodilution-induced enhancement of coagulation is attenuated in vitro by restoring antithrombin III to predilution concentration. Anaesth Intesive Care 29:489-93
32. Ng KFJ, Lam CCK, Chan IC (2002) In vivo effect of haemodilution with saline on coagulation: a randomized controlled tril. Br J Anaesth 88:475-80
33. Janvrin SB, Davies G, Greenhalgh RM (1980) Postoperative deep vein thrombosis caused by intravenous fluids during surgery. Br J Surg 67:690-3
34. Kramer GC, Perron PR, Lindsey DC, Ho HS, Gunther RA, Boyle WA et al (1986) Small-volume resuscitation with hypertonic saline dextran solution. Surgery 100:239-47
35. Layon J, Duncan D, Gallagher TJ, Banner MJ (1987) Hypertonic saline as a resuscitation solution in hemorrhagic shock: effects on extravascular lung water and cardiopulmonary function. Anesth Analg 66:154-8
36. Whinney RR, Cohn SM, Zacur SJ (2000) Fluid resuscitation for trauma patients in the 21st century. Curr Opin Crit Care 6:395-400
37. Maningas PA, Bellamy RF (1986) Hypertonic sodium chloride solutions for the prehospital management of traumatic hemorrhagic shock: a possible improvement in the standard of care? Ann Emerg Med 15:1411-4
38. Wade CE, Kramer GC, Grady JJ, Fabian TC, Younes RN (1997) Efficacy of hypertonic 7.5% saline and 6% dextran- 70 in treating trauma: a meta-analysis of controlled clinical studies. Surgery 122:609-16
39. Bunn F, Roberts I, Tasker R, Akpa E (2002) Hypertonic versus isotonic crystalloid for fluid resuscitation in critically ill patients (Cochrane Review). Cochrane Database Syst Rev CD002045

How to Maintain and Restore Fluid Balance: Colloids

4

Felice Eugenio Agrò, Dietmar Fries and Maria Benedetto

4.1 Colloids

Colloids are high molecular weight molecules that do not dissolve completely in water, nor do they pass freely through the capillary membrane. According to their molecular size, structure and vessel permeability, colloids determine the oncotic pressure.

4.1.1 Classification

Many colloids are currently available. They include natural colloids (human albumin, HA) and synthetic colloids (dextrans, gelatins, hydroxyethyl starches), differing in their physicochemical properties, pharmacokinetics, clinical effects and safety. Colloids also can be classified according to their electrolyte composition and tonicity. Consequently, there are balanced and unbalanced colloids, plasma-adapted and non-plasma-adapted colloids.

4.1.2 Physiological Properties of the Main Colloids

The table below describes the main properties of some colloids used in clinical practice (Table 4.1).

M. Benedetto (✉)
Postgraduate School of Anesthesia and Intensive Care, Anesthesia, Intensive Care and Pain Management Department, University School of Medicine Campus Bio-Medico of Rome, Rome, Italy
e-mail: m.benedetto@unicampus.it

F. E. Agrò (ed.), *Body Fluid Management*,
DOI: 10.1007/978-88-470-2661-2_4 © Springer-Verlag Italia 2013

Table 4.1 Main properties of some colloids used in clinical practice

Electrolyte or parameter	Plasma	Venofundin® 6%	Gelofusin® 4%	Tetraspan® 6%
Colloid-osmotic pressure (mmHg)	25	37.8	33.3	37.8
Osmolality (mOsm/Kg)	287	308	274	296
Colloid	Albumin	HES 130/0.42	MFGel	HES 130/0.42
Sodium (mEq/L)	142	154	154	140
Potassium (mEq/L)	4.5	-	-	4
Magnesium (mEq/L)	1.25	-	-	1
Calcium (mEq/L)	2.5	-	-	2.5
Chloride (mEq/L)	103	154	120	118
Bicarbonate (mEq/L)	25	-	-	-
Acetate/Malate (mEq/L)	-	-	-	24/5

4.1.3 Pharmacokinetics: Distribution and Duration of Action

The colloid-osmotic pressure influences the vascular expansion effect: the higher the oncotic pressure, the greater the initial volume increase in the intravascular space (IVS) [1] The volume effect is also determined by molecular weight (MW); the higher the MW, the greater the IVS volume expansion [1]. However, the plasma half-life of colloids, which is determined by MW and organ elimination (mainly by the kidneys), limits the duration of the volume effect. Thus, different colloids have different duration of volume effects [1].

Isotonic and iso-oncotic colloids have poor volume-replacing power, in contrast to hypertonic and hyperoncotic colloids. Based on previous evidence [2], Mcllroy et al. [3] found that, given its colloid-osmotic pressure, an isotonic colloid is distributed only within the IVS (Fig. 4.1). The efficiency of this solution to expand the plasma volume is 100%.

However, in physiological terms, this is not significant, since iso-oncotic, isosmotic colloids rapidly leave the vascular tree, through extravasation or metabolism [4, 5], especially during certain conditions, such as systemic inflammation, sepsis, capillary leak syndrome, and third-space syndrome.

4.2 Natural Colloids: Human Albumin (HA)

For many years, HA was considered to be the gold-standard in hypovolemia treatment. HA is made up of 585 amino acids with a molecular mass of 69,000 Daltons. It is the main plasma protein (50–60%), accounting for 80% of normal oncotic pressure [1-6]. Furthermore, HA contributes to the formation of a normal anion gap and acid-base balance, while being a charged protein.

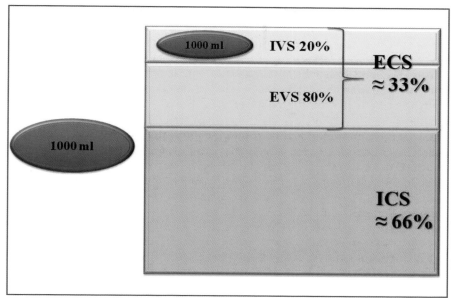

Fig. 4.1 Isotonic colloid distribution. *IVS*, Intravascular space; *ECS*, extracellular space; *EVS*, extravascular space; *ICS*, intracellular space

4.2.1 Composition and Concentration

Current HA solutions consist of 96% albumin, with the remaining 4% being globulins. Different concentrations of HA are commercially available: 20% and 25% HA (hyperoncotic), 5% HA (iso-oncotic), 4% HA (hypo-oncotic).

4.2.2 Pharmacokinetics: Distribution, Elimination and Duration of Action

A 5% HA solution can be reasonably considered for volume replacement, leading to an 80% initial volume expansion, whereas HA 25% leads to a 200–400% volume increase within 30 min. The volume effect lasts for 16–24 h [8-9]. The decrease in plasma HA concentration is firstly due to passage from IVS to EVS through the transporter albondin (transcapillary exchange) and secondly to the fractional degradation rate [6].

4.2.3 Clinical Use

The primary use of HA is the treatment of acute hypovolemia, especially following trauma, surgical hemorrhage and cardiac surgery. Additional applications are other clinical conditions, such as systemic inflammatory response syndrome, sepsis, and capillary leakage syndromes, even if the true indications for HA are actually not well defined. Based on the results of the SAFE [10] study, HA has been mainly used to treat low plasma protein levels, especially in Austrian and German hospitals. The rationale is to prevent fluid extravasation by increasing the intravascular colloid-oncotic pressure (COP) [11] in patients at high risk of hypoalbuminemia. However, HA is not exclusively retained in the IVS; rather, 10% of the administered dose leaves the IVS within 2 h. It is therefore likely to leak into the interstitial space (ISS), potentially aggravating interstitial edema and hypoalbuminemia, without clinical benefits [6-12]. Low serum albumin (< 2 g/dL) was shown to be a marker of poor outcome [13-15], with a mortality of approximately 100% [16]. Albumin is often used in hypoalbuminemic cardiac surgery patients, even if the clinical benefits are not yet clear.

4.2.4 Potential Risks and Side Effects

4.2.4.1 Pulmonary Edema
Several lines of evidence explain why HA supplementation may worsen the condition of critically ill patients. In fact, after rapid volume replacement, cardiac failure may occur, causing or worsening pulmonary edema, especially in capillary leak syndrome [17].

4.2.4.2 Coagulation and Homeostasis
Furthermore, HA may impact coagulation and hemostasis by enhancing antithrombin III activity and inhibiting platelet function [18-20].

Tobias et al. [21] found that albumin may also lead to hypocoagulability. Dietrich et al. showed an in vitro increase in bleeding time [22], which may increase blood loss in post-surgical or trauma patients. Finally, albumin administration may impair the efficiency of endothelial cell adhesion. The importance of this effect is uncertain, since increased plasma levels of endothelial adhesion molecules may be markers of mortality [17].

4.2.4.3 Electrolytic and Acid-Base Balance
Currently available HA solutions are prepared as NaCl solutions, which can lead to hyperchloremia and interfere with sodium and water excretion, thus impairing renal function, especially in hypovolemic shock patients. In acute renal failure, HA may accumulate after its massive administration [17].

4.2.4.4 Immunologic Reactions
HA is generally well tolerated, but immediate allergic reactions characterized by fever, nausea, vomiting, pruritus, hypotension and even cardio-respiratory collapse, are possible.

4.2.5   Indications

HA use is guided by absolute and relative indications.

The administration of HA is indicated in acute conditions requiring plasma expansion and in chronic conditions characterized by low albumin plasma levels [23]. There is widespread consensus in the literature and clinically regarding absolute indications. Relative indications refer to settings in which HA is indicated when other specific criteria are satisfied.

Absolute indications are:

- paracentesis: > 5 L or > 5 g albumin/L in ascites fluid;
- therapeutic plasmapheresis: plasma exchange > 20 mL/kg;
- spontaneous bacterial peritonitis in cirrhosis: associated with antibiotic administration.

Relative indications are:

- cardiac surgery: third choice after crystalloids and synthetic colloids;
- major surgery: only if albuminemia < 2 g/dL and after the restoration of normovolemia;
- cirrhosis: diuretic-resistant ascites with albuminemia < 2 g/dL;
- hemorrhagic shock: only when not responsive to crystalloids and synthetic colloids;
- hepatorenal syndrome: in association with vasoconstrictors;
- nephrotic syndrome: in the presence of albuminemia < 2 g/dL associated with hypovolemia and/or pulmonary edema;
- organ transplantation: in the presence of albuminemia < 2 g/dL and hematocrit $> 30\%$, in postoperative liver transplant patients, in order to control ascites and peripheral edema;
- burns: $> 30\%$ of the body surface after the first 24 h;

In these situations the adequate HA dose can be calculated as follows:

Dose (g) = [targeted albuminemia (2.5 g/dl) – real albuminemia (g/dL)] × plasmatic volume (0.8 × body weight in kg).

There are a few conditions in which albumin is administered routinely, albeit improperly [24, 25]:

- albuminemia > 2.5 g/dL (excluding the situations mentioned above);
- hypoalbuminemia in the absence of peripheral edema or acute hypotension;
- malnutrition and malabsorption;
- wound healing;
- non-hemorrhagic shock;
- diuretic-responsive ascites;
- acute and chronic pancreatitis;
- hemodialysis;
- ischemic stroke;
- acute normovolemic hemodilution in major surgery.

4.3   Synthetic Colloids

Synthetic or artificial colloids (dextrans, gelatins, hydroxyethyl starches) are produced from biological, non-human molecules. Their assessment criteria include (Table 4.2):

- concentration;
- initial volume effect;
- duration of the volume effect.

Table 4.2 Comparison between main therapeutic and side effects of synthetic colloids

Colloid	Volemic effect		Side effect		
	Efficacy	Duration	AKI	Coag.	Anaf.
Dextrans	+++	+++	+++(40)	+++(70)	++
Gelatins	+	+	+	+	+++
HES high MW	+++	+++	++	+++	+
HES low MW	+++	++	+	++	+

+, mild; ++, moderate; +++, high; *MW*, molecular weight; *AKI*, acute kidney injury.

4.4   Dextrans

Dextrans are glucose polymers of different sizes, derived from *Leuconostoc mesenteroides*, a bacteria originally isolated from contaminated sugar beets.

4.4.1   Classification

Dextrans are mainly used in the USA, as they are no longer available in European countries, including Germany and Austria. The most widely used dextran solutions are dextran 40 (a 10% solution with 40,000 MMW) and dextran 70 (a 6% solution with 70,000 MMW) (Table 4.3).

Table 4.3 Characteristics of dextran solutions

Characteristics of Dextran Solutions	6% Dextran 70	10% Dextran 40
Mean Molecular Weight (Dalton)	70,000	40,000
Volume efficacy (%) (approx.)	100	175-(200)
Volume effect (hours) (approx.)	5	3-4
Maximum Daily Dose (g/kg)	1.5	1.5

4.4.2 Pharmacokinetics: Distribution, Elimination and Duration of Action

Dextrans are endowed with a high COP, due to their high water-binding capacity. They lead to a 100–150% volume increase of the IVS [9].

Dextrans are mainly eliminated by the kidney, while only a small fraction transiently passes into the ISS or is eliminated by the gastrointestinal tract. In particular, smaller molecules (14,000–18,000 kDa) are excreted by the kidney within 15 min, whereas larger molecules are excreted after several days. At 12 hours from administration, 60% of dextran 40 and 30% of dextran 70 have already been eliminated [9, 26, 27].

4.4.3 Clinical Use

Dextran solutions have positive effects on the macro- and microcirculation. In fact, they have been mainly used to maintain hemodynamics in different kinds of shock and to ameliorate tissue perfusion and microcirculation. At the same degree of hemodilution, rheological effects are mainly correlated with the use of dextran 40 rather than with any other plasma substitute [28]. Moreover, dextran protects against ischemia-reperfusion injury by reducing the harmful interactions between activated leukocytes and the microvascular endothelium.

4.4.4 Potential Risks and Side Effects

Dextran is no longer used because of its side effects.

4.4.4.1 Anaphylaxis
Dextran administration may lead to anaphylactoid reactions more frequently and more severely than other colloids. This is due to the massive production of vasoactive mediators triggered by anti-dextran antibodies. These reactions may be prevented by pretreatment with 20 mL hapten solution (dextran 1000) few minutes before infusion [29].

4.4.4.2 Nephrotoxicity
Another possible side effect is renal dysfunction and acute renal failure, through the production of hyperviscous urine leading to swelling and vacuolization of tubular cells and tubular plugging [1]. This is especially true in patients with advanced age, hemodynamic alterations, pre-existing renal disease, and dehydration [30, 31].

4.4.4.3 Coagulation and Hemostasis
Finally, dextrans may alter platelet function, decrease factor VIII levels, and increase fibrinolysis, with significant bleeding disorders, especially after the

administration of high doses [9, 32, 33]. These side effects resulted in maximum daily dose recommendation of approximately 1.5 L [34, 35].

4.5   Gelatins

Gelatins are polydispersed peptides derived from bovine collagen [6, 11]. First-generation gelatins had a high MW and high viscosity, with very high oncotic power but also the tendency to gel when stored at low temperatures. Thus, lower MW gelatins have been produced; while they gel more slowly, they also have a reduced oncotic power [36].
Gelatin solutions are available in most European and Asian countries.

4.5.1   Classification

Three types of gelatins are currently available: cross-linked or oxypolygelatins (e.g., Gelofundiol), urea-cross-linked gelatins (e.g. Haemacell), and succinylated or modified fluid gelatins (e.g., Gelofusine) (Table 4.4).

Gelatins are produced in an apyrogenic and sterile formulation. They do not contain preservatives and have a shelf-life of a few years (if stored at temperatures below 30°C). Their average MW is 30–35,000 and they are based on unbalanced, hypotonic solutions. In particular, polygelines are dispersed in a 3.5% polyelectrolyte solution generally containing: Na+ 145, K+ 5.1, Ca++ 6.25, and Cl– 145 mmol/l. Thus, they may increase serum calcium, in particular after large volume infusions. Succinylated gelatins are dispersed in a 4% polyelectrolyte solution generally containing: Na+ 154, K+ 0.4, Ca++ 0.4, and Cl –120 mmol/l. Their low chloride content reduces the risk of hyperchloremic acidosis and may be helpful in patients with acid-base alterations. They are compatible with blood transfusions because of their low calcium content [1, 36-38].

Table 4.4 Characteristics of gelatin solutions

Characteristics of gelatin solutions	Succinylated gelatin	Cross-linked gelatin	Urea cross-linked gelatin
Concentration (%)	4.0	5.5	3.5
Mean Molecular Weight (Dalton)	30,000	30,000	35,000
Volume efficacy (%) (approx.)	80	80	80
Volume effect (hours) (approx.)	1-3	1-3	1-3
Osmolarity (mOsm/L)	274	296	301

4.5.2   Pharmacokinetics: Distribution, Elimination, and Duration of Effect

Gelatins have similar IVS volume-expanding power and a half-life of about 2.5 h. 24 h post-administration, 13% remains in the IVS, 16% has passed into the ISS, 71% is rapidly cleared by the kidney, and a small amount has been cleaved by proteases in the reticuloendothelial system (RES). Notably, the volume expansion is lower than the infused volume (about 70–80%). Gelatins have a shorter duration of effect than any other colloid. Therefore, repeated infusions are required and allowed, as there are no dose limitations, in contrast to other colloids [1, 21, 34, 35].

4.5.3   Potential Risks and Side Effects

Compared to starch solutions, gelatins are associated with a lower risk of acute kidney injury. They are not stored in the RES or in other tissues, but there is a higher incidence of anaphylactic reactions than is the case with natural colloid albumin [33, 36].

4.5.3.1 Hemodynamic
In patients with ascites, after massive paracentesis, gelatin infusion may cause hemodynamic impairment due to increased plasma aldosterone and renin activity [39].

4.5.3.1 Coagulation and Hemostasis
Gelatins were classically thought not to significantly impair coagulation. However, recently, there has been evidence of their causing platelet dysfunction and clotting disorders. In a study comparing the effects of progressive hemodilution with gelatins, saline, hydroxyethyl starch, and albumin on blood coagulation, significant changes in the thromboelastogram were found after the infusion of gelatin solutions [40]. Nonetheless, in clinical practice, they seem to impair fibrin polymerization less than the "modern" medium-weight starches. Thus, in critically ill patients and in patients with severe hemorrhagic shock, who need large intravascular volume replacement, gelatin solutions are still widely adopted because of the absence of significant side effects on either the coagulation system/fibrinogen polymerization or kidney function, the lack of accumulation in the RES, and the unlimited dose.

4.6   Hydroxyethyl Starches

Hydroxyethyl starches (HES) are modified natural polysaccharides derived from amylopectin, a highly branched starch similar to glycogen that is found

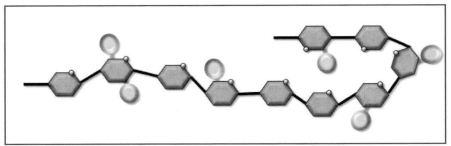

Fig. 4.2 HES are obtained substituting hydroxyl groups of natural starches with hydroxyethyl groups (*big grey round*) at carbon position C2, C3 and C6 of the anhydroglucose residues

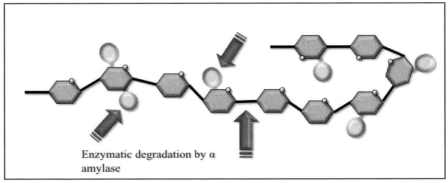

Fig. 4.3 Hydrolyzation by circulating amylase. The *arrows* represent the site of action of the enzyme. The hydroxhyethil group block two of the three site of hydrolisis

in maize or potatoes (Fig. 4.2). Polymerized D-glucose units are connected by 1-4 linkages with one 1-6 branching linkage every 20 glucose units.

Natural starches cannot be used in clinical routine since they are rapidly hydrolyzed by circulating amylase (Fig. 4.3). HES are obtained by replacing the hydroxyl groups of natural starches with hydroxyethyl groups at the C2, C3, and C6 carbon positions of anhydroglucose residues. This results in greater solubility and less amylase degradation especially for hydroxyethyl groups at the C2 position [1, 41].

4.6.1   Classification

The first HES, Hespan, was produced in the 1970s in the USA. Since then, further generations have been produced.

HES are designated by a series of numeric parameters (e.g., HES 10% 200/0.5/5) reflecting their pharmacokinetics. The first number relates to the solution concentration, the second represents the mean MW, the third is the molar substitution rate (MSR), and the fourth is the C2/C6 ratio. Thus, HES may be classified according to:

- concentration (3%, 6%, 10%);
- mean MW (low molecular weight: 70 kDa; medium-molecular weight: 130–270 kDa; high-molecular weight: > 450 kDa);
- molar substitution (low MS: 0.4–0.5; high MS: 0.62–0.7);
- C2/C6 ratio.

4.6.1.1 Concentration

The volume expansion power of HES is firstly influenced by the concentration. HES at 6% concentration are iso-oncotic and have a 100% volume-expanding power (1 L infused fluid = 1L plasma volume expansion). HES at 10% concentration are hyperoncotic and have a volume-expanding power > 100% (1 L infused fluid = > 1 L plasma volume expansion) [1, 6].

4.6.1.2 Mean Molecular Weight

The arithmetic mean of the MW of all HES molecules dispersed in a solution is referred to as the mean molecular weight (MMW). HES are polydispersed solutions made up of different-sized molecules. Particles with a low MW (45–70 kDa) have a rapid enzymatic degradation and a fast renal excretion because their size is under the renal threshold. Particles with high MW (> 70 kDa) have a longer half-life, according to both their size and their rate of enzymatic degradation [6, 33].

4.6.1.3 Molar Substitution

The molar ratio of the total number of hydroxyethyl groups to the total number of glucose units is termed the molar substitution. The MS impacts human α-amylase degradation and thus the break down of the starch: the higher the MS, the slower the degradation, the longer the volume effect and the higher the incidence of side effects [1, 6, 33].

4.6.1.4 C2:C6 Ratio

The quotient of the total number of hydroxyethyl groups on carbon atom 2 and the total number of hydroxyethyl groups on carbon atom six yields the C2:C6 ratio (Fig. 4.4). For example, a C2:C6 ratio of 9 to 1 means that substitution with hydroxyethyl groups at position C2 is nine times higher than at position C6 [33].

The C2 hydroxyethyl group hinders the action of α-amylase, delaying HES degradation and increasing the volume-expanding power. A higher C2:C6 ratio means lower α-amylase degradation, with a longer and greater volume effect.

4.6.1.5 HES Electrolyte Composition

HES can also be classified according to the electrolyte features of the carrier solution, yielding balanced or unbalanced, plasma-adapted, and non-plasma-adapted HES solutions.

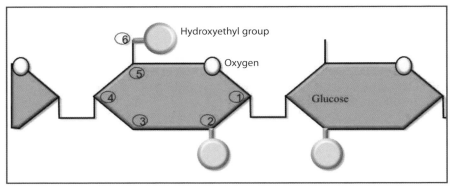

Fig. 4.4 Representation of the C2:C6 ratio. A higher C2:C6 ratio means lower α-amylase degradation, with a longer and greater volume effect

Table 4.5 Differences between the three different generations of HES

Concentration	Origin	Solvent	Mean Molecular Weight	Molar (Mw) Substitution	C2:C6 Ratio
3% (hyponcotic)	Potato-derived HES	Unbalanced	Low (LMW) 70 KD	Low MS: < 0.5	9:1
6% (normoncotic)	Waxy maize-derived HES	Balanced	Medium (MMW) from 130 to 370 KD	Medium MS: 0.5	6:1
10% (hyperoncotic)	-	-	High (HMW) > 450 KD	High MS: > 0.5	4:1

Three successive generations of HES have been commercialized (Table 4.5):
- First-generation: MW > 450 kDa, MS > 0.7, and high C2:C6 ratio
- Second-generation: lower MW (200 kDa), MS (0.5), and lower C2:C6 ratio
- Third-generation: MW = 130 kDa, MS < 0.5, and lower C2:C6 ratio.

Thus, HESs widely differ with respect to the extent and duration of their volume-expansion power and their impact on the clotting system, renal function, inflammation, itching, and storage.

4.6.2   Pharmacokinetics: Distribution, Elimination, and Duration of Action

The water-binding capacity of HES varies between 20 and 30 mL/g. As previously described, small molecules are rapidly excreted by the kidney (up to 50% of the administered dose within 24 h), whereas larger molecules are retained for longer amounts of time. The oncotic effect of HES is due solely to the number of particles, and not to their size. While renal elimination of the small molecules reduces the oncotic power, this is compensated by the enzymatic degradation of the large molecules. Consequently, the expanding power of HES is greater than that of other synthetic colloids, particularly gelatins. The duration of the expanding power equals the time interval of HES retention in the vascular bed, usually 8–12 h. A minor amount of the small molecules passes into the ISS, for later redistribution and elimination. Another fraction is trapped by reticuloendothelial cells, which slowly break down the starch (tissue storage). Thus, HES can be detected for several days after their infusion [42].

As mentioned above, there are potato- and maize-derived HES. They have the same oncotic power and plasma-expanding effects, even if the former have a more rapid elimination due to their lower amylopectin content (about 80%) [43].

In the subsequent HES generations, MMW, MS and the C2:C6 ratio have been modified to allow α-amylase degradation, in order to reduce the retention of residual fractions, and to prolong the volume effect, with less accumulation and side effects (Table 4.6).

HES molecules are generally dispersed in unbalanced, non-plasma-adapted solutions (first-, second-, and third-generations). The first balanced HES solution (Hextend) had high MMW (550 kDa) and MS (0.7). However, it resulted in tissue storage, impaired coagulation, and platelet dysfunction. Consequently, the latest generation HES have a lower MMW and MSR and are dissolved in balanced solutions (Fig. 4.5).

Nowadays the best HES for clinical practice are the latest generation HES, such as HES 130/042. It is available in two different carrier solutions: 9% saline solution (Venofundin) and a solution very similar to plasma (Tetraspan) (Table 4.7).

Table 4.6 Characteristics of HES

Characteristics	HES 70/0.5	HES 130/0.4	HES 200/0.5	HES 200/0.5	HES 200/0.62	HES 400/0.7
Concentration (%)	6	6	6	10	6	6
Mean Molecular Weight (KD)	70	130	200	200	200	450
Volume effect (hours) (approx.)	1-2	2-3	3-4	3-4	5-6	5-6
Volume efficacy (%) (approx.)	100	100	100	130	100	100
Molar Substitution (MS)	0.5	0.4	0.5	0.5	0.62	0.7
C2:C6 ratio	4:1	9:1	6:1	6:1	9:1	4.6:1

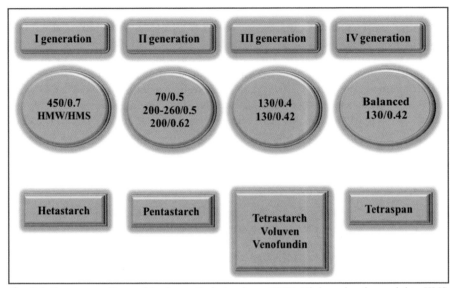

Fig. 4.5 Four generations of hydroxyethyl starches. *HMW*, High molecular weight; *HMS*, high molar substitution

Table 4.7 Comparison between Venofundin® and Tetraspan® composition

Electrolyte or parameter	Venofundin® 6%	Tetraspan® 6%
Colloid-osmotic pressure (mmHg)	37.8	37.8
Osmolality (mOsm/Kg)	308	296
Colloid	HES 130/0.42	HES 130/0.42
Sodium (mEq/L)	154	140
Potassium (mEq/L)	-	4
Magnesium (mEq/L)	-	1
Calcium (mEq/L)	-	2.5
Chloride (mEq/L)	154	118
Bicarbonate (mEq/L)	-	-
Acetate/Malate	-	24/5

4.6.3   Clinical Use

The various preparations of HES have been successfully used to improve the macro- and microcirculation of hypovolemic patients. Their effects are determined by their high hemodilutional power in combination with a specific action on red cells, platelets, plasma viscosity, and the endothelium. A lower blood viscosity means reduced vascular resistance, increased venous return, and improved cardiac index. This ameliorates tissue perfusion and oxygenation, with fewer infectious complications, especially in critically ill patients. The anti-inflammatory action of HES may play a role in maintaining the gut microcirculation in endotoxemia [44]. Third-generation HES result in improved tissue oxygenation in patients undergoing major abdominal surgery. However, patients treated with HES in 0.9% NaCl experienced greater dilution and hyperchloremic acidosis than patients treated with HES in balanced solutions [45].

4.6.4 Potential Risks and Side Effects

4.6.4.1 Coagulation and Hemostasis

Coagulation
There is broad debate about whether HES impair coagulation. Observed decreases in von Willebrand factor, fibrinogen levels, and thrombin generation presumably alter the coagulation time (normal value: 100–240 s), clot formation time (normal value: 30–110 s) and maximum clot firmness (normal value: 50–72 mm), as shown in intrinsic thromboelastography. In animal experiments, MMW was determined to not be a key factor in impaired coagulation. Previous reports in the literature showed a severe increase in the bleeding risk with high MMW and high MSR HSE (i.e., Heptastich: MW 450 kDa, MSR: 0.7). This is due to a von-Willebrand-like syndrome, with decreased factor VIII activity and reduced levels of von Willebrand factor antigen and factor VIII-related ristocetin cofactor [46-49].

HES also impairs fibrin polymerization, although HES with a medium MMW and a low MS probably do not strongly affect the coagulation system.

Platelet Function
Another side effect of HES is impaired platelet function. The reduction of factor-VIII-related ristocetin cofactor leads to its reduced binding to platelet membrane receptor glycoproteins GPIb and GPIIb/IIIa, resulting in decreased platelet adhesion. HES with a high MMW, high MS, and high $C2/C6$ ratio (e.g., HES 450/0.7 or HES 200/0.62) alter platelet function to a greater extent than HES with a lower MMW and a lower MS, as mentioned above for coagulation [50-53].

Franz et al. [54] studied the effects of IV infusion of saline solution and four HES preparations with different MWs and MSs on platelet function. HES 450/0.7, HES 200/0.6, and HES 70/0.5 prolonged platelet function analyzer (PFA)-100 closure times. All of the tested HES preparations reduced platelet GPIIb/IIIa expression. By contrast, the newest-generation HES seem to have no negative effects on platelets. Stögermüller et al. [55] reported that the expression of platelet GP IIb/IIIa was reduced after the infusion of non-balanced HES 200. However, according to in vitro studies, GP IIb/IIIa expression increases with high MMW, high MSR HES in balanced solutions. This unexpected result was obtained with a solvent containing calcium chloride dehydrate (2.5 mmol/L) [55, 56]. By contrast, HES in balanced plasma-adapted solutions were shown to have fewer effects on platelets. Many reports confirmed the importance of the solvent in determining potential adverse effects of HES solutions [54].

HES and Fibrin Polymerization Disturbances

In a mathematical model it was shown that in the case of normovolemic dilution with an initial fibrinogen level of ≤ 300 mg/dl critical fibrinogen concentration of 150 mg/dl is reached before a critical hematocrit value would require the administration of erythrocytes [57]. Several clinical studies in orthopedics, cardiac surgery, and pediatric surgery have shown that even relatively moderate dilution with HES above all disturbs fibrin polymerization.

Clinical Evidence

Gallandat et al. [58] found that in cardiac surgery patients new-generation HES increase von Willebrand factor levels to a greater extent than HES 200/0.5, resulting in a reduction of bleeding risk and transfusion need. Similar results were found in patients undergoing orthopedic surgery [59] and major surgery [60]. However, negative effects of modern HES preparations on coagulation and platelets have also been reported. For example, Scharbert et al. [61] found an impairment of platelet function by HES 130 similar to that of HES 200 in patients with chronic back pain undergoing epidural anesthesia. Nevertheless, HES 130 produced a not clinically significant platelet alteration. Similar results were reported for minor elective surgery [62].

4.6.4.2 Nephrotoxicity

Another clinical concern about HES use is the risk of kidney failure. All colloids can induce kidney injury. Some studies showed an increased incidence of kidney dysfunction in patients treated with high MMW and high MS HES [62, 63].

Risk Factors and Mechanisms

The proposed risk factors for HES-related kidney dysfunction are: age (older patients have a higher risk), hypovolemia, previous kidney alterations (chronic or acute injury due to other causes), and others comorbidities (such as diabetes and others conditions causing direct or indirect renal alterations). Other risk factors are the type of HES administered (higher MMW and MS) and the total amount per kg body weight.

The most likely mechanism of renal dysfunction is a tubular obstruction caused by hyperoncotic urine formation with the storage of colloidal molecules filtered by the glomeruli. This mechanism is further impaired by a condition of dehydration. Another suggested mechanism is an increase in plasma oncotic pressure, with secondary renal macromolecules accumulation [64].

Adequate hydration using crystalloids may prevent this injury. The anatomic feature of renal damage is an *osmotic nephrosis-like lesion*. In fact histological studies conducted after HES infusion revealed a reversible swelling of renal tubular cells due to the reabsorption of colloidal molecules [65].

Clinical Evidence

Clinical evidence of the renal effects of HES are not uniform and there is still intense debate in the literature as to whether there is truly a critical creatinine level for HES administration.

In a retrospective study on transplanted kidneys from brain-dead donors, Legendre et al. [66] found an 80% rate of renal injury after the infusion of HES 200/0 [62]. However, these anatomic alterations did not cause adverse effects in kidney transplant recipients. A similar study found that the use of 6% HES 200/0.62 caused renal dysfunction after transplantation [63].

In a prospective multicenter study, patients with sepsis or septic shock were treated with HES 200/0.62 or gelatin [67]. In the HES group, 42% of the patients developed acute renal failure, while in the gelatin group only 23% of the patients showed kidney alterations. Neither the need for renal replacement therapy nor mortality were significantly different between the two groups. In another study, the use of 10% HES 200/0.5 was compared with lactated Ringer (LR). The HES group showed a higher incidence of late acute kidney dysfunction [68]. In two meta-analyses [69, 70] HES were related to a higher significant risk of renal damage and dysfunction. On the other hand, large doses (> 2 L) of HES solutions with low MMW and low MS, such as HES 130/0.4 or HES 200/0.5, have been safely used [71-72]. Moreover, in a large observational study, intensive-care patients receiving HES (type not specified) had the same incidence of acute renal dysfunction and similar renal failure scores as patients receiving other plasma substitutes [73].

In the recent literature, the administration of the latest generation HES was suggested to reduce the risk of short-term and long-term renal injury [1].

In a study on brain-dead kidney donors, Blasco et al. [74] compared two HES of different generations: HES 130/0.4 and HES 200/0.62. At one month and one year post-administration, they found better effects on renal function (lower serum creatinine) with HES 130/0.4 than with HES 200/0.62. In neurosurgical patients, the infusion of high doses of HES 6%/130/0.4 was not associated with a deterioration of renal function [72].

The use of fourth-generation HES seems to cause much less harm than older-generation HES, even in patients with previous renal impairment. The infusion of 500 mL of HES 6%/130/0.4 did not cause any kidney damage in volunteers with mild-to-severe renal dysfunction [75].

In a review comprising 34 studies (2607 patients), HES were compared with other fluids [76]. The results evidenced an increased risk of acute renal dysfunction with HES, especially in patients with sepsis.

Conclusions

According to the recent literature, the latest generation HES seems to be the better colloidal solutions to protect the kidney from oncotic damage, while assuring an adequate volume replacement. However, the influence of HES on kidney function remains controversial and large studies are still needed to evaluate the incidence of acute kidney injury with HES in patients without sepsis, directly applying the RIFLE criteria, which distinguish worsening levels of acute kidney function (risk of injury and failure, loss of kidney function, and end-stage kidney function) by precisely measuring the GFR and urine output together with creatinine and neutrophil gelatinase-associated lipocalin (NGAL).

4.6.4.3 Anaphylaxis

All colloidal plasma substitutes can cause anaphylactic/anaphylactoid reactions due to specific or non-specific histamine release. In a trial comprising approximately 20,000 patients, Laxenaire et al, found a decreased incidence of anaphylaxis with HES compared to other colloids [77]. Histamine release seems to be induced by the starch itself; thus, it is unlikely that recent modifications of the MMW, MS, or C2/C6 ratio are the cause of the increased anaphylactic power.

4.6.4.4 Storage

HES are stored in either the reticuloendothelial or the mononuclear phagocyte system, depending on their chemical features, without causing phagocyte dysfunction. High MMW HES have an elevated rate of storage, especially after prolonged or repetitive administrations. By contrast, in animal studies, the newest-generation HES were found to cause less storage, even after multiple uses [78, 79]. One day after the infusion of HES 130/0.4, the percentage remaining in the plasma is approximately 2%, rather than the 8% after the infusion of HES 200/0.5 [78]. Moreover, in a prospective crossover study on healthy volunteers, HES 130/0.42 showed slight accumulation after repeated administration, whereas HES 200/0.5 was stored in significant amounts [79].

4.6.4.5 Itching

Itching occurs after the prolonged administration of large amounts of HES, especially those of the older generations [80, 81]. In some cases, pruritus has been reported after a single large HES dose ($\geq$ 2 L) [80]. Itching induced by HES is of late onset (weeks or even months after their administration) and long lasting. It is due to storage of the material in small peripheral nerves [81]. In a prospective multicenter study, 500 patients were observed 3–9 weeks postoperatively; no differences were found in terms of itching between patients treated with HES and control patients [82].

4.6.4.6 Hyperglycemia

Since HES are similar to glycogen they have the potential to interfere with blood glucose levels. In a study of 150 non-diabetic, ASA class I (American Society of Anesthesiologists) patients undergoing elective surgery, blood sugar levels significantly increased in patients receiving HES 450/0.7 and in those receiving HES 200/0.5 [83]. Although this increase was statistically significant, blood sugar concentration always remained within the normal range. Large clinical trials including patients with established diabetes mellitus and receiving the newest HES preparations are needed to finally address this issue.

Key Concepts
- Advantages and disadvantages of albumin administration
- Properties of dextran solutions: advantages and disadvantages
- Gelatins: limited by the short duration of their volume expansion
- Hydroxyethyl starches (HESs): good plasma volume expanders
- HES effect on coagulation, platelets, and renal function
- Clinical differences between new and old HES

Key Words
- Natural colloids
- Synthetic colloids
- Volume effect
- Albumin
- Dextrans
- Gelatins
- Hydroxyethyl starches (HES)
- Renal impairment
- Clotting disorders

Focus on…
- Dart AB, Mutter TC, Ruth CA, Aback SP (2010) Hydroxyethyl starch (HES) versus other fluid therapies: effects on kidney function. Cochrane Database Syst Rev 1:CD007594

References

1. Mitra S, Khandelwal P (2009) Are all colloids same? How to select the right colloid? Indian Journal of Anaesthesia 53(5):592
2. Nadler SB, Hidalgo JU, Bloch T (1962) Prediction of blood volume in normal human adults. Surgery 51:224–32
3. McIlroy DR, Kharasch ED (2003) Acute intravascular volume expansion with rapidly administered crystalloid or colloid in the setting of moderate hypovolemia Anesth Analg 96(6):1572-7
4. Chappell D, Jacob M, Hofmann-Kiefer K, Conzen P, Rehm M (2008) A rational approach to perioperative fluid management Anesthesiology 109(4):723-40
5. Roberts JS, Bratton SL (1998) Colloid volume expanders. Problems, pitfalls and possibilities Drugs 55(5):621-30
6. Dubois MJ, Vincent JL (2007) Colloid Fluids. In: Hahn RG, Prough DS, Svensen CH (eds) Perioperative Fluid Therapy, 1 edn. New York, Wiley, pp 153-611
7. Nicholson J, Wolmaris M, Park G (2000) The role of albumin in critical illness. Br J Anaesth 85:599-610
8. Mitra S, Khandelwal P (2009) Are all colloids same? How to select the right colloid? Indian J Anaesth 53(5):592–607
9. Schnitzer JE, Carley WW, PAlade GE (1988) Specific albumin binding to microvascular endothelium in culture. Am J Physiol 254:H425-27
10. SAFE Study Investigators, Finfer S, McEvoy S, Bellomo R, McArthur C, Myburgh J, Norton R (2011) Impact of albumin compared to saline on organ function and mortality of patients with severe sepsis. Intensive Care Med 37(1):86-96
11. Martino P (2007) Colloid and crystalloid resuscitation. The ICU Book, 3 edn. Philadelphia, Churchill Livingstone 233-54
12. Randolph L, Takacs M, Davis K (2002) Resuscitation in the pediatric trauma population: Admission base deficit remains an important prognostic indicator. J Trauma 53:838-842
13. Fleck A, Raines G, Hawker F, Trotter J, Wallace PI, Ledingham IM et al (1985) Increased vascular permeability. Major cause of hypoalbuminaemia in disease and injury. Lancet 1:781-3
14. Marik PE (1993) The treatment of hypoalbuminemia in the critically ill patient. Heart Lung 22:166-70
15. Margarson MP, Soni N (1998) Serum albumin: touchstone or totem? Anaesthesia 53:789-803
16. Rubin H, Carlson S, deMeo M, Ganger D, Craig RM (1997) Randomized, double-blind study of intervenous human albumin in hypoalbuminemic patients receiving total parenteral nutrition. Crit Care Med 25:249-52
17. Kaminski MV, Williams SD (1990) Review of the rapid normalization of serum albumin with modified total parenteral nutrition solutions. Crit Care Med 18:327-35
18. Rajnish K J et al (2004) Albumin: an overview of its place in current clinical practice. J Indian An
19. Jorgensen KA, Stofferson E (1979) Heparin-like activity of albumin. Thrombos Res 16:573-8
20. Jorgensen KA, Stofferson E (1980) On the inhibitory effects of albumin on platelet aggregation. Thrombos Res 17:13-8
21. Tobias MD, Wambold D, Pilla MA, Greer F (1998) Differential effects of serial hemodilution with hydroxyethyl starch, albumin, and 0.9% saline on whole blood coagulation. J Clin Anesth 8:366-71
22. Dietrich G, Orth D, Haupt W, Kretschmer V (1990) Primary hemostasis in hemodilution-infusion solutions. Infusionstherapie 17:214-6
23. Vincent JL, Dubois MJ, Navickis RJ, Wilkes MM (2003) Hypoalbuminemia in acute illness: is there a rationale for intervention? A meta-analysis of cohort studies and controlled trials. Ann Surg 237:319-34
24. Prinoth O, Strada P (2002) Proposta di linee guida al corretto uso dell'albumina. Il Servizio Trasfusionale 3:5-10

25. Prinoth O (2007) Servizio Aziendale di Immunoematologia e Trasfusione - Comprensorio Sanitario di Bolzano. Terapia con emocomponenti e plasmaderivati: linee guida ed aspetti medico-legali

26. Arthurson G, Granath K, Thoren L, Wallenius G (1964) The renal excretion of LMW dextran. Acta Clin Scand 127:543-51

27. Atik M (1967) Dextran-40 and dextran-70, a review. Arch Surg 94:664-67

28. Menger MD, Sack FU, Hammersen F, Messmer K (1989) Tissue oxygenation after prolonged ischemia in skeletal muscle: therapeutic effect of prophylactic isovolemic hemodilution. Adv Exp Med Biol 248:387-95

29. Allhoff T, Lenhart FP (1993) Severe dextran-induced anaphylayctic/ anaphylactoid reaction inspite of hapten prophylaxis. Infusionsther Transfusionsmed 20:301–6

30. Baron JF (2000) Adverse effects of colloids on renal function. In: Vincent JL (ed) Yearbook of intensive care and emergency medicine. Springer, Berlin, pp 486-93

31. Moran M, Kapsner C (1987) Acute renal failure associated with elevated plasma oncotic pressure. N Engl J Med 317:150-3

32. Linder P, Ickx B (2006) The effects of colloid solutions on haemostasis. Can J Anesth 53:s30–39

33. Barron ME, Wilkes, Navickis RJ (2004) A systematic review of the comparative safety of colloids. Arch Surg 139:552-563

34. Levi M, Jonge E (2007) Clinical relevance of the effects of plasma expanders on coagulation. Semin Thromb Haemost 33:810–815

35. Kato A, Yonemura K, Matsushima H et al (2001) Complication of oliguric acute renal failure in patients treated with low-molecular weight dextran. Ren Fail 23:679–684

36. Roberts J, Nightingale P (2003) Properties and use of gelatines. In: Webb AR (ed) Therapeutics. Germany, Braun, pp 45-52

37. Lobo DN, Stanga Z, Simpson JA et al (2001) Dilution and redistribution effects of rapid 2-litre infusions of 0.9% (w/v) saline and 5 % (w/v) dextrose on haematological parameters and serum biochemistry in normal subjects: A double-blind crossover study. Clin Sci 101:173-179

38. Zander R (2009) Fluid Management. Bibliomed, Medizinische Verlagsgesellschaft mbH, Melsungen

39. Gines A, Fernandez-Esparrach G, Monescillo A et al (1996) Randomized trial comparing albumin, dextran-70 and polygeline in cirrhotic patients with ascitis treated by paracentesis. Gastroenterology 111:1002-10

40. Adamson JW (2008) New blood, old blood, or no blood? N Engl J Med 358:1295-1296

41. Wilkes NJ, Wolf RL, Powanda MC et al (2002) Hydroxyethil starch in balanced electrolyte solution (Hextend®)-pharmacokinetic and pharmacodynamic profiles in healthy volunteers. Anesth Analg 94:538-44

42. Solanke TF, Khwaja MS, Kadomemu EL (1971) Plasma volume studies with four different plasma volume expanders. J Surg Res 11:140-43

43. Lehmann G, Marx G, Forster H (2007) Bioequivalence comparison between hydroxyethyl starch 130/0.42/6:1 and hydroxyethyl starch 130/0.4/9:1. Drugs R D 8:229–40

44. Schaper J et al (2008) Volume therapy with colloid solutions preserves intestinal microvascular perfusion in endotoxaemia. Eur J Heart Failure 76:120-128

45. Wilkes NJ, Woolf R, Mutch M et al (2001) The effect of balanced versus saline-based hetastarch and crystalloid solutions on acid-base and electrolyte status and gastric mucosal perfusion in elderly surgical patients. Anesth Analg 93:811-816

46. DeJonge E, Levi M (2001) Effects of different plasma substitutes on blood coagulation: a comparative review. Crit Care Med 29:1261–7

47. Sanfelippo MJ, Suberviola PD, Geimer NF (1987) Development of a von Willebrand-like syndrome after prolonged use of hydroxyethyl starch. Am J Clin Pharmacol 88:653–5

48. Treib J, Baron JF, Grauer MT, Strauss RG (1999) An international view of hydroxyethyl starches. Intensive Care Med 25:258–68

49. Madjdpour C, Dettori N, Frascarolo P, Burki M, Boll M, Fisch A, Bombeli T, Spahn DR (2005)

Molecular weight of hydroxyethyl starch: is there an effect on blood coagulation and pharmacokinetics? Br J Anaesth 94:569–76

50. Kozek-Langenecker SA (2005) Effects of hydroxyethyl starch solutions on hemostasis. Anesthesiology 103:654–60

51. Strauss RG, Pennell BJ, Stump DC (2002) A randomized, blinded trial comparing the hemostatic effects of pentastarch versus hetastarch. Transfusion 42:27–36

52. Haynes GH, Havidich JE, Payne KJ (2004) Why the Food and Drug Administration changed the warning label for hetastarch. Anesthesiology 101:560 –1

53. Treib J, Haass A, Pindur G (1997) Coagulation disorders caused by hydroxyethyl starch. Thromb Haemost 78:974–83

54. Franz A, Bräunlich P, Gamsjäger T, Felfernig M, Gustorff B, Kozek-Langenecker SA (2001) The effects of hydroxyethyl starches of varying molecular weights on platelet function. Anesth Analg 92:1402–7

55. Stögermüller B, Stark J, Willschke H, Felfernig M, Hoerauf K, Kozek-Langenecker SA (2000) The effect of hydroxyethylstarch 200 kD on platelet function. Anesth Analg 91:823–7

56. Deusch E, Thaler U, Kozek-Langenecker SA (2004) The effects of high molecular weight hydroxyethyl starch solutions on platelets. Anesth Analg 99:665–8

57. Felfernig M, Franz A, Bräunlich P, Fohringer C, Kozek-Langenecker SA (2003) The effects of hydroxyethyl starch solutions on thromboelastography in preoperative male patients. Acta Anaesthesiol Scand 47:70–3

58. Gallandat Huet RCG, Siemons AW, Baus D, van Rooyen-Butijn WT, Haagenaars JA, van Oeveren W, Bepperling F (2000) A novel hydroxyethyl starch (Voluven®) for effective perioperative plasma volume substitution in cardiac surgery. Can J Anaesth 47:1207–15

59. Jungheinrich C, Sauermann W, Bepperling F, Vogt NH (2004) Volume efficacy and reduced influence on measures of coagulation using hydroxyethyl starch 130/0.4 (6%) with an optimised in vivo molecular weight in orthopaedic surgery: a randomised, double-blind study. Drugs R D 5:1–9

60. Kozek-Langenecker SA, Jungheinrich C, Sauermann W, Van der Linden P (2008) The effects of hydroxyethyl starch 130/0.4 (6%) on blood loss and use of blood products in major surgery: a pooled analysis of randomized clinical trials. Anesth Analg 107:382–90

61. Scharbert G, Deusch E, Kress HG, Greher M, Gustorff B, Kozek-Langenecker SA (2004) Inhibition of platelet function by hydroxyethyl starch solutions in chronic pain patients undergoing peridural anesthesia. Anesth Analg 99:823–7

62. Chen G, Yan M, Lu QH, Gong M (2006) Effects of two different hydroxyethyl starch solutions (HES200/0.5 vs.HES130/0.4) on the expression of platelet membrane glycoprotein. Acta Anaesthesiol Scand 50:1089–94

63. Cittanova ML, LeBlanc I, Legendre C, Mouquet C, Riou B, Coriat P (1996) Effects of hydroxyethyl starch in braindead kidney donors on renal function in kidney-transplant recipients. Lancet 348:1620-2

64. Rozich JD, Paul RV (1989) Acute renal failure precipitated by elevated colloid osmotic pressure. Am J Med 87:358–60

65. Kief H, Englelhart K (1966) Reabsorptive Vacuolisation der gewundenen Nierenhauptstuecke (sog. osmotische Nephrose). Frank Zeitschr Path 75:53–9

66. Legendre C, Thervet E, Page B, Percheron A, Noe`l LH, Kreis H (1993) Hydroxyethylstarch and osmotic-nephrosis-like lesions in kidney transplantation. Lancet 342:248–9

67. Schortgen F, Lacherade JC, Bruneel F, Cattaneo I, Hemery F, Lemaire F, Brochard L (2001) Effects of hydroxyethylstarch and gelatin on renal function in severe sepsis: a multicenter randomized study. Lancet 357: 911–6

68. Brunkhorst FM, Englel C, Bloos F, Meier-Hellmann A, Ragaller M, Weiler N, Moerer O, Gruendling M, Oppert M, Grond S, Olthoff D, Jaschinski U, John S, Rossaint R, Welte T, Schaefer M, Kern P, Kuhnt E, Kiehntopf M, Hartog C, Natanson C, Loeffler M, Reinhart K. German competence network sepsis (SepNet) (2008) Intensive insulin therapy and pentastarch resuscitation in severe sepsis. N Engl J Med 358:125–39

69. Wiedermann CJ (2008) Systematic review of randomized clinical trials on the use of hydroxyethyl starch for fluid management in sepsis. BMC Emerg Med 24:8-1
70. Davidson IJ (2006) Renal impact of fluid management with colloids: a comparative review. Eur J Anaesthesiol 23:721–38
71. Vogt NH, Bothner U, Lerch G, Lindner KH, Georgieff M (1996) Large-dose administration of 6% hydroxyethyl starch 200/0.5 for total hip arthroplasty: plasma homeostasis, hemostasis, and renal function compared to use of 5% human albumin. Anesth Analg 83:262-8
72. Neff TA, Doelberg M, Jungheinrich C, Sauerland A, Spahn DR, Stocker R (2003) Repetitive large-dose infusion of the novel hydroxyethyl starch 130/0.4 in patients with severe head injury. Anesth Analg 96:1453-9
73. Sakr Y, Payen D, Reinhart K, Sipmann FS, Zavala E, Bewley J, Marx G, Vincent JL (2007) Effects of hydroxyethyl starch administration on renal function in critically ill patients. Br J Anaesth 98:216–24
74. Blasco V, Leone M, Antonini F, Geissler A, Albanese J, Martin C (2008) Comparison of the novel hydroxyethylstarch 130/0.4 and hydroxyethylstarch 200/0.6 in brain-dead donor resuscitation on renal function after transplantation. Br J Anaesth 100:504–8
75. Jungheinrich C, Scharpf R, Wargenau M, Bepperling F, Baron JF (2002) The pharmacokinetics and tolerability of an intravenous infusion of the new hydroxyethyl starch 130/0.4 (6%, 500 mL) in mild-to-severe renal impairment. Anesth Analg 95:544–51
76. Dart AB, Mutter TC, Ruth CA, Taback SP (2010) Hydroxyethyl starch (HES) versus other fluid therapies: effects on kidney function. Cochrane Database Syst Rev 20(1):CD007594
77. Laxenaire M, Charpentier C, Feldman L (1994) Reactions anaphylactoides aux subitutes colloidaux du plasma: incidence, facteurs de risque, mecanismes. Ann Fr Anest Reanimat 13:301–10
78. Jungheinrich C, Neff TA (2005) Pharmacokinetics of hydroxyethyl starch. Clin Pharmacokinet 44:681–99
79. Waitzinger J, Bepperling F, Pabst G, Opitz J (2003) Hydroxyethyl starch (HES) [130/0.4], a new HES specification: pharmacokinetics and safety after multiple infusions of 10% solution in healthy volunteers. Drugs R D 4:149–5
80. Lehmann GB, Asskali F, Boll M, Burmeister MA, Marx G,Hilgers R, Forster H (1995) HES 130/0.42 shows less alteration of pharmacokinetics than HES 200/0.5 when dosed repeatedly.Br J Anaesth 2007;98:635–44
81. Spittal MJ, Findlay GP. The seven year itch. Anaesthesia 50:913–4
82. Metze D, Reimann S, Szepfalusi Z, Bohle B, Kraft D, Luger TA (1997) Persistent pruritus after hydroxyethyl starch infusion therapy: a result of long-term storage in cutaneous nerves. Br J Dermatol 136:553–9
83. Murty SS, Kammath S, Chaudhari LS (2004) Effects of hydroxyethyl starches on blood sugar levels: a randomized double blind study. Indian J Anaesth 48:196–200

Clinical Treatment: The Right Fluid in the Right Quantity

5

Felice Eugenio Agrò, Dietmar Fries and Marialuisa Vennari

5.1   A Little Bit of History

One of the most important questions about fluid management is what kind of fluid to use. Historically, the debate was developed around the dispute crystalloids vs. colloids. In its course, the medical literature has largely demonstrated the difference in the pharmacokinetics and pharmacodynamics of these two classes of plasma substitutes (see Chapters 3 and 4). Consequently, crystalloids should no longer be considered as an alternative to colloids and viceversa. Instead, they must be considered as the two faces of the same coin, and their use as part of an integrative fluid management.

The electrolyte composition of fluids (crystalloid or colloid) is another source of controversy. The debate on balanced, plasma-adapted solutions started in the 1970s, when their features were first described. A new definition was proposed in 2000 in "Avoiding iatrogenic hyperchloremic acidosis: Call for a new crystalloid fluid", published in *Anesthesiology* [1], which referred to the classic need for "a solution containing sodium bicarbonate" because it was clear that "...the predominate physiologic deficit is metabolic acidosis...". Subsequent developments were summarized in 2003 by Reid et al [2], who highlighted that scientists and clinicians must inevitably reach a compromise in their long-standing attempts to find the ideal physiological solution.

On the other hand, the Hamletic doubt fluid management is "to fill or not to fill" the patient? Many studies have tried to answer the question, resulting in a 50-year ongoing debate in which many strategies have been proposed, especially in surgical patients.

M.Vennari (✉)
Postgraduate School of Anesthesia and Intensive Care, Anesthesia, Intensive Care and Pain Management Department, University School of Medicine Campus Bio-Medico of Rome, Rome, Italy
e-mail: m.vennari@unicampus.it

F. E. Agrò (ed.), *Body Fluid Management*,
DOI: 10.1007/978-88-470-2661-2_5 © Springer-Verlag Italia 2013

The initial evidence supported the use of large amounts of IV fluids ("liberal" approach). Subsequently, a "restricted" approach was proposed, especially in major abdominal surgery. The more recent literature has emphasized rational and guided fluid management in the context of a hemodynamic evaluation of each patient (Goal-Directed Fluid Therapy), optimizing tissue oxygenation and avoiding acid-base disequilibrium and electrolytic alterations.

5.2   What Fluid for What Purpose?

5.2.1   Clinical Settings

The effects of the different fluids should take into account organ function, endothelial leakage, inflammation, organ tissue/perfusion, comorbidities of the patient, and her/his clinical situation (major surgery, critically ill, pediatric, pregnancy, etc.).

The most frequent fluid deficits are due to:
- acute blood loss;
- dehydration.

5.2.1.1 Acute Blood Loss
The main physiological reaction to acute blood loss is the activation of the Sympathetic Nervous System (SNS) and of the renin-angiotensin-aldosterone axis, with increased ADH levels (Fig. 5.1).

All these responses lead to a fluid shift from the extravascular space (EVS) into the intravascular space (IVS), resulting in blood volume restoration and a concomitant decrease in colloid-oncotic pressure (COP). The return to normal values of the plasma protein concentration (80% COP) is reached within 24 h, from a blood loss of 30%. This observation suggests that the body replaces a blood loss ≤ 15% in about 24 h, even in the absence of intravenous fluid administration [3-5].

The amount of blood volume loss determines the clinical manifestations of hemorrhage. Blood losses up to 15% of blood volume are compensated by the hormonal and autonomic response to hypovolemia, with minor clinical manifestations. Consequently, they can optionally be replaced with crystalloid. Blood loss > 15% (about 750 mL) should be treated with colloid infusion, as should major blood loss (> 30%) which may also require red blood cells transfusion [6, 7].

Comparison Between Colloids and Crystalloids
Theoretically, we expect greater advantages in blood volume expansion with isotonic colloids than with isotonic crystalloids. This is due to many reasons:
- Crystalloids are mainly distributed in the interstitial space (ISS), with less effectiveness in maintaining plasma volume, because they do not contain oncotic particles (Fig. 5.2). Their duration of action is short, with a rela-

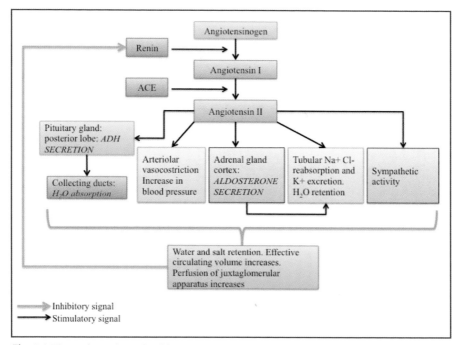

Fig. 5.1 The renin-angiotensin-aldosterone system: hypovolemia reduces perfusion of the juxaglomerular apparatus, with renin release. Circulating renin coverts angiotensinogen to angiotensin I, while ACE (angiotensin converting enzyme) acts on angiotensin I converting it to angiotensin II. This hormone increases sympathetic nervous system activity and the reabsorption of Na^+ and water directly by the kidneys and through aldosterone action, which causes vasoconstriction and ADH secretion

tively large volume needed for a specific target volume expansion. Their infusion dilutes plasma proteins, thus reducing the COP. Consequently, there is a diffusion of fluids from the IVS to the ISS. This fluid shift increases when vascular permeability is altered, causing interstitial edema.

- Colloids are distributed in the IVS, with a larger increase in plasma volume because they contain oncotic particles. They have a longer duration of action, with smaller volumes needed for a specific target volume expansion. If endothelial permeability is intact, colloids are retained in the IVS, with a subsequent increase of the plasma oncotic pressure and the diffusion of fluids from the ISS to the IVS (Fig. 5.2).

When using colloids, it is important to remember that they have a "contest volume effect" [8]. In hypovolemic patients, they have a volume effect > 90% of the infused volume; in normovolemic patients, two-thirds of the infused volume shifts to the ISS within minutes [9, 10]. Consequently, they

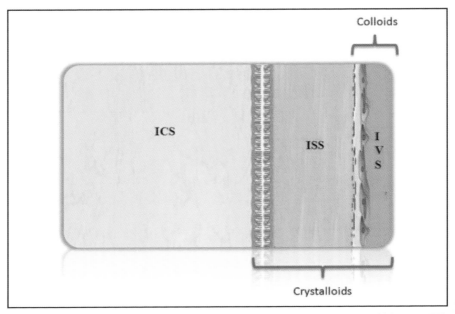

Fig. 5.2 Crystalloids and colloids distribution. *ICS*, intracellular space; *ISS*, interstitial space; *IVS*, intravascular space

should be used only in hypovolemia, even when there is capillary membrane damage. In fact, in this case hypovolemia is connected to the shift into the ISS of protein-rich fluids, with a plasma COP reduction. Colloids that are able to increase COP are needed: their use reduces ISS overload [8].

In 2001, Jarvela [11] reported that intravascular volume expansion was significantly higher after HES than after crystalloids infusion. In 2006, Verheij [12] showed that volume expansion and Cardiac Index (CI) following cardiac surgery were significantly higher after colloid infusion than after the administration of crystalloids.

However, in 2004, Jones [13] found no significant differences between colloids and crystalloids in pre-load (Central Venous Pressure, CVP; Pulmonary Arterial Occlusion Pressure, PAOP), post-load (Systemic Vascular Resistence, SVR), Heart Rate (HR) and CI during acute normovolemic hemodilution.

Concerns about Colloids
Debates about hemodynamic effects exist also with respect to the different isotonic colloids. Verheij [12] found no significant difference in hemodynamic state and COP registration after the infusion of 6% HES 450/0.7, 5% HA, or 6% dextran.

For the same solutions, Jones [13] demonstrated no significant differences in hemodynamic power. On the other hand, Niemi [14] found that CI increases immediately after the infusion of 6% HES 130/0.4, whereas over the long term the increase of CI in the studied HES group was comparable to that of the group treated with 4% HA. In 2006, Palumbo [15] found that after the infusion of crystalloids, CVP (pre-load!) does not significantly change and that CI significantly increases after the infusion of 6% HES 130/0.4 but not after the infusion of 20% HA. In addition, Van der Linden [16]. showed that the quantity of colloids necessary to maintain target values of CI, O_2 saturation, and diuresis did not significantly change ($p > 0.05$) between 6% HES 200/0.5 and gelatins.

Another issue is the hemodynamic effects of the different isotonic HES, depending on their metabolism. The enzymatic degradation of HES has two opposing effects on volemic expansion: (1) a reduction in volume expansion, because it improves renal excretion; (2) an increase in hemodynamic power, by increasing the number of active osmotic particles. Most studies report similar hemodynamic effects between HES with higher MMW and MSR, and HES with lower MMW and MSR [17, 18]. However, according to a report on a small sample population (20 patients) plasma volume expansion induced by an HES with low MMW and MS (HES 130/0.4) is longer lasting than that achieved with the infusion of an HES with high MMW and MS (HES 670/0.75) [19].

Concerns about Crystalloids
Hypertonic crystalloids induce a greater and a more rapid increase of the plasma volume than isotonic solutions, for the same infused volume. However, hypertonic crystalloids induce a short-lasting volemic expansion, probably because of their strong diuretic effect (see Chapter 3).

5.2.1.2 Dehydration
Dehydration derives from an imbalance between water intake and losses. It consists of a reduction of ISS and ICS water. Common causes are:
- diarrhea;
- vomiting;
- fever;
- excessive sweating;
- prolonged fasting;
- renal loss.

Even in case of dehydration, the organism uses compensatory mechanisms. The most important reactions to dehydration are ADH release by the neurohypophysis and hypothalamic stimulation of thirst (Fig. 5.3).

Mild to moderate dehydration can be resolved by oral water intake (excepted for the patient who cannot drink); severe dehydration needs immediate medical treatment. The safest approach is prevention, by monitoring fluid balance (water balance = 0).

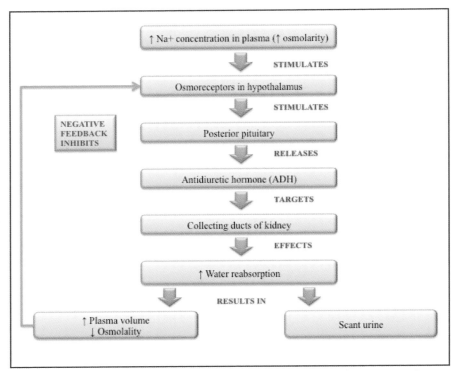

Fig. 5.3 Mechanism of ADH secretion: hypothalamic osmo-receptors are stimulated by IVS water losses with increased plasmatic osmolarity. The hypothalamus then stimulates the posterior pituitary gland to release antidiuretic hormone (ADH), which increases free water reabsorption by the renal distal tubules, in order to maintain fluid balance. ADH secretion is more sensitive to plasma osmolarity than to that of the circulating blood

Water losses are associated with sodium losses, with a modification of plasma osmolarity. Thus, with respect to water losses/sodium losses we can distinguish among three types of dehydration:
- hypotonic (water losses < sodium losses);
- hypertonic (water losses > sodium losses);
- isotonic (water losses = sodium losses).

Fluid therapy must be adapted to the specific needs of the patient. In case of hypotonic dehydration, a hypertonic solution should be carefully (slow infusion) administered, in order to allow the restoration of plasma sodium, reducing the risk of an ICS fluid shift and cellular death (see Chapter 1). In case of hypertonic dehydration, a dextrose solution may be indicated in order to restore plasma sodium. In fact, dextrose is distributed throughout the body spaces as free water (free from the osmolar effect of sodium) allowing dilution of the hypernatremia and body water restoration (Fig. 5.4).

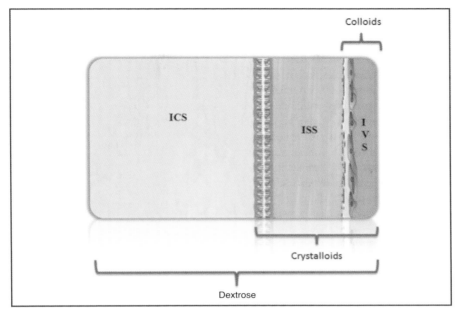

Fig. 5.4 Dextrose distribution compared to crystalloids and colloids

In case of isotonic dehydration, isotonic electrolyte solutions should be used in order to restore water and sodium balances, with no significant effects on plasma osmolarity and electrolytes.

5.2.1.3 To Summarize
Evidence [8] suggests that fluid management must be adapted to the specific loss of body water (Fig. 5.5).
- Use crystalloids to restore urinary loss, *perspiratio insensibilis*, and physiologic fluid circulation between the ISS and the IVS.
- Use colloids to restore blood loss and the ISS shift of protein-rich fluid when the vascular barrier is damaged.
- Use hypertonic or dextrose solutions when water loss is accompanied by significant alteration of plasma osmolarity (i.e., alterations in plasma sodium concentration).

5.2.2   Goal-Directed Fluid Therapy: An Overview

Goal-directed therapy (GDT) is a complex strategy for fluid infusions aimed at optimizing tissue perfusion and oxygenation; it is guided by hemodynamic variables. Through hemodynamic monitoring, GDT allows physicians to

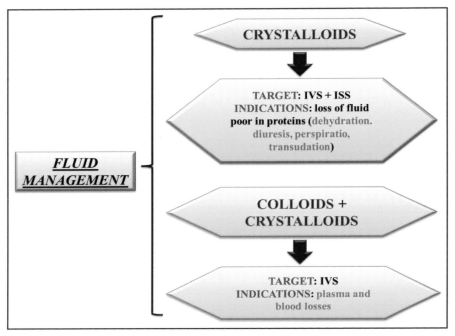

Fig. 5.5 Specific treatment according to affected body water space

administer fluids, and/or use other therapies, such as inotropic or vasoactive drugs, only to those patients who need them, in order to assure oxygen delivery sufficient to fulfill the metabolic requirement of the particular patient. With GDT, hemodynamic management is therefore personalized.

5.2.2.1 GDT: Physiological Basis

Management of both critically ill and elective surgery patients is mainly aimed at assuring adequate tissue perfusion and oxygenation. Physiologically adequate oxygen delivery (DO_2) is assured by the cardiovascular and respiratory systems and it corresponds to the quantity (in mL) of oxygen per minute carried to the tissues [20].

DO$_2$ is defined by the following equation:

$$DO_2 \ (mL/min) = cardiac \ output \ (CO) \times arterial \ oxygen \ content \ (CaO_2)$$
$$(Eq. \ 5.1)$$

DO$_2$ physiologically corresponds to 900–1100 mL/min or to 500–600 mL/min/m^2 if reported as body surface area (DO$_2$I).

Considering the factors determining CO and CaO_2, Eq. 5.1 can be rewritten as:

$$DO_2 \ (mL/min) = (HR \times SV) \times [(1.34 \ x \ Hb \ x \ SaO2) + (0.003 \times paO_2)]$$
(Eq.5.2)

where:
- HR is the heart rate;
- SV is the stroke volume;
- 1.34 is the number of mL of oxygen carried by hemoglobin at 100% saturation;
- Hb is the amount of hemoglobin in g/dl;
- SaO_2 is the O_2 saturation in arterial blood;
- 0.003 is the solubility coefficient of oxygen;
- PaO_2 is the partial O_2 pressure of arterial blood;
  Thus, oxygen delivery can be improved by modifying:
- SV, by using inotropic (heart contractility) or vasoactive drugs (post-load) and fluid administration (pre-load);
- Hb, by the transfusion of red cells;
- SaO_2 and paO_2, by O_2 therapy and in some cases by mechanical ventilation.
  Oxygen demand-consumption (VO_2) is the quantity (in mL) of oxygen consumed by the tissue per minute. It depends on the metabolic state and is increased by surgical stress and critical conditions. VO_2 may be described by the following relationship:

$$VO_2 \ (mL/min) = caridac \ outpout \ (CO) \times [arterial \ O_2 \ content \ (CaO_2)$$
$$- venous \ O_2 \ content \ (CvO_2) \ (Eq. \ 5.3)$$

Equation 5.3 can be rewritten as:

$$VO_2 \ (mL/min) = (FC \times SV) \times [(1.34 \times Hb \times SaO_2) + (0.003 \times paO_2) -$$
$$(1.34 \times Hb \times SvO_2) + (0.003 \times pvO_2)] \ (Eq. \ 5.4)$$

where:
- CO and CaO_2 are described by the same factor as in Eq. 5.2;
- SvO_2 is the saturation of mixed venous blood;
- PvO_2 is the partial O_2 pressure in mixed venous blood.
  VO_2 is about 200–300 mL/min (110–160 mL/min/m^2 if reported as body surface area) at basal metabolism. Under stress conditions it may increase of four- to six-fold.
  O_2 extraction (O_2ER) is the fraction of DO_2 released to the tissues per minute. It is a tissue oxygenation index, expressed as:

$$O_2ER = VO_2/DO_2 \ (Eq. \ 5.5)$$

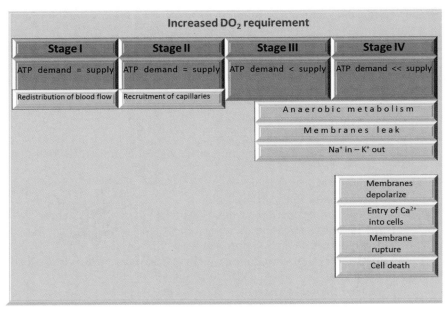

Fig. 5.6 Relation between DO_2, VO_2 and O_2ER: VO_2 is assured despite wide-ranging values of DO_2, through an increase in O_2 extraction (O_2ER). Below a critical value of DO_2 (critical DO_2), O_2ER can no longer increase and VO_2 becomes flow dependent. Tissue hypoxia appears and anaerobic metabolism starts

Under basal conditions, the ratio is 0.25, but it can increases in order to assure VO_2. In fact, normally, VO_2 is maintained despite wide-ranging DO_2 values, through an increase of O_2ER. Below a critical value of DO_2 (critical DO_2), O_2ER can no longer increase and VO_2 becomes flow dependent (Fig. 5.6). Tissue hypoxia appears and anaerobic metabolism is initiated [20].

The tissue hypoxia causes a disequilibrium between ATP production and ATP demand. A reduction in cAMP and cGMP levels activates the endothelium, reducing its barrier function and causing the release of pro-inflammatory cytokines, leading to capillary leak syndrome. Disruption of the endothelial barrier exposes the blood to pro-coagulant factors and leukocyte adhesion molecules. Leukocytes and complement are activated, leading to a systemic inflammation with organ hypoperfusion and failure (multi-organ failure). The detection and prevention of tissue hypoxia is therefore crucial [20].

A rational approach to fluid therapy (GDT) is the most readily available and simplest tool to assure adequate DO_2.

Some patients are lacking in compensatory mechanisms when VO_2 increases, because of comorbidities (cardiovascular or pulmonary diseases), and thus have a higher probability of reaching the critical DO_2 under stress conditions. These are high-risk patients who are likely to benefit from a GDT approach.

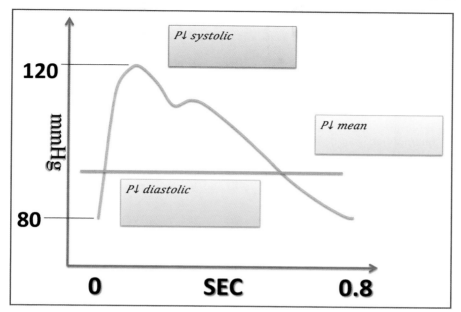

Fig. 5.7 Pulse pressure variation (PPV). The determination of PPV requires an invasive system to measure arterial blood pressure.
Pulse pressure = systolic pressure – diastolic pressure

5.2.2.2 Hemodynamic Variables in GDT

The rational approach to fluid administration in GDT is based on the prediction of fluid responsiveness. It refers to a strategy aimed at identifying fluid responders, i.e., patients who, according to Starling's law, will benefit from fluid loading in terms of hemodynamic stability and DO_2, avoiding the administration of unnecessary fluid boluses. Defined hemodynamic variables are necessary to test fluid responsiveness. These can be divided into static and dynamic. Static variables indicate hemodynamic status at a specific time, for the pre-load value at that time. An example of static variable is the value of Cardiac Index obtained in a single thermodilution through Swan-Ganz catheter. Dynamic variables indicate hemodynamic changes in response to a periodic variation in pre-load. Static indexes are comparable to a picture, while dynamic ones to a movies. Dynamic variables are better indicators of fluid responsiveness than static ones [20].

Historically, cardiac filling pressures (CVP and PAOP) were used to guide intravascular volume therapy. Indeed, CVP measurement is still widely used. However, recent studies have shown that CVP does not adequately reflect pre-load and fails to predict fluid responsiveness [21, 22]. At the same time, other parameters have been considered, such as the Pulse Pressure Variation (PPV), defined as the difference between systolic and diastolic pressure for each heart beat (Fig. 5.7).

PPV is the variation in pulse pressure at different heart beats induced by variations of the intra-thoracic pressure due to mechanical ventilation (MV) and caused by a variation in pre-load value (Fig. 5.8). Its use in guiding volume therapy has been demonstrated, suggesting a possible improvement in outcome after high-risk surgery [23].

Pulse wave analysis allows the assessment of other functional hemodynamic parameters, such as Stroke Volume Variation (SVV) and CI (Fig. 5.9).

Intermittent transpulmonary thermodilution, according to the monitoring system applied, can be used to calibrate pulse wave analysis, which enhances the reliability of CI measurements.

It can also be used to measure Stroke Volume Variation (SVV), Extravascular Lung Water (EVLW), and Global End Diastolic Volume (GEDV). SVV, GEDV, and EVLW (the "golden triangle") may be used in combination for GDT assessment.

SVV is based on cyclic changes in the SV due to intrathoracic pressure during mechanical ventilation and caused by a variation in pre-load value (Fig. 5.9).

$$SVV = (SV\ max - SV\ min)/SV\ mean$$

It is conceptually similar to PPV, but more precise and reliable.

SVV and other dynamic variables may indicate the actual position on the Frank–Starling curve. When the heart operates on the ascending limb of the curve, the intrathoracic pressure variation with MV induces large changes in pre-load and SV (SVV > 13%), indicating a preserved pre-load reserve and CI improvement after fluid administration (fluid responders). By contrast at the plateau of the Frank-Starling curve, there are minimal or no CI improvement after fluid administration. In this case small change in SV (SVV < 13%) are registered in response to intrathoracic pressure variation, indicating a minimum pre-load reserve (Fig. 5.10). In this case inotropes may be required.

SVV has been found to consistently predict fluid responsiveness, with threshold values of 11–13% [24, 25]. However, there are some limitations that may exclude a valid use of SVV:
- right ventricular failure;
- arrhythmias;
- spontaneous breathing;
- ratio heart rate/respiratory rate < 3.6;
- low tidal volume (< 8 mL/kg).

GEDV (total cardiac filling volume) is a better marker of cardiac pre-load than CVP [26]. However, it is a static parameter that does not allow the evaluation of cardiac responsiveness to fluid loading.

In case of left ventricular failure or acute lung injury, the EVLW (index of lung edema) can be used. EVLW is an independent predictor of survival. In GDT, use of the EVLW accelerates the resolution of lung edema, whether due to increased vascular permeability or to an increase in hydrostatic pressure [27, 28].

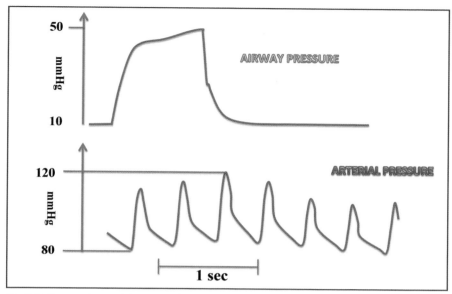

Fig 5.8 Changes in arterial pressure in response to respiration. When the intrathoracic pressure increases in the inspiratory phase of mechanical ventilation, pre-load decreases, with a transitory reduction of CO and consequently of systolic pressure and PPV. In expiration, intrathoracic pressure decreases and pre-load increases, with a transitory increase of CO and consequently of systolic pressure and PPV

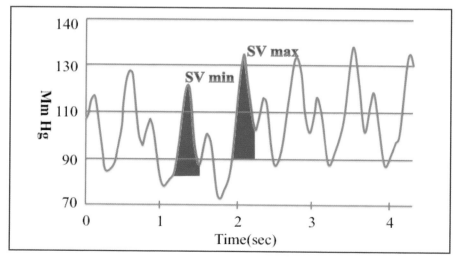

Fig. 5.9 Pulse wave analysis: the area under the curve corresponds to the stroke volume (SV). Knowing the heart rate, the cardiac index may be calculated continuously. The variation of the area under the curve, and consequently of SV (SVV), reflects through the time CI variation in response to pre-load variation due to intrathoracic pressure variation in mechanical ventilated patients

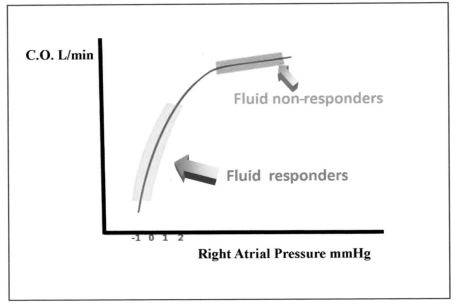

Fig 5.10 Fluid responders and fluid non-responders according to the Frank–Starling curve. Fluid responders: On the ascending limb (*pink*) of the curve, intrathoracic pressure changes induce large changes in pre-load (right atrial pressure) and SV (SVV > 13%). Fluid non-responders: On the plateau (*red* of the curve) only small SV changes are observed (SVV < 13%) in response to intrathoracic pressure variation

In cardiac surgery patients, the use of a goal-directed protocol (GEDV > 800 ml/m^2, EVLW = 10–12 ml/kg) resulted in an enhanced post-operative outcome [29]. In patients with subarachnoid hemorrhage, CI was maximized using GEDV and EVLW (targets: CI $\geq$ 3 L/min/m^2, indexed GEDV >= 700 ml/m^2, EVLW >= 14 ml/kg) in order to prevent secondary brain injury: no congestive heart failure was observed using the goal-directed protocol [30].

5.2.2.3 Monitoring Systems in GDT

The use of GDT requires hemodynamic assessment and monitoring. The ideal system should be simple, non- or hardly invasive, safe, and precise, allowing immediate therapeutic intervention. Unfortunately, however, this system has not yet been invented, although many systems have been proposed for hemodynamic assessment, especially recently.

All these systems have to be compared to the Swan-Ganz or Pulmonary Artery Catheter (PAC), which remains the gold standard, despite its limits. In fact, a PAC is not recommended when GDT is performed in the routine perioperative setting, as demonstrated by multiple clinical trials. Its use is further discouraged by the invasiveness of the procedure, which exposes patients to complications. In addition, PAC cannot be used without adequate training and experience. Finally, its performance mainly refers to filling pressure values (PVC, PAOP), which may be affected by valvular pathologies and alterations in cardiac compliance. Consequently, its fame in the literature and in clinics has decreased over the years. Moreover, less invasive systems with similar precision have been introduced [20].

Modern technologies provide filling volume values that are more reliable as pre-load and fluid responsiveness indices. Current and less invasive flow-monitoring techniques include Doppler technologies or arterial pressure waveform analysis, which measure changes in stroke volume or cardiac output.

The Esophageal Doppler (ED) allows measurement of blood velocity at the level of the descending aorta. The flow time in the descending aorta, corrected for HR (FTc normally 330–360 ms) corresponds to the SV. According to the chosen probe, the correspondence is obtained through a nomogram calculated from comparative studies performed with a PAC or through the measurement of the vessel cross-section. At lower FTc, hypovolemia should be suspected. ED requires less operator training than other systems and does not require calibration, but it is difficult to use in awake patients and the results may be operator-dependent. GDT using ED was shown to improve patient outcomes [31]. Chytra et al. have shown that the optimization of fluid management using ED in trauma patients reduces blood lactate levels, the incidence of infections, and the duration of the intensive-care unit (ICU) and hospital stay [32]. A meta-analysis showed that patients undergoing major abdominal surgery who received ED GDT had a reduction in complications, requirement of inotropes, ICU admissions, and hospital stay, with a rapid gastrointestinal function recovery [31].

Today, less invasive hemodynamic monitoring devices, such as the PiCCO (Pulsion Medical System) and the new EV1000 system, provide parameters that may improve the monitoring of fluid therapy. These devices combine pulse wave analysis and trans-pulmonary thermodilution, with the former based on data obtained by the latter. For this reason, the validity of pulse pressure analysis depends on periodic recalibration through thermodilution [33, 34]. These systems require invasive arterial lines and a central venous catheter, but they are less invasive than PAC.

The PICCO system yields the GEDV and EVLW through thermodilution curves, while EV1000 uses the maximum slope of the thermodilution curve's ascent and descent to calculate GEDV. This method can reduce the interference potential of the indicator with the thermic recirculation. Recently, the results of a first validation study on animal models showed that the performance of the two devices is comparable [35]. SVV evaluated by the PiCCO plus system (an evolution of PiCCO) adequately indicates fluid-responders in various clinical settings.

Another system based on pulse wave analysis is the FloTrac/Vigileo (Edwards Lifesciences, Irvine, CA, USA; SVVFloTrac) system. It uses Langewouters' algorithm to perform the wave analysis and does not require thermodilution for calibration. Consequently, it can be used only with a normal invasive arterial line connected to the FloTrac sensor [20].

A study on 40 patients undergoing cardiac surgery compared the SVV measured with FloTrac/Vigileo and the PiCCOplus and found no significant difference in the prediction of fluid responsiveness [36].

Mayer et al. showed that the use of a GDT protocol through FloTrac/Vigileo in high-risk patients undergoing major abdominal surgery resulted in a reduction of both hospital stay and the incidence of complications [37]. In similar patients, Benes et al. found that intraoperative fluid optimization through the Vigileo/FloTrac system decreased the incidence of postoperative complications, reducing hospitalization time [25]. The limits of Vigileo involve the validity of the wave pressure analysis and SVV values only in mechanically ventilated patients.

A new, non-invasive monitor for the measurement of continuous CO is the Nexfin HD monitor. It measures CO continuously completely non-invasively by an inflatable finger cuff. The Nexfin HD using volume clamp technology, continuously measures finger blood pressure and converts the value into a blood pressure wave of the brachial artery. The truly non-invasive nature of the Nexfin HD allows the measurement of CO and can be used in awake, not mechanically ventilated patients.

5.2.2.4 Current Results of GDT in Critically Ill Patients. A Systematic Review

Our group has evaluated the current results of hemodynamic monitoring and manipulation in critically ill patients [38]. In a systematic review and meta-analysis of randomized controlled trials (RCTs), GDT was compared with the standard of care. Studies were searched in MEDLINE, EMBASE and Cochrane Library databases. RCTs included in the analysis were:

I.   Those in which the effects of hemodynamic GDT on mortality or morbidity in critically ill patients was the main research topic. GDT was defined as the monitoring and manipulation of hemodynamic parameters to reach normal or supranormal values using fluids and/or vasoactive therapy. Studies with no description of GDT, no difference between groups in the optimization protocol, with therapy titrated to the same goal in both groups were excluded.

II. The control group comprised patients treated according to the standard of care.

III. The study population consisted of critically ill, non-surgical patients, or postoperative patients with already established sepsis or organ failure. Studies involving mixed populations or surgical patients undergoing non-cardiac or cardiac surgery were excluded.

A random effects model was chosen for all analyses, since it involves the assumption that the effects estimated in different studies are not identical but follow certain distributions and that studies represent a random sample of the relevant distribution of effects. The combined effects estimate is the mean effect of this distribution. Several sensitivity and subgroup analyses for the main outcome were planned on the basis of: *clinical setting, treatment, therapeutic goals, nor-*

mal and supranormal hemodynamic optimization, monitoring tools.

Among the 3060 patients randomized in the 14 included studies, hospital mortality was recorded in 966 cases (31%). Of these deaths, 518 occurred in the control group (34%), and 448 in the experimental group (29%). Table 5.1 shows the overall responses (ORs) and 95% confidence intervals for the observed in-hospital mortality in each trial as well as the pooled estimate. The overall effect when combining the studies was a significant reduction in mortality for the experimental group [pooled OR of 0.74 (0.57–0.96); $p = 0.02$], with a significant heterogeneity among studies ($p = 0.01$; $I^2 = 52\%$).

The experimental protocol significantly reduced mortality in studies with homogeneous populations, including patients with sepsis or trauma patients only, but this advantage was not observed in studies including mixed populations (test for subgroup difference $p = 0.002$; Table 5.2). A supranormal target as opposed to a normal target ($p = 0.38$), the use of a PAC as opposed to other monitoring devices ($p = 0.68$) and CI/oxygen delivery as the end point as opposed to other end points ($p = 0.22$) were not superior in reducing hospital mortality in the experimental group. Fluids and inotropes as opposed to fluids alone did not provide any significant advantage on hospital mortality ($p = 0.87$) but fluids alone in the experimental protocol were used in one study only.

In conclusion, hemodynamic optimization can reduce mortality in non surgical critically ill patients. However subgroup analysis showed that such a benefit was relevant for septic or trauma patients only meanwhile it was no longer observed when this therapy was applied to a mixed population of critically ills. In patients receiving hemodynamic optimization, supranormal target as opposed to normal target, using a pulmonary artery catheter as opposed to other monitoring devices and cardiac index/oxygen delivery as the end point as opposed to other end points and fluids and inotropes as opposed to fluids alone were not superior in reducing hospital mortality.

5.2.2.5 Conclusions

Pre-load assessment and hemodynamic optimization by assessing fluid responsiveness represent the main hemodynamic goal in critically ill patients. In patients with reduced circulating volume, but fluid responders, management with intravenous fluid is required. Colloids are needed when a fast hemodynamic improvement is necessary [39]. The volume effect of colloids depends on the volume and hydration state of the patient. Giving fluids, not before but when relative hypovolemia occurs, seems to be more rational because the volume effects of colloids have been demonstrated to be more sensitive [40]. Furthermore, treating relative hypovolemia with colloids in patients undergoing surgery or in the critically ill who need sedation ignores the indirect vasodilatory effect of anesthetic drugs. Thus, when vascular tone is restored, a relative hypervolemia can occur, in some cases causing post-operative pulmonary edema, especially in patients who have undergone major visceral surgery, and in those with abdominal hypertension and intracranial trauma. The kidneys do not seem to compensate this overload [41].

Table 5.1 Effect of hemodynamic optimization on hospital mortality in the experimental group versus the control group

Study	Experimental Group	Control Group	Weight	Odds Ratio (95%CI)
Bishop (1995)	9/50	24/65	5.8	0.38 [0.16, 0.90]
Chytra (2007)	13/80	18/82	6.6	0.69 [0.31, 1.52]
De Oliveira (2008)	8/51	21/51	5.3	0.27 [0.10, 0.68]
Durham (1996)	3/27	3/31	2.1	1.17 [0.22, 6.33]
Fleming (1992)	8/33	15/34	4.6	0.41 [0.14, 1.15]
Gomersall (2000)	44/104	48/106	9.5	0.89 [0.51, 1.53]
Holm (2004)	8/25	10/25	3.9	0.71 [0.22, 2.25]
Lin (2006)	58/108	83/116	9.4	0.46 [0.27, 0.80]
Rhodes (2002)	40/130	62/133	10.1	0.51 [0.31, 0.84]
Rivers (2001)	46/95	50/106	9.4	1.05 [0.60, 1.83]
Santhanam (2008)	13/74	13/73	6.0	0.98 [0.42, 2.30]
Takal (2011)	52/199	39/187	10.6	1.34 [0.84, 2.16]
Velmahos (2000)	6/40	4/35	3.1	1.37 [0.35, 5.30]
Wheeler (2006)	140/513	128/487	13.6	10.5 [0.80, 1.39]
Overall	448/1529	518/1531	100	0.74 [0.57, 0.96]

Heterogeneity: $I^2 = 52\%$; $\chi^2 = 27$; P = 0.01, Overall effect: Z = 2.26; P = 0.02

Bishop (1995) J Trauma 38:780–787; *Chytra* (2007) Critical Care 11:R24; *De Oliveira* (2008) Intensive Care Med 34:1065–1075; *Durham* (1996) J Trauma 41(1):32–40; *Fleming* (1992) Arch Surg 127(10):1175–1181; *Gomersall* (2000) Crit Care Med 28(3):607-614; *Holm* (2004) Burns 30:798–807; *Lin* (2006) Shock 26:551-557; *Rhodes* (2002) Intensive Care Med 28:256–264; *Rivers* (2001) N Engl J Med 345:1368-77; *Santhanam* (2008) Pediatric Emergency Care 24:647-55; *Takala* (2011) Critical Care 15:R148; *Velmahos* (2000) Ann Surg 232:409-418; *National Heart, Lung, and Blood Institute Acute Respiratory Distress Syndrome (ARDS) Clinical Trials Network, Wheeler et al.* (2006) N Engl J Med 354:2213-24.

Table 5.2 Effect of hemodynamic optimization on hospital mortality in the experimental group versus the control group, based on the underlying disease of the study population

Study	Experimental Group	Control Group	Weight	Odds Ratio (95%CI)
Sepsis				
De Oliveira (2008)	8/51	21/51	5.3	0.27 [0.10, 0.68]
Lin (2006)	58/108	83/116	9.4	0.46 [0.27, 0.80]
Rivers (2001)	46/95	50/106	9.4	1.05 [0.60, 1.83]
Santhanam (2008)	13/74	13/73	6.0	0.98 [0.42, 2.30]
Overall	*119/363*	*179/374*		*0.50 [0.34, 0.74]*
Trauma				
Bishop (1995)	9/50	24/65	5.8	0.38 [0.16, 0.90]
Chytra (2007)	13/80	18/82	6.6	0.69 [0.31, 1.52]
Fleming (1992)	8/33	15/34	4.6	0.41 [0.14, 1.15]
Velmahos (2000)	6/40	4/35	3.1	1.37 [0.35, 5.30]
Overall	*36/203*	*61/216*		*0.56 [0.34, 0.92]*
Mixed				
Durham (1996)	3/27	3/31	2.1	1.17 [0.22, 6.33]
Gomersall (2000)	44/104	48/106	9.5	0.89 [0.51, 1.53]
Rhodes (2002)	40/130	62/133	10.1	0.51 [0.31, 0.84]
Takal (2011)	52/199	39/187	10.6	1.34 [0.84, 2.16]
Overall	*285/938*	*268/917*		*1.08 [0.88, 1.32]*
Burn				
Holm (2004)	8/25	10/25	3.9	0.71 [0.22, 2.25]
Overall	*448/1529*	*518/1531*	*100*	*0.74 [0.57, 0.96]*

Heterogeneity: $I^2 = 52\%$; $\chi^2 = 27$; $P = 0.01$ Overall effect: $Z = 2.26$; $P = 0.02$

Bishop (1995) J Trauma 38:780–787; *Chytra* (2007) Critical Care 11:R24; *De Oliveira* (2008) Intensive Care Med 34:1065–1075; *Durham* (1996) J Trauma 41(1):32–40; *Fleming* (1992) Arch Surg 127(10):1175–1181; *Gomersall* (2000) Crit Care Med 28(3):607–614; *Holm* (2004) Burns 30:798–807; *Lin* (2006) Shock 26:551-557; *Rhodes* (2002) Intensive Care Med 28:256–264; *Rivers* (2001) N Engl J Med 345:1368-77; *Santhanam* (2008) Pediatric Emergency Care 24:647-55; *Takala* (2011) Critical Care 15:R148; *Velmahos* (2000) Ann Surg 232:409-418.

Goal-directed therapy has been proven to be an effective strategy for rational fluid administration, based on the hemodynamic valuation of the patient, improving outcome in different clinical settings.

Key Concepts
- Management of hypovolemia
- Management of dehydration
- Physiology and pathophysiology of O_2 delivery
- Goal-directed therapy
- Fluid responsiveness

Key Words
- Hypovolemia
- Dehydration
- DO_2
- VO_2
- O_2ER
- Starling's law
- PPV
- SVV
- GEVD
- EVLW

Focus on...
- Giglio et al (2009) Goal-directed haemodynamic therapy and gastrointestinal complications in major surgery: a meta-analysis of randomized controlled trials. Br J Anaesth 103(5):637-46
- Forget et al (2010) Goal-directed fluid management based on the pulse oximeter–derived Pleth variability index reduces lactate levels and improves fluid management. Anesth Analg 111:910-914
- Reinhart K, Perner A, Sprun CL, Jaeschke R, Schortgen F, Johan Groenveld AB, Beale R, Hartog CS (2012) Consensus statement of the ESICM task force on colloid volume therapy in critically ill patients. Intensive Care Med 38(3):368-83

References

1. Dorje P, Adhikary G, Tempe DK (2000) Avoiding iatrogenic hyperchloremic acidosis: Call for a new crystalloid fluid. Anesthesiology 92:625-626
2. Reid F, Lobo DN, Williams RN et al (2003) (Ab)normal saline and physiological Hartmann's solution: A randomized double-blind crossover study. Clin Sci 104: 17-24
3. Sjostrand F, Hahn RG (2004) Volume kinetics of glucose 2.5% solution during laparoscopic cholecystectomy. Br J Anaesth 92:485–92
4. Länne T, Lundvall J (1989) Very rapid net transcapillary fluid absorption from skeletal muscle and skin in man during promounced hypovolaemic circulatory stress. Acta Physiol Scand 136: 1-6
5. Lundvall J, Länne T (1989) Large capacity in man for effective plasma volume control in hypovolaemia via fluid transfer from tissue to blood. Acta Physiol Scand 137: 513-520
6. Garrioch MA (2004) The body's response to blood loss. Vox Sanguinis 87 (Suppl. 1):S74–S76
7. Riddez L, Hahn RG, Brismar B et al (1997) Central and regional hemodynamics during acute hypovolemia and volume substitution in volunteers. Crit Care Med 25:635-640
8. Chappell D, Jacob M, Hofmann-Kiefer K, Conzen P, Rehm M (2008) A rational approach to perioperative fluid management. Anesthesiology 109:723-40
9. McCrae AF, Wildsmith JA (1993) Prevention and treatment of hypotension during central neural block. Br J Anaesth 70:672–80
10. Rehm M, Haller M, Orth V, Kreimeier U, Jacob M, Dressel H, Mayer S, Brechtelsbauer H, Finsterer U (2001) Changes in blood volume and hematocrit during acute preoperative volume loading with 5% albumin or 6% hetastarch solutions in patients before radical hysterectomy. Anesthesiology 95:849–56
11. Jarvela K, Koobi T, Kauppinen P, Kaukinen S (2001) Effects of hypertonic 75 mg/ml (7.5%) saline on extracellular water volume when used for preloading before spinal anaesthesia. Acta Anaesthesiol Scand. 45:776-81
12. Verheij J, van Lingen A, Beishuizen A, Christiaans HM, de Jong JR,Girbes AR et al (2006) Cardiac response is greater for colloid than saline fluid loading after cardiac or vascular surgery. Intensive Care Medicine 32:1030–8
13. Jones SB, Whitten CW, Monk TG (2004) Influence of crystalloid and colloid replacement solutions on hemodynamic variables during acute normovolemic hemodilution. J Clin Anesth 16:11-7
14. Niemi T, Schramko A, Kuitunen A, Kukkonen S, Suojaranta-Ylinen R (2008) Haemodynamics and Acid-base equilibrium after cardiac surgery: comparison of rapidly degradable hydroxyethyl starch solutions and albumin. Scandinavian Journal of Surgery 97:259–65
15. Palumbo D, Servillo G, D'Amato L, Volpe ML, Capogrosso G, De Robertis E, Piazza O, Tufano R (2006) The effects of hydroxyethyl starch solution in critically ill patients. Minerva Anestesiol 72:655-664
16. Van der Linden PJ, De Hert SG, Daper A, Trenchant A, Schmartz D, Defrance P, Kimbimbi P (2004) Can 3.5% urea-linked gelatin is as effective as 6% HES 200/0.5 for volume management in cardiac surgery patients.J Anaesth 51:236-41
17. Gandhi SD, Weiskopf RB, Jungheinrich C et al (2007) Volume replacement therapy during major orthopedic surgery using Voluven® (hydroxyethyl starch 130/0.4) or hetastarch. Anesthesiology 106: 1120–1127
18. Ickx BE, Bepperling F, Melot C, Schulman C, Van der Linden PJ (2003) Plasma substitution effects of a new hydroxyethyl starch HES 130/0.4 compared with HES 200/0.5 during and after extended acute normovolaemic haemodilution. Br J Anaesth 91:196–202
19. James MF, Latoo MY, Mythen MG et al (2004) Plasma volume changes associated with two hydroxyethyl starch colloids following acute hypovolaemia in volunteers. Anaesthesia 59:738–742
20. Lees et al (2009) Clinical review: Goal-directed therapy in high risk surgical patients. Critical Care 13:231 (doi:10.1186/cc8039)

21. Cavallaro F et al (2008) Functional hemodynamic monitoring and dynamic indices of fluid responsiveness. Minerva Anestesiol 74:123–35
22. Marik PE, Baram M, Vahid B (2008) Does central venous pressure predict fluid responsiveness. A systematic review. Chest 134:172-8
23. Lopes et al (2007) Goal-directed fluid management based on pulse pressure variation monitoring during high-risk surgery: a pilot randomized controlled trial. Critical Care 11:R100
24. Marik PE, Cavallazzi R, Vasu T et al (2009) Dynaminc changes in arterial wayforme derived variables and fluid responsivensess in mechanically ventilated patients: a systematic review. Crit Care Med 37:2642-2647
25. Benes J, Cgytra I, Altmann P et al (2010) Intaoperative fluid optimization using stroke volume variation in high risk surgical patients: result of prospective randomized study. Crit Care 14:R118
26. Michard F, Alaya S, Zarka V et al (2003) Global-end diastolic volume as an indicator of cardiac preload in patients with septic shock. Chest 124:1900-8
27. Sakka SG, Klein M, reinhart K et al (2003) A prognostic value of extravascular lung water in critically ill patients. Chest 122:2080-6
28. Mitchell JP, Schuller D, Calandrino FS et al (1992) Improved outcome based on fluid management in critically ill patient requiring pulmonary artery catheterization. Am Rev Respir Dis 145:990-8
29. Goepfer MS, Reuter DA, Akyiol D et al (2007) Goal-directed fluid management reduces vasopressor and cathecolamine use in cardiac surgery patients. Intensive Care Med 33:96-103
30. Mutho T, Kazumata L, Ajiki M et al (2007) Goal-directed fluid management by bedside transpulmonary hemodynamic monitoring after subarachnoid haemorrhage. Stroke 38:18-24
31. Abbas SM et al (2008) Systematic review of the literature for the use of oesophageal Doppler monitor for fluid replacement in major abdominal surgery. Anaesthesia 63:44-51
32. Chytra I et al (2007) Esophageal Doppler-guided fluid management decreases blood lactate levels in multiple-trauma patients: a randomized controlled trial. Crit Care 11(1):R24
33. Marik PE, Cecconi M, Hofer CF (2011) Cardiac output monitoring: an integrative perspective. Crit Care 15:214
34. Reuter DA, Huang C, Edrich T et al (2010) Cardiac output monitoring using indicator-dilution techniques: basic, limits and perspectives. Anesth Analg 110:799-811
35. Bendjelid K, Giraud r, Siegenthaler N et al (2010) Validation of a new transpulmonary thermodilution systemto assess global end-diatolic volume and extravascular pulmonary water. Crit Care 14:R209
36. Hofer et al (2008) Assessment of stroke volume variation for prediction of fluid responsiveness using the modified FloTrac™ and PiCCOplus™ system. Critical Care 12:R82
37. Mayer et al (2010) Goal-directed intraoperative therapy based on autocalibrated arterial pressure waveform analysis reduces hospital stay in high-risk surgical patients: a randomized, controlled trial. Critical Care 14:R18
38. Agrò FE, Benedetto U, Cocomello L, Benedetto M. A systematic review and meta-analysis of randomized controlled trials on the comparison between hemodynamic optimization versus standard care in non-surgical critically ill patients. Submitted
39. Voga G (2010) Preload assessment and optimization in critically ill patients. Lijec Vjesn 132 Suppl 1:28-30
40. Jacob M, Chappell D, Rehm M (2007) Clinical update: Perioperative fluid management. Lancet 369:1984–6
41. Arieff AI (1999) Fatal postoperative pulmonary edema: Pathogenesis and literature review. Chest 115:1371–7

Body Fluid Management in Abdominal Surgery Patients

6

Felice Eugenio Agrò, Carlo Alberto Volta and Maria Benedetto

6.1 Major Abdominal Surgery

6.1.1 Introduction

Perioperative intravenous fluid therapy is a fundamental part of the management of any surgical procedure and a daily challenge for anesthesiologists. While historically it has been quite neglected in clinical practice, in the last few years fluid administration has received suitable interest, following several studies demonstrating its influence on the outcome of perioperative fluid management [1, 2].

6.1.2 Physiopathology

Major surgery is associated with a significant systemic inflammatory response (SIRS) that is responsible for an increase in oxygen demand.

An important goal of perioperative fluid therapy is to maintain a safe range of DO_2, which may be compromised by both surgery and general conditions of the patient. In fact, the risk of postoperative multi-organ failure severely affects the prognosis of surgical patients.

Thus, it is necessary to identify high-risk surgical patients (based on surgery and patient-related risk factors) [3], to modify preoperatively the possible causes of tissue hypoxemia and to optimize intraoperative fluid management [4] (Fig. 6.1).

M. Benedetto (✉)
Postgraduate School of Anesthesia and Intensive Care, Anesthesia, Intensive Care and Pain Management Department, University School of Medicine Campus Bio-Medico of Rome, Rome, Italy
e-mail: m.benedetto@unicampus.it

F. E. Agrò (ed.), *Body Fluid Management*,
DOI: 10.1007/978-88-470-2661-2_6 © Springer-Verlag Italia 2013

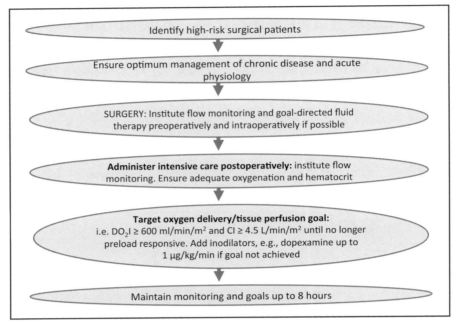

Fig 6.1 Perioperative management of high-risk surgical patients (data from Lees [2009], N Crit Care 13:231)

6.1.3   History

Fluid administration during surgery has been a matter of debate for 50 years. Francis Moore was one of the first authors to focus attention on the need to limit the amount of water and sodium used in the intraoperative and early postoperative phase [5], taking into account that the metabolic and hormonal responses ("stress response") to surgical injury are targeted "to save" salt and water. In the early 1960s, Shires [6] introduced the concept known as the "third space loss," i.e. to compartments not available for restoration of lost plasma volume (traumatized tissues, intracellular and interstitial spaces), the amount of which was dependent on the degree of surgical injury and not on blood losses. Although debated, this concept became the theoretical structure for the liberal approach to intravenous fluid therapy, leading to the administration of fluid volumes often exceeding the effective volume deficit.

6.1.4   Clinical Management of Fluids

Recently, there has been renewed controversy regarding the "optimal" perioperative fluid therapy [10-12]. Starting from 2000, many randomized controlled trials (RCT) began to consider different fluid regimens in elective open abdominal surgery and their effects on the outcome of the procedure. Several trials emphasized the superiority of a "restrictive" fluid strategy [7-9]. Moreover, a recent meta-analysis [10] showed the importance of assuring fluid balance throughout the perioperative period. In fact, those results proved that water and salt overload, resulting in a 2.5- to 3-kg weight increase, impaired clinical outcome.

6.1.4.1 Which Kind of Fluid?

The controversy between the use of crystalloids vs. colloids in major surgery is not yet resolved.

Balanced Plasma-Adapted Solutions

There is, however, large consensus on the importance of the type of fluid infused and not only the administered volume [13-15].

As fully explained in other sections of this book, in the recent literature there is evidence favoring balanced solutions with an electrolyte concentration similar to plasma. Many trials have suggested that hyperchloremic acidosis caused by the infusion of large volumes of normal saline should be avoided due to its effects on splanchnic perfusion [16]. In addition, 0.9% saline is retained in the ISS for longer than balanced crystalloids [15, 17]. Even so, an overload of balanced solutions should be avoided [15] because it may cause mucosal edema, thus impairing the efficacy of the intestinal anastomosis [18].

6.1.4.2 How Much Fluid?

An appropriate volume of the correct fluid allows physicians to establish proper blood volume and organ function [1]. Fluid overload and underhydration can compromise an adequate fluid balance, resulting in adverse clinical outcomes [2].

Fluid Overload

Nature has provided humans with efficient mechanisms to save salt and water in order to preserve the effective circulating volume against injury. Excess dietary salt and water is a phenomenon linked to modern life and prosperity. Therefore, constant suppression of the renin–angiotensin–aldosterone axis has become the most important mechanism to excrete eventual overload and it is largely unproductive [14, 19] (Fig. 6.2).

Infusions of 0.9% saline, commonly used in clinical practice, may cause hyperchloremic acidosis, with renal vasoconstriction and reduction of the glomerular filtration rate [20].

A load of 2 L of normal saline over 25 min may require over 2 days to be excreted by a healthy person [21]. Most of the retained fluid after acute infusions accumulates in the ISS, leading to edema [13-15]. In particular, splanchnic edema can result in increased intra-abdominal pressure, ascites, and even abdominal compartment syndrome [22, 23]. The worst effect of this intra-abdominal hypertension is the reduction in mesenteric blood flow, with conse-

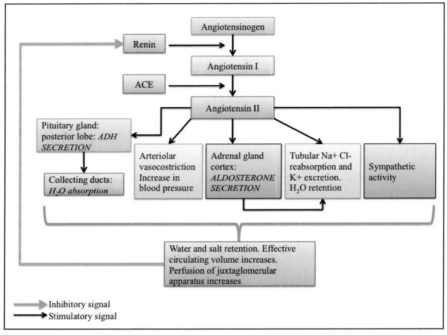

Fig. 6.2 Renin-angiotensin-aldosterone system

quent intestinal failure, increased intestinal permeability, and ileus. The decrease in mesenteric blood flow, along with tissue edema, may lead to tissue hypoxia. This can impair the anastomotic capability, up to obstruction and/or anastomotic dehiscence [23-25].

Another undesirable effect of hyperchloremic acidosis, as a result of saline infusions, is reduction of gastric blood flow and a decrease of gastric intramucosal pH in elderly surgical patients [26]. Besides macroscopic effects, salt and water overload can result in disorders at tissue and cell levels, such as membrane hyperpolarization, disordered neurotransmitter metabolism, and impairment of the mitochondrial activity [26].

Fluid Restriction
Similarly harmful effects occur with fluid restriction, as it causes a state of underhydration with potential hemodynamic effects (reduction in venous return and cardiac output, which negatively impact tissue perfusion and DO_2).

Fluid restriction can also increase blood viscosity, with multiple effects, e.g., decreased saliva production, with a predisposition to post-operative parotitis and an increased viscosity of pulmonary secretions, with a predisposition to mucous plug formation and lung atelectasis [27].

Goal-Directed Therapy

There are two main strategies in perioperative fluid management: fixed regimens with estimation of fluid losses conducted without monitoring systems [11], and goal-directed therapy (GDT) based on fluid responsiveness and optimization of hemodynamic parameters [28, 29]. As is well-known, perioperative fluid restriction has been found to improve clinical outcomes, with faster recovery and decreased mortality [7-9, 18; 30, 31]. Furthermore, it seems to ameliorate the microcirculation of perianastomotic tissues [32].

As previously stated, there are many unwanted results of both fluid overload (tissue edema, low tissue oxygenation and even anastomotic breakdown) [7, 12, 18, 30, 31] and underhydratation (hypovolemia, organ hypoperfusion and dysfunction) [22, 32, 33]. Nevertheless, a physician's aim should be to preserve the volume in the intravascular space (IVS) in order to ensure adequate organ perfusion while limiting the increased endothelial permeability resulting from surgical trauma [12]. With an individualized GDT approach, hypovolemia and fluid overload can be prevented [34, 40]. Recent data suggest that early signs of tissue hypoxia should be considered in the management of surgical patients, [41-43], since hypovolemia (with reduced $ScvO_2$) enhances the incidence of postoperative complications [44]. A study by Holte et al. on elective laparoscopic patients, and another study on hysterectomy patients, found a more rapid removal of fluids administered during surgery than those administered postoperatively [45, 46].

Randomized trials by Kehlet et al. have shown the ability of GDT to improve clinical outcomes such as postoperative nausea and vomiting, ileus, and the rapidity of recovery [34, 47-49], while taking into account the need to consider the particular patient's cardiovascular capability [34, 47, 50].

Special Settings

Although maintaining patients in a state of fluid balance should be one of the main goals of the anesthesiologist, there are particular cases and contexts in which this is neither possible nor desirable. Hemorrhagic shock and sepsis are characterized by a reduction in effective circulatory volume, which is often dramatic. In these situations, resuscitation procedures should include the administration of relatively large amounts of fluids (crystalloids, colloids, or blood) in order to replace the intravascular volume lost and guarantee tissue perfusion and oxygen delivery. Thus, fluid overload may be an inevitable but tolerated consequence to avoid the impairment of tissue oxygen delivery, organ failure, and adverse clinical outcomes. In these extreme situations, a restriction of salt and water intake in the post-acute phase can aid in the excretion of fluid excess, thus improving recovery and convalescence [51, 52].

Intestinal fistula is another peculiar condition characterized by huge losses of fluids and electrolytes. It may require the administration of large amounts of fluids, both in terms of volume and electrolytes [53].

6.1.4.3 What and How Much Fluid Over Time?

Preoperative Management

Three principles explain the need for preoperative fluid infusion [12]:

1. Preoperative fasting causes hypovolemia, since it is associated with diuresis and perspiration.
2. Perspiration dramatically increases after skin incision.
3. The shift of fluids into the third space requires an appropriate fluid replacement.

According to the British Consensus Guidelines, if the patient undergoes a bowel preparation, disorders of fluid balance and electrolytes may occur. These must be prevented and corrected with balanced fluid therapy [4].

Extreme gastric losses should be treated preoperatively with crystalloids containing an appropriate load of potassium (balanced solution). A solution of 0.9% saline is indicated in cases of hypochloremia, but with attention paid not to produce hypernatremia. Fluid losses from ileostomy, diarrhea, and small bowel fistulae should be replaced with balanced solutions [4].

Hypovolemia can occur even preoperatively and should be appropriately monitored. When advanced monitoring systems are not available, hypovolemia should be clinically diagnosed, based on arterial pulse pressure, capillary refill time, Glasgow Coma Scale, and diuresis, together with acid-base and lactate measurements [4].

In case of acute blood loss, absolute hypovolemia should be first treated with balanced crystalloids and colloids, until blood is available.

In cases of sepsis, peritonitis, or pancreatitis, relative hypovolemia should be treated with balanced crystalloids and colloids [4].

In clinical settings, fluid overload must be minimized. In fact, critically ill patients are not able to excrete excess water and sodium, thus being at risk of tissue edema.

Given clinical uncertainty regarding the presence of hypovolemia and an inability to determine central venous pressure (CVP), fluid responsiveness to a bolus of a 200 mL colloids or crystalloids 15 minutes post-infusion should be tested. Fluid infusion should be reiterated until there is no further hemodynamic improvement [4].

Intraoperative Management

In patients undergoing major surgery, fluid therapy should be given in order to optimize cardiac function and to decrease both the incidence of post-operative complications as well as the lengths of the ICU and hospital stays. Patients should receive intravenous fluids in order to achieve an optimal stroke volume from the beginning of surgery to the first 8 h after surgery [4].

For decades, fluids have been liberally infused during surgery and general anesthesia in order to treat both relative hypovolemia due to anesthetic drugs and absolute hypovolemia due to fasting, perspiration, and blood losses [11, 12]. However, fluid overload impairs the efficacy of the vascular barrier, thus causing pulmonary and peripheral tissue edema, despite a restrictive fluid

Table 6.1 Adverse effects of restrictive vs. liberal approach to perioperative fluid management in patients undergoing colorectal surgery [4]

Restrictive fluid use	Liberal fluid use
Hypotension	Interstitial edema
Increased postoperative nausea	Poor wound healing
Inadequate organ perfusion	Prolonged/resumption in bowel function
Impaired tissue oxygenation	Delayed gastric emptying
	Fluid overload resulting in heart failure

strategy that seems to reduce cardiopulmonary and bowel complications, thus reducing the length of hospital stay [12]. Liberal approaches to fluid management in surgical patients are becoming the subject of discussion, particularly in colorectal surgery patients. The varies reports in the literature mostly encourage a restrictive approach (Table 6.1) [54].

According to the recent literature, GDT is the best way to manage high-risk surgical patients undergoing major surgery. The evidence recommends giving fluids to patients who need them, in the quantity they need! A systematic review of patients undergoing major abdominal surgery revealed improved hemodynamic outcomes after fluid therapy guided by esophageal Doppler monitoring instead of the conventional parameters, such as arterial blood pressure, heart rate, CVP, and diuresis. This alternative form of monitoring results in a decreased need of inotropes, a faster return to normal intestinal function, shorter hospital stays, and fewer ICU admissions [47].

Buettner et al. found that, compared with routine care, intraoperative GDT was associated with slightly increased fluid administration whereas there was no difference in organ perfusion [48].

Another study, performed by Lopes et al., showed that GDT during high-risk surgery decreases the incidence of postoperative complications as well as the duration of mechanical ventilation, time of ICU stay, and hospital stay [49].

Finally, in high-risk major abdominal surgery patients, intraoperative GDT using the Vigileo/FloTrac monitor increased hemodynamic stability during the operation, decreased lactate concentration at the end of the operation, and was associated with a lower rate of postoperative complications and length of ICU stay [55].

Postoperative Management

After the patient leaves the operating room, the amount and type of fluids used in the perioperative phase must be assessed and then compared with intraoperative blood, urinary, and insensible losses.

Maintenance fluids must contain low levels of sodium and chloride and must not cause volume overload. They are essential to ensure adequate oxygen delivery. In edematous patients, hypovolemia should be treated only if it is truly present, followed by a gradual negative balance of sodium and water. The plasma concentration of potassium should also be carefully monitored.

Malnourished patients should be carefully re-nourished, as soon as possible, by enteral or parenteral nutrition, including foods rich in potassium, phosphate, and thiamine. If edema is present, the diet must be low in sodium and water. The surgical patient should be evaluated in terms of nutrition on the basis of guidelines for perioperative nutritional support [4].

Key Concepts
- Effects of fluid restriction and fluid overload
- Fluid management in the preoperative, intraoperative, and postoperative periods

Key Words
- Balanced plasma-adapted solutions
- Fluid overload
- Fluid restriction
- Goal-directed therapy

Focus on...
- Soni N (2009) British Consensus Guidelines on Intravenous Fluid Therapy for Adult Surgical Patients (GIFTASUP): Cassandra's view. Anaesthesia 64:235-8
- Abbas SM, Hill AG (2008) Systematic review of the literature for the use of oesophageal Doppler monitor for fluid replacement in major abdominal surgery. Anaesthesia 63:44–51

References

1. Holte K, Sharrock NE, Kehlet H (2002) Pathophysiology and clinical implications of perioperative fluid excess. Br J Anaesth 89:622–32
2. Holte K, Kehlet H (2002) Compensatory fluid administration for preoperative dehydration – does it improve outcome? Acta Anaesthesiol Scand 46:1089–93
3. Moonesinghe SR, Mythen MG, Grocott MPW (2011) High risk surgery: epidemiology and Outcomes. Anesth Analg 112:891-901
4. Soni N (2009) British Consensus Guidelines on Intravenous Fluid Therapy for Adult Surgical Patients (GIFTASUP) Cassandra's view. Anaesthesia 64(3):235-8
5. Moore FD (1959) Metabolic care of the surgical patient. Saunders, Philadelphia
6. Shires T, Williams J, Brown F (1961) Acute changes in extracellular fluids associated with major surgical procedures. Ann Surg 154:803-810
7. Lobo DN, Bostock KA, Neal KR et al (2002) Effect of salt and water balance on recovery of gastrointestinal function after elective colonic resection: a randomised controlled trial. LANCET 359:1812-1818
8. Brandstrup B, Tonnesen H, Beier-Holgersen R et al (2003) Effects of Intravenous fluid restriction on postoperative complications : comparison of two perioperative fluid regimens. Ann Surg 238:641-648
9. Nisanevich V, Felsenstein I, Almogy G et al (2005) Effect of intraoperative fluid management on outcome after intraabdominal surgery. Anesthesiology 103:25-32
10. Van Der Linden P (2007) Volume optimization in surgical patients Wet or Dry? Acta Anaesth Belg 58:245-250
11. Jacob M, Chappell D, Rehm M (2007) Clinical update: perioperative fluid management. Lancet 369(9578):1984-1986
12. Chappell D, Jacob M, Hofmann-Kiefer K, Conzen P, Rehm M (2008) A rational approach to perioperative fluid management. Anesthesiology 109(4):723-740
13. Lobo DN, Stanga Z, Simpson JAD et al (2001) Dilution and redistribution effects of rapid 2-litre infusions of 0.9% (w/v) saline and 5% (w/v) dextrose on haematological parameters and serum biochemistry in normal subjects: a double-blind crossover study. Clin Sci (Lond) 101:173–179
14. Lobo DN, Stanga Z, Aloysius MM et al (2010) Effect of volume loading with 1 liter intravenous infusions of 0.9% saline, 4% succinylated gelatine (Gelofusine) and 6% hydroxyethyl starch (Voluven) on blood volume and endocrine responses: a randomized, three-way crossover study in healthy volunteers. Crit Care Med 38:464–470
15. Reid F, Lobo DN, Williams RN et al (2003) (Ab)normal saline and physiological Hartmann's solution: a randomized double-blind crossover study. Clin Sci (Lond) 104:17–24
16. Lang K, Boldt J, Suttner S, Haisch G (2001) Colloids versus crystalloids and tissue oxygen tension in patients undergoing major abdominal surgery. Anesth Analg 93:405-409
17. Awad S, Allison SP & Lobo DN (2008) The history of 0.9% saline. Clin Nutr 27:179–188
18. Marjanovic G, Villain C, Juettner E et al (2009) Impact of different crystalloid volume regimes on intestinal anastomotic stability. Ann Surg 249:181–185
19. Drummer C, Gerzer R, Heer M et al (1992) Effects of an acute saline infusion on fluid and electrolyte metabolism in humans. Am J Physiol 262:F744–F754
20. Hansen PB, Jensen BL & Skott O (1998) Chloride regulates afferent arteriolar contraction in response to depolarization. Hypertension 32:1066–1070
21. Shoemaker WC, Wo CC, Thangathurai D et al (1999) Hemodynamic patterns of survivors and nonsurvivors during high risk elective surgical operations. World J Surg 23:1264-1271
22. Mayberry JC, Welker KJ, Goldman RK et al (2003) Mechanism of acute ascites formation after trauma resuscitation. Arch Surg 138:773–776
23. Balogh Z, McKinley BA, Cocanour CS et al (2003) Supranormal trauma resuscitation causes more cases of abdominal compartment syndrome. Arch Surg 138:637–642

24. Sheridan WG, Lowndes RH & Young HL (1987) Tissue oxygen tension as a predictor of colonic anastomotic healing. Dis Colon Rectum 30, 867–871

25. Lobo DN (2004) Sir David Cuthbertson medal lecture. Fluid, electrolytes and nutrition: physiological and clinical aspects. Proc Nutr Soc 63:453–466

26. Wilkes NJ, Woolf R, Mutch M et al (2001) The effects of balanced versus saline-based hetastarch and crystalloid solutions on acid-base and electrolyte status and gastric mucosal perfusion in elderly surgical patients. Anesth Analg 93:811–816

27. Lobo DN & Allison SP (2005) Fluid, electrolyte and nutrient replacement. In: Burnand KG, Young AE, Lucas J et al (eds) The New Aird's Companion in Surgical Studies. Churchill Livingstone, London, pp 20–41

28. Donati A, Loggi S, Preiser JC et al (2007) Goal-directed intraoperative therapy reduces morbidity and length of hospital stay in high-risk surgical patients. Chest 132:1817-1824

29. Rahbari NN, Zimmermann JB, Schmidt T, Koch M, Weigand MA, Weitz J (2009) Meta-analysis of standard, restrictive and supplemental fluid administration in colorectal surgery. Br J Surg 96:331-341

30. Walsh SR, Tang TY, Farooq N, Coveney EC, Gaunt ME (2008) Perioperative fluid restriction reduces complications after major gastrointestinal surgery. Surgery 143:466-468

31. Holte K, Kehlet H (2006) Fluid therapy and surgical outcomes in elective surgery: a need for reassessment in fast-track surgery. J Am Coll Surg 202:971-989

32. Kehlet H, Bundgaard-Nielsen M (2009) Goal-directed perioperative fluid management: why, when, and how? Anesthesiology 110:453-455

33. Jonsson K, Jensen JA, Goodson WH III, West JM, Hunt TK (1987) Assessment of perfusion in postoperative patients using tissue oxygen measurements. Br J Surg 74:263-267

34. Bundgaard-Nielsen M, Holte K, Secher NH, Kehlet H (2007) Monitoring of peri-operative fluid administration by individualized goal-directed therapy. Acta Anaesthesiol Scand 51(3):331-340

35. Wilson J, Woods I, Fawcett J et al (1999) Reducing the risk of major elective surgery: randomised controlled trial of preoperative optimisation of oxygen delivery. BMJ 318(7191):1099-1103

36. Venn R, Steele A, Richardson P, Poloniecki J, Grounds M, Newman P (2002) Randomized controlled trial to investigate influence of the fluid challenge on duration of hospital stay and perioperative morbidity in patients with hip fractures. Br J Anaesth 88(1):65-71

37. Sinclair S, James S, Singer M (1997) Intraoperative intravascular volume optimisation and length of hospital stay after repair of proximal femoral fracture: randomised controlled trial. BMJ 315(7113):909-912

38. Tote SP, Grounds RM (2006) Performing perioperative optimization of the high-risk surgical patient. Br J Anaesth 97(1):4-11

39. Wakeling HG, McFall MR, Jenkins CS et al (2005) Intraoperative oesophageal Doppler guided fluid management shortens postoperative hospital stay after major bowel surgery. Br J Anaesth 95(5):634-642

40. Sinclair S, Singer M (1995) National Confidential Enquiry into Perioperative Deaths. Perioperative haemodynamic monitoring and fluid management: NCEPOD revisited. Br J Hosp Med 53(4):166-168

41. Collaborative Study Group on Perioperative ScvO2 Monitoring. (2006) Multicentre study on peri- and postoperative central venous oxygen saturation in high-risk surgical patients. Crit Care 10(6):R158

42. Pearse R, Dawson D, Fawcett J, Rhodes A, Grounds RM, Bennett ED (2005) Changes in central venous saturation after major surgery, and association with outcome. Crit Care 9(6):R694-R699

43. Pearse RM, Hinds CJ (2006) Should we use central venous saturation to guide management in high-risk surgical patients? Crit Care 10(6):181

44. Futier E, Constantin JM, Petit A, Chanques G, Kwiatkowski F, Flamein R, Slim K, Sapin V, Jaber S, Bazin JE (2010) Conservative vs restrictive individualized goal-directed fluid replacement strategy in major abdominal surgery: A prospective randomized trial. Arch Surg 145(12):1193-200

45. Holte K et al (2007) Influence of "liberal" versus "restrictive" intraoperative fluid administration on elimination of a postoperative fluid load. Anesthesiology 106(1):75-9
46. Strandberg P et al (2005) Volume kinetics of glucose 2.5% solution and insulin resistance after abdominal hysterectomy. Br J Anaesth 94:30–8
47. Abbas SM, Hill AG (2008) Systematic review of the literature for the use of oesophageal Doppler monitor for fluid replacement in major abdominal surgery. Anaesthesia 63:44–51
48. Buettner M et al (2008) Influence of systolic-pressure-variation-guided intraoperative fluid management on organ function and oxygen transport. Br J Anaesth 101:194–9
49. Lopes MR et al (2007) Goal-directed fluid management based on pulse pressure variation monitoring during high-risk surgery: A pilot randomized controlled trial. Crit Care 11:R100–9
50. Spahn DR, Chassot PG: CON (2006) Fluid restriction for cardiac patients during major non-cardiac surgery should be replaced by goal-directed intravascular fluid administration. Anesth Analg; 102:344–6
51. Plank LD, Connolly AB & Hill GL (1998) Sequential changes in the metabolic response in severely septic patients during the first 23 days after the onset of peritonitis (see comments). Ann Surg 228:146–158
52. Lobo DN, Bjarnason K, Field J et al (1999) Changes in weight, fluid balance and serum albumin in patients referred for nutritional support. Clin Nutr 18:197–201
53. Varadhan KK, Lobo DN (2010) A meta-analysis of randomised controlled trials of intravenous fluid therapy in major elective open abdominal surgery: getting the balance right. Proc Nutr Soc 69(4):488-98
54. Bamboat ZM et al (2009) Perioperative fluid management. Clin Colon Rectal Surg 22(1):28-33
55. Benes J et al (2010) Intraoperative fluid optimization using stroke volume variation in high risk surgical patients: results of prospective randomized study. Crit Care 14(3):R118. Epub 2010 Jun 16

Fluid Management in Thoracic Surgery

7

Edmond Cohen, Peter Slinger, Boleslav Korsharskyy,
Chiara Candela and Felice Eugenio Agrò

7.1 Thoracic Surgery

7.1.1 Introduction

Fluid and electrolyte balance is of paramount importance for patients undergoing major non-cardiac intrathoracic surgery. The intravenous fluid resuscitation profoundly influences perioperative morbidity and mortality [1]. Despite significant differences in anesthetic techniques during these operations, the approach to the fluid therapy seems to follow the same direction.

7.1.2 How Much Fluid?

7.1.2.1 Pulmonary Resection Surgery

Specific areas of concern in the management of patients undergoing one-lung ventilation (OLV) for pulmonary resection include fluid management, intraoperative tidal volume, and acute lung injury post-surgery, which together lead to the concept of protective lung ventilation [2].

Fluid administration after major lung resection remains an issue. In an early retrospective report by Zeldin et al. [3], the authors evaluated the risk factors for the development of Acute Lung Injury (ALI) after pulmonary resection, more specifically evaluating the incidence of post-pneumonectomy pulmonary edema. They concluded that a right-sided pneumonectomy is associated with an increased incidence of postoperative pulmonary edema (6.9%

C. Candela (✉)
Postgraduate School of Anesthesia and Intensive Care, Anesthesia, Intensive Care and Pain Management Department, University School of Medicine Campus Bio-Medico of Rome, Rome, Italy
e-mail: chiaracandela@yahoo.it

F. E. Agrò (ed.), *Body Fluid Management*,
DOI: 10.1007/978-88-470-2661-2_7 © Springer-Verlag Italia 2013

post-pneumonectomy vs. 2.1% post-lobectomy). This procedure was also shown to be associated with increased perioperative intravenous fluid administration and increased urine output in the postoperative period. In anesthetized dogs, the same study demonstrated that, following a pneumonectomy, blood flow can increase up to six-fold. Therefore, any increase in blood volume, following excessive fluid administration, would injure the capillary endothelium, with the leakage of protein-rich fluid into the alveolar space. A more recent study by Licker et al. consisted of a retrospective analysis of 879 patients, showing that ALI was associated with four risk factors: high ventilatory pressure, excessive administration of intravenous fluid in thoracic surgical patients (in that case more than 3L in the first 24 h), pneumonectomy, and preoperative alcohol abuse [4]. Thus, an excessive amount of fluid can lead to ALI, which, after pneumonectomy, has a high mortality rate [5].

In patients undergoing pneumonectomy, respiratory failure is one of the most significant causes of postoperative morbidity and mortality. In most cases, it is associated with a decrease in respiratory function (FEV1 or DLCO) in those patients who are particularly at risk [6]. A significant correlation between ALI and high tidal volume was previously reported. A retrospective report [7] by Fernandez-Perez, involving 170 pneumonectomy patients, showed that patients receiving median tidal volumes higher than 8 mL/kg had a major risk of developing respiratory failure following pneumonectomy compared to patients who received tidal volumes < 6 mL/kg.

Schilling et al [8] reported that a tidal volume of 5 mL/kg during OLV significantly reduces the inflammatory response induced by alveolar cytokines.

The incidence of ALI after pneumonectomy is only 4, but the mortality rate is 30–50%.

The clinical picture of post–pneumonectomy pulmonary edema is usually related to other complications, such as aspiration, bronchopleural fistula, and surgical complications. Currently, only symptomatic management is appropriate. This includes fluid restrictions, use of diuretics, low ventilatory pressures and tidal volumes (when mechanical ventilation is used), and measures to reduce pulmonary arterial pressure. Even if pulmonary resection results in a slight postoperative pulmonary hypertension during exercise, right ventricular systolic function is normally minimally affected [9].

A serious concern for anesthesiologists is that fluid restriction in thoracic surgery may contribute to postoperative renal dysfunction, previously reported as being associated with a very high (19%) mortality [10]. In a recent review by Reimer et al., of over 100 pneumonectomies acute kidney injury (AKI), as defined by the RIFLE classification, occurred in 22% of the patients [11]. However, there was no association between AKI and fluid balance; neither was there an increased mortality of AKI patients. AKI is associated with preoperative hypertension and complex surgical procedures such as extrapleural pneumonectomy.

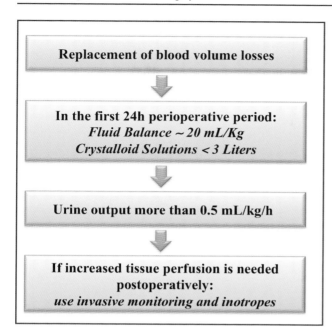

Fig. 7.1 Suggested fluid management for pneumonectomy patients

In patients undergoing pneumonectomy restricted intraoperative fluid administration should be performed, while being careful to preserve renal function. Some patients may require inotropes/vasopressors to maintain hemo-dynamic balance while under fluid restriction (Fig. 7.1).

This balance between fluid administration and the use of inotropes should be closely monitored, particularly in the patient who received a thoracic epidural for postoperative pain management. The vasodilatation caused by the epidural may initially have a "protective effect" from fluid overload. However, it should be interpreted with caution since weaning of the epidural effect may significantly increase the intravascular volume, placing the patient at risk for pulmonary edema. In summary, close monitoring of fluid administration is part of a protective lung ventilation strategy together with limiting the tidal volume and the peak airway pressure during OLV.

7.1.2.2 Transplanted Lung

A brief discussion of the management of the transplanted lung is warranted.

The interruption of lymphatic drainage in the graft may predispose the patient to peri-operative pulmonary interstitial fluid overload. Since it is unsure when and to what extent lymphatic channels are restored in human lung transplants, careful management and monitoring of intrathoracic fluids are rec-ommended, at least in the early post-transplantation period [12]. If large quan-tities of crystalloids/colloids are needed, interstitial pulmonary edema can be prevented by intraoperative ventilation with moderate-to-high PEEP. However, excessive fluid replacement becomes harmful after tracheal extubation, because the increase in venous return, as the mechanical ventilation is withdrawn, may determine pulmonary congestion. If the PiCCO system has been used for hemodynamic monitoring, it will probably show an increased intrathoracic blood volume with a significant expansion of extravascular lung water [13]. Quite often, the presence of renal dysfunction, associated with lung transplantation, complicates peri-operative fluid management, rendering these patients more vulnerable to fluid retention.

7.1.2.3 Procedures Involving the Esophagus

Fluid requirements change widely depending on the patient and the type of surgical procedure, such that ultimately the chosen strategy represents the sum of preoperative deficits, maintenance requirements, and ongoing losses. Preoperative fluid deficits in patients undergoing esophageal surgery may be relevant, although they have not been well defined [14]. In these patients, it should be taken into account that esophageal obstruction or dysphagia may limit fluid intake; in addition, there will be perioperative losses such as urinary and gastrointestinal losses, bleeding, and interstitial fluid shifts. Indeed, a fluid shift from the intravascular space into the interstitial space follows surgical trauma and is likely to reflect vascular damage.

"Third space" losses describe fluid loss into non-interstitial extracellular spaces that are not in equilibrium with the vascular compartment and thus considered to comprise a "non-functional" extracellular fluid compartment. However, this space has not been well characterized and its existence has been recently questioned [15]. Fluid management for esophageal resection is particularly challenging because thoracic epidural analgesia has been shown to improve outcome for these patients [16], but its use tends to contribute to hypotension, and in turn to ischemia of the gut anastomosis [17]. Treatment with excessive fluids is likely to exacerbate the problem due to swelling of the mucosa [18]. Many surgeons have expressed concern about the effects of vasopressors on the gut blood flow [19]. Often, the surgeon will ask the anaesthesiologist to refrain from administering vasopressors because of the fear of bowel ischemia. However, several recent animal studies suggested that the treatment of intraoperative hypotension with norepinephrine does not cause any reduction of gut blood flow [20, 21].

For major surgeries, including esophageal procedures, the best choice for fluid management is an individualized strategy, optimizing cardiac output and oxygen delivery. There is some evidence that fluid therapies designed to achieve individualized and specific flow-related hemodynamic endpoints, such as stroke volume, cardiac output, or measures of fluid responsiveness, such as stroke volume variation (Goal-Directed Therapy, GDT), may be a better choice than fixed regimens [22, 23]. Most practitioners would at least measure central venous pressure in patients administered a thoracic epidural.

In addition to the importance of the timing and amount of fluid administered, several authors argue that patient outcome is strongly influenced by the choice of the kind of fluid [24]. Intravascular colloid retention during the treatment of hypovolemia may approach 90%, vs. 40% during normovolemia [15].

The relationship between hydrostatic and oncotic pressure in the determination of fluid flux across a semi-permeable membrane was described in an equation developed in 1896 by Starling. However, it does not clearly explain several clinical observations, such as the relative resistance of the intact organism to the development of edema. This discrepancy is now attributed to the glycocalyx, a microcilial layer that lines the endothelium and acts as a molecular sieve [15]. This layer tends to decrease leukocyte and platelet adhesion to the endothelium while increasing the oncotic pressure on its inner surface. The glycocalyx deteriorates during ischemia-reperfusion and in the presence of a wide variety of inflammatory mediators, and thus probably contributes to the increased vascular permeability seen in these situations. Also, the glycocalyx is disrupted in the presence of atrial natriuretic peptide, which may explain the increase in plasma protein filtration seen following the administration of colloid boluses. Thus, protecting the glycocalyx may be among the anesthesiologist's most important duties perioperatively.

In summary, several new important guidelines are:
- the fasting deficit in most patients is very small or nil [25];
- basal fluid loss during a major procedure such as esophagectomy is probably only 1mL/kg/h;
- hypotension (mean BP < 70) is probably harmful to gastric tube blood flow;
- treatment of hypotension with excess fluids is probably harmful;
- treatment of hypotension with sympathomimetic vasopressors (norepinephrine or epinephrine) is probably beneficial [26].

7.1.3 Which Kind of Fluid?

The controversy between the use of crystalloid vs. colloid in thoracic surgery patients includes the propensity of each fluid to cause pulmonary edema. Crystalloids are safe and inexpensive. However, thoracic surgery, and lung surgery in particular, poses a significant problem of fluid overload and pulmonary edema. In fact, compared with colloids, a very large volume of crystalloids is needed to achieve the same amount of volume expansion. As already seen, this can easily lead to fluid overload.

In a study comparing the effects of saline vs. colloids administration in patients with ALI undergoing thoracic surgery, it was found that neither one altered capillary permeability (when fluid overloading was avoided), although, it was observed that hydroxyethyl starch (HES) may improve the increased permeability [27].

Some data are currently available that favor using colloids for the replacement of volume losses due to fluid shifting and/or bleeding. It is likely that the greater effectiveness of colloids in this context reflects their better effect on volume expansion [28] and their minimized shifting of liquid through potentially damaged capillary membranes [29, 30].

In patients undergoing esophagectomy, the choice of crystalloids versus colloids as intraoperative fluid therapy and its effect on intestinal anastomotic healing remains a matter of debate.

Marjanovic et al. [31] reported intriguing findings in an experimental model in which the treatment group received more colloids than the controls. This was not the initial intention of the investigators, but rather a result of the study design. Nevertheless, in contrast to a similar volume of crystalloid, colloids showed positive effects on intestinal anastomotic healing.

In animal models, only goal-directed colloid, and not crystalloid, therapy increased intestinal microcirculatory blood flow and tissue oxygen tension after abdominal surgery [32].

Ultimately, according to the type of fluid loss/deficit, a goal-directed approach with the appropriate fluid might improve the surgical outcome [15]. Nonetheless, based on the above-described evidence, colloids are increasingly being used to compensate the reduction in plasma volume related to blood losses during major surgery [33].

Older, high-molecular-weight preparations of HES exhibited prolonged hemodynamic effects but their used was hindered by major side effects in terms of renal impairment, clotting disorders, and anaphylactoid reactions. [34-36]. As explained elsewhere in this monograph, the latest-generation HES, with a lower molecular weight, were shown to be associated with fewer side effects while maintaining the desirable properties of plasma expansion [36, 37].

A recent study [38] compared the use of HES 130/0.4, HES 200/0.5, and modified fluid gelatin for volume replacement in patients undergoing major thoracic surgery. Fluid infusion was guided by transesophageal Doppler. The study found comparable hemodynamic stabilization effects for all three solutions, but fewer side effects in terms of hemostasis and kidney impairment with HES 130/0.4.

Key Concepts
- Strategy of fluid administration in pulmonary resection
- Strategy of fluid administration in esophageal procedures
- What kind of fluid in thoracic surgery?

Key Words
- Acute lung injury
- Pulmonary edema
- Fluid restriction
- Third space
- Goal-directed fluid therapy

Focus on...
- Hiltebrand LB, Koepfli E, Kimberger O et al (2011) Hypotension during fluid restricted abdominal surgery. Anesthesiology 114:557-64
- Klijn E, Niehof S, de Jong J et al (2010) The effect of perfusion pressure on gastric tissue blood flow in an experimental gastric tube model. Anesth Analg 110:541-546
- Hamilton MA (2009) Perioperative fluid management: Progress despite lingering controversies. Cleveland Clin J Med 76 Suppl 4 S28-S31

References

1. Mark A. Hamilton (2009) Perioperative fluid management: Progress despite lingering controversies. Cleveland Clinic Journal of Medicine 76 Suppl 4 S28-S31
2. Slinger P (2009) Update on anesthetic management for pneumonectomy. Curr Opinion Anaesth 22:31-7
3. Zeldin RA, Normadin D, Landtwig BS et al (1984) Postpneumonectomy pulmonary edema. J Thorac Cardiovasc Surg 87:359-64
4. Licker M, Perrot M, Spiliopoulos A et al (2003) Risk factors for acute lung injury after thoracic surgery for lung cancer. Anesth Analg 97:1558-65
5. Slinger PD (2006) Postpneumonectony pulmonary edema: good news, bad news. Anesthesiology 105:2-4
6. Alam N, Park BJ, Wilton A et al (2007) Incidence and risk factors for lung injury after lung cancer resection. Ann Thorac Surg 84:1085-91
7. Fernandez-Perez ER, Keegan MT, Brown DR et al (2006) Intraoperative tidal volume as a risk factor for respiratory failure after pneumonectomy. Anesthesiology 105:14-18
8. Schilling T, Kozian A, Huth C et al (2005) The pulmonary immune effects of mechanical ventilation in patients undergoing thoracic surgery. Anesth Analg 101:957-62

9. Heerdt PM (2003) Cardiovascular adaptation to lung resection. In: Thoracic Anesthesia 3 edn. Philadelphia, Churchill Livingston, pp 423-35

10. Gollege G, Goldstraw P (1994) Renal impairment after thoracotomy: incidence, risk factors and significance. Ann Thorac Surg 58:524-8

11. Reimer C, McRae K, Seitz D et al (2010) Perioperative acute kidney injury in pneumonectomy: a retrospective cohort study. Can J Anesth:A802743

12. Baker CS, Yost CU, Niemann (2005) Organ transplantation. In: Miller RD (ed) Miller's Anesthesia, 6 edn. Elsevier, Philadelphia, p 2271

13. Della Rocca MG, Costa (2005) Volumetric monitoring: principles of application. Minerva Anestesiol 71:303–306

14. Blank RS et al (2011) Anesthesia for Esophageal Surgery. In: Slinger P (ed) Principles and practice of anesthesia for thoracic surgery. Springer, New York

15. Chappell D, Jacob M, Hofmann-Kiefer K et al (2008) A rational approach to perioperative fluid management. Anesthesiology 109:723-740

16. Cense HA, Lagarde SM, de Jong K et al (2006) Association of no epidural analgesia with postoperative morbidity and mortality after transthoracic esophageal cancer resection. J AM Coll Surg 202:395-400

17. Al-Rawi OY, Pennefather S, Page RD et al (2008) The effect of thoracic epidural bupivacaine and an intravenous adrenalin infusion on gastric tube blood flow during esophagectomy. Anesth Analg 106:884-7

18. Holte K, Sharrock NE, Kehlet H (2002) Pathophysiology and clinical implications of perioperative fluid excess. Br J Anaesth 89:622-632

19. Theodorou D, Drimousis PG, Larentzakis A et al (2008) The effects of vasopressors on perfusion of gastric graft after esophagectomy. J Gastrointest Surg 12:1497

20. Klijn E, Niehof S, de Jong J et al (2010) The effect of perfusion pressure on gastric tissue blood flow in an experimental gastric tube model. Anesth Analg 110:541-6

21. Hiltebrand LB, Koepfli E, Kimberger O et al (2011) Hypotension during fluid restricted abdominal surgery. Anesthesiology 114:557-64

22. Oohashi S, Endoh H (2005) Does central venous pressure or pulmonary capillary wedge pressure reflect the status of circulating blood volume in patients after extended transthoracic esophagectomy? J Anesth 19:21-25

23. Kobayashi M, Ko M, Kimura T et al (2008) Perioperative monitoring of fluid responsiveness after esophageal surgery using stroke volume variation. Expert Rev Med Devices 5:311-6

24. Wei S, Tian J, Song X, Chen Y (2008) Association of perioperative fluid balance and adverse surgical outcomes in esophageal cancer and esophagogastric junction cancer. Ann Thorac Surg 86:266-272

25. Jacob M, Chappell D, Conzen P et al (2008) Blood volume is normal after pre-operative overnight fasting. Acta Anaesthesiol Scand 52:522-9

26. Van Brommel J, De Jonge J, Buise AP et al (2010) The effects of nitroglycerine and norepinephrine on gastric mucosal microvascular perfusion in an experimental model of gastric tube reconstruction. Surgery 148:71-7

27. van Lingen VA, Raijmakers PGHM, Rijnsburger ER, Veerman DP, Wisselink W, Girbes ARJ, Groeneveld ABJ (2006) Effect of fluid loading with saline or colloids on pulmonary permeability, edema and lung injury score after cardiac and major vascular surgery. British Journal of Anaesthesia 96:21–30

28. McIlroy DR, Kharasch ED (2003) Acute intravascular volume expansion with rapidly administered crystalloid or colloid in the setting of moderate hypovolemia. Anesth Analg 96:1572–7

29. Matharu NM, Butler LM, Rainger GE, Gosling P, Vohra RK, Nash GB (2008) Mechanisms of the anti-inflammatory effects of hydroxyethyl starch demonstrated in a flow-based model of neutrophil recruitment by endothelial cells. Crit Care Med 36:1536-42

30. Jacob M, Bruegger D, Rehm M, Welsch U, Conzen P, Becker BF (2006) Contrasting effects of colloid and crystalloid resuscitation fluids on cardiac vascular permeability. Anesthesiology 104:1223-31

31. Marjanovic G, Villain C, Timme S et al (2010) Colloid vs. crystalloid infusionsin gastrointestinal surgery and their different impact on the healing of intestinal anastomoses. Int J Colorectal Dis 25:491-498
32. Hiltebrand LB, Kimberger O, Arnberger M et al (2009) Crystalloids versus colloids for goal-directed fluid therapy in major surgery. Crit Care 13:R
33. Bunn F, Alderson P, Hawkins V (2001) Colloid solutions for fluid resuscitation (Cochrane Review). Cochrane Database Syst Rev: 2.1
34. Kannan S, Milligan KR (1999) Moderately severe anaphylactoid reaction to pentastarch (200/0.5) in a patient with acute severe asthma. Intensive Care Med 25:220
35. Kozek-Langenecker SA (2005) Effects of hydroxyethyl starch solutionson hemostasis. Anesthesiology 103:654–60
36. Brunkhorst FM, Engel C, Bloos F et al (2008) German Competence Network Sepsis (Sep-Net). Intensive insulin therapy and pentastarch resuscitation in severe sepsis. N Engl J Med 358:125–39
37. Ickx B, Bepperling F, Melot C et al (2003) Plasma substitution effects of a new hydroxyethyl starch HES 130/0.4 compared with HES 200/0.5 during and after extended acute normovolaemic haemodilution. Br J Anaesth 9:1–7
38. Abdallah MS, Assad OM (2010) Randomized study comparing the effect of Hydroxyethyl Starch HES 130/0.4, HES 200/0.5 and modified fluid gelatin for perioperative volume replacement in thoracic surgery: guided by transesophageal doppler EJCTA - Volume 4 Number 2

Fluid Management in Loco-Regional Anesthesia

8

Laura Bertini, Annalaura Di Pumpo and Felice Eugenio Agrò

8.1 Regional Anesthesia

8.1.1 Introduction

In regional anesthesia, only a specific part of the body is anesthetized. The pain signal coming from the anesthetized area is blocked at the level of the central or peripheral nervous system and does not reach the brain. There is also a reduction in tactile sensitivity and the movement ability of the muscles is abolished.

Regional anesthesia allows faster recovery and causes fewer side effects than general anesthesia.

The three types of regional anesthesia are:

- peripheral nerve block: in which local anesthetic is injected around the nerve such that the supplied area loses sensitivity;
- spinal block: in which a small dose of anesthetic is injected into the subarachnoid space, thus blocking all stimuli from the nerves that go to the brain (Fig. 8.1);
- epidural anesthesia: in which the anesthetic is injected into the extradural space (Fig. 8.1).

Regional anesthesia is frequently used in obstetric-gynecologic procedures and in orthopedic surgery, but it can be used also for:

- urologic surgery;
- vascular limb surgery;
- inguinal hernia repair;
- proctologic surgery;

A. Di Pumpo (✉)
Postgraduate School of Anesthesia and Intensive Care, Anesthesia, Intensive Care and Pain Management Department, University School of Medicine Campus Bio-Medico of Rome, Rome, Italy
e-mail: annalaurad.p@live.it

F. E. Agrò (ed.), *Body Fluid Management*,
DOI: 10.1007/978-88-470-2661-2_8 © Springer-Verlag Italia 2013

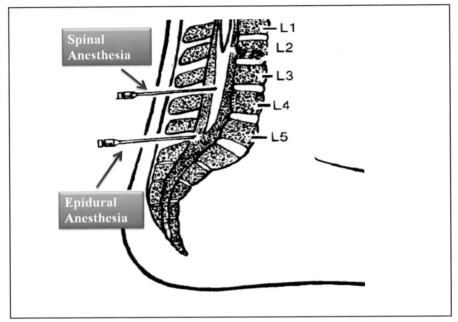

Fig. 8.1 Spinal and epidural anesthesia

- eye surgery;
- some operations on the nose and ears.

8.1.2   Cesarean Section

Neuraxial anesthesia causes a preganglionic blockade of the fibers of the sympathetic nervous system innervating smooth muscle of arteries and veins; this causes vasodilation and thus blood pooling, with a decrease in venous return to the heart. There may even be significant changes in systemic blood pressure, especially in patients who are intravascularly depleted. Some studies have determined a passage of fluids from the intravascular to the interstitial space, based on measurements of hemoglobin [1, 2]. The ensuing hypotension typically occurs about 30 min after the administration of epidural anesthesia and earlier in spinal anesthesia. These hemodynamic effects are not due to a reduction of blood volume per se, but rather to vasodilatation, which causes a relative "functional" hypovolemia [2].

One of the most debated issues in regional anesthesia is the prevention of hypotension following spinal anesthesia. This is one of the most common complications during elective cesarean delivery under spinal anesthesia, with an incidence up to 80% [3].

The effects of preinduction fluid administration to reduce the incidence and severity of spinal-induced hypotension have been extensively studied over the past few decades. In fact, the administration of colloid or cristalloid volume preload before induction has become a widespread practice. However, not all studies have found a difference in mean arterial pressure and heart rate in preload and non-preload situations in which crystalloid was administered. The only difference was a greater time to reach the sensory block [4]. This is of importance in the elderly population, as it is important to avoid hypotension and reduce unnecessary fluid infusion. Coe et al. compared two different regimens of crystalloid infusion but failed to find any difference in the incidence of hypotension in the normovolemic elderly [5]. Additionally, crystalloids infusion 20 min before the induction of spinal anesthesia may induce the secretion of atrial natriuretic peptide (ANP) [6], resulting in peripheral vasodilatation followed by an increased rate of preloaded fluid excretion, if renal function is preserved, as in the normal population. In elderly patients with impaired renal status, however, this may be the cause of fluid retention. A more physiological approach may be to administer a fluid preload at the beginning of the anesthetic block. This practice has been termed "coload" [7]. Yet, several authors [8] did not find any difference between standard preload and "coload" protocols in terms of blood pressure, vasopressor requirements, and neonatal outcome [9] in an obstetric population. Instead, they suggested the use of a modest colloid preload (no more than 500 mL) plus phenylephrine support to maintain blood pressure close to the baseline, claiming a better final outcome [8, 10]. Both the administration of fluids and vasoactive drugs can play the same role in restoring hemodynamic balance.

Intravascular fluid administration of colloids and crystalloid differs in terms of their half-life and thus also in altering osmotic pressure and cardiac output (CO) [3].

A study by Holte et al. [2] examined the effects of ephedrine vs. HES administration 90 min after the administration of an epidural block. The hemodynamic effects in the two groups were equal, but a reduction in hemoglobin concentration was recorded with HES. The authors, therefore, concluded that ephedrine administration is preferred for the treatment of hypotension after epidural anesthesia, above all, when there are contraindications to its use or when there is harmful fluid overload (as in cardiopulmonary diseases).

Regional anesthesia should be followed by a decrease in fluid requirements due to a perioperative decrease in blood loss [11]. Over the last 20 years, the mean intraoperative fluid administration in orthopedic surgery has fallen from 3108 to 1563 mL [12]. In high epidural anesthesia, when hypotension is more likely, CO may be improved by increasing preload in the form of increased fluid intake, or by sympathomimetic drugs, acting on myocardial contractility, with unchanged fluid balance. Low spinal or epidural anesthesia, below T10, is usually the cause of minor circulatory impairment due to compensatory vasoconstriction in the upper part of the body. This compensation generally is enough to counteract the vasodilatation in the anesthetized area.

8.1.3 Orthopedic Surgery

In the last few years, fluid administration has received suitable interest because several studies have demonstrated the influence on outcome of perioperative fluid management. In fact, it was recently found that the optimization of fluid management has an important impact in reducing postoperative complications and mortality [13, 14].

In patients undergoing spinal surgery, it was demonstrated that the administration of excessive amounts of liquid causes an increase in respiratory complications [15]. Some authors proposed hypertonic 75 mg/mL (7.5%) saline as an alternative for preloading before spinal anesthesia in patients affected by comorbidities in which excess free water administration is not desired. It is effective in small doses of 1.6 mL/kg, which increase the extracellular water, plasma volume and CO, and thus maintains hemodynamic stability during spinal anesthesia [16].

8.1.3.1 Assessment of Liquid Request

Patients undergoing major surgery, such as orthopedic surgery, are more likely to develop complications if they have a limited supply of physiological fluids. Proper fluid administration can reduce the stress of the surgical trauma in addition to improving outcome and reducing hospital stay [17-19].

In the past few years, attempts to optimize fluid therapy has led to a more thorough examination of the fluids requested in the hospital setting. Previously, fluid administration was often based on non-specific parameters, such as urine output, which are not adequate to indicate subclinical hypovolemia. Nowadays, parameters such as stroke volume (SV) and CO guide volemic filling. These parameters have been shown to be related to outcome and are predictive for both survival and complications [20-22].

One of the easiest ways to monitor invasive cardiovascular parameters is esophageal Doppler, which uses Doppler ultrasonography to measure blood flow in the descending aorta. This technique allows the administration of repeated boluses of fluids or vasoactive drugs on the basis of ongoing assessments of SV and preload indices. For example, the control of CO by esophageal Doppler in patients undergoing hip surgery reduced the hospital stay from 17 to 12 days [12, 23].

Parker et al., in a study on hip fracture surgery, compared the effects of two fluid strategies: 500 mL gelatin solution and conventional crystalloid solution. Since no difference emerged with respect to the outcome of these two groups of patients, the authors concluded that invasive monitoring of hemodynamic functions in the perioperative period is desirable, in order to identify patients in whom a more precise fluid control will generate actual benefits [22]. The effects of invasive techniques on other important, longer-term outcomes have yet to be studied [12].

In orthopedic surgery performed under regional anesthesia, an invasive evaluation of CO is not always possible because the patients are awake and obviously cannot tolerate an esophageal probe. Instead, new techniques, such as thoracic electrical impedance cardiography can be utilized to measure CO and SV [24]. CO data obtained with bio-impedance seem to correlate with those obtained from more invasive techniques [25, 26].

Techniques such as Esophageal Doppler ultrasonography or central venous pressure monitoring and non-invasive advanced techniques, such as plethysmographic pulse volume determination, may be used in awake patients; while techniques involving arterial wave analysis (pulse contour, pulse power), measuring variations in pulse-pressure, systolic blood pressure, and SV induced by mechanical ventilation, are useful during general anesthesia [27, 28]. However, the optimal protocol has not been determined and further studies are needed.

8.1.3.2 How Much Fluid?

The choice of the amount of fluid to be administered has always been more difficult and controversial than the choice of the type of fluid to be administered. Currently, very few studies are available concerning the amount of fluid to be administered during the perioperative period; moreover, these studies are not uniform, instead covering different types of surgery and patients.

Available data, however, show that in patients undergoing minor surgery the perioperative administration of 1–2 L of fluids (mainly crystalloids) is a rational strategy to correct dehydration. In addition, it can reduce postoperative complications such as drowsiness, dizziness, nausea, vomiting, and postsurgical pain [29-31].

In major surgery, there are three major strategies for fluid administration: liberal, restricted, and goal-directed therapy (GDT). Studies comparing liberal vs. restricted strategies have not provided unanimous results. In fact, some support restrictive fluid administration (approximately 3–3.6 L), arguing that it reduces postoperative complications [32, 33] whereas other authors argue for a liberal approach (approximately 5–5.9 L) [34].

A recent study on knee arthroplasty [35] found better results with a liberal (median 4250 mL) than with a restrictive (median 1740 mL) approach in terms of improving pulmonary function 6 h postoperatively and reducing the incidence of vomiting, but it did induce significant hypercoagulability (although with unknown clinical implications) 24–48 h postoperatively. No further differences were found with respect to outcome and functional recovery.

In a recent review based on currently available evidence, Holte could not offer definitive recommendations on the optimal fluid in elective surgery while the IV administration of > 5 L of fluids is not indicated as it can lead to postoperative problems [36].

The results of studies on GDT are more consistent. GDT is a strategy of fluid administration specific and highly individualized for each patient. Its purpose is to optimize perfusion and tissue oxygenation under the guidance of hemodynamic variables that suggest the need for fluids or other therapies (such as vasoactive inotropic drugs). Many studies have shown that GDT is a valid approach for managing patients undergoing major surgery, reducing both hospital stay and postsurgical complications [37, 38]. However, there are some limitation of GDT studies: many of them had a small sample size and there has been a lack of standardization, in addition to concerns of inappropriate goal selection [39]. GDT also requires increased fluid administration compared to standard approaches, but there are as yet no data on postoperative weight gain. Other rapid rehabilitation techniques might also allow a good outcome.

8.1.3.3 Which Kind of Fluid?

In fluid management, it is important to identify the compartments vulnerable to fluid loss and to restore those losses with a suitable fluid. In an acute emergency, the priority is to restore circulating volume, suggesting the need for colloids or crystalloids. In other conditions, such as prolonged surgery with evaporative loss, water, in the form of 5% glucose, is needed.

Patients undergoing orthopedic surgery, especially major surgery such as the repair of hip fractures and major joint replacements, are at risk of important fluid losses due to decreased intake, bleeding before and after surgery, medications that promote fluid losses (elderly patients on diuretic therapy), among others.

Hypovolemia is the most important conditions that may occur during major orthopedic surgery and must be prevented during the perioperative period. Hypovolemia due to bleeding must be promptly treated with balanced crystalloid associated with a colloid rather than crystalloids alone [40]. Several authors have shown that volume expansion is greater with colloids than with crystalloids [16, 41]. Furthermore, fluid infusion reduces the possibility of hypercoagulability [42] and vomiting in the post-operative period [35]. Nevertheless, it is also important to consider the effects of colloids on coagulation.

Many studies comparing the effects of colloids and crystalloids on clotting showed that colloids interfere with clotting more than crystalloids [43, 44]. The alterations in the coagulation system are due to interference with fibrinogen/fibrin polymerization. Different fluids can worsen the coagulation state. For example, in stressful situations or when hyperfibrinolysis is either suspected or detected by thromboelastography and in the presence of colloids, clot disintegration is faster than clots formed in the presence of Ringer's lactate. Thus, clot strength and clot resistance to fibrinolysis will be better preserved by administering crystalloids rather than colloids to maintain normovolemia under these conditions [45].

This effect is particularly pronounced for HES. The main advantage of HES over crystalloid infusions is a faster restoration of the intravascular volume deficit using smaller amounts of fluids; however HES can significantly affect blood coagulation. Consequently, in patients in whom copious blood losses are expected crystalloids and gelatin solutions should be used instead of HES [45].

The exception may be the latest-generation HES, which differ from older HES formulations in their impact on coagulation. Studies carried out in vivo and in vitro, comparing HES 130/0.4 (Voluven) with an older-generation HES, showed much less pronounced effects on coagulation by the former [46-49].

Probably this effect is due to Voluven faster removal from the body although it has the same efficacy in restoring plasma volume. Langeron et al. suggested that the use of Voluven is appropriate in patients undergoing surgery in which a large blood loss is expected [45, 46]. Gandhi et al. obtained the same results comparing the safety of Voluven and HES 670/0.75 for volume replacement in orthopedic surgery [50]. Thromboelastographic analysis of healthy male patients also demonstrated less compromise of thromboelastogram parameters with HES 130/0.4 than with other HES solutions [50, 51]. Recent studies focus on HES diluted in balanced solutions [52]. Finally, a controlled, randomized, double-blind, multicenter trial confirmed that both solutions have positive effects on volume replacement, but Voluven has less adverse effects on coagulation.

Papakitsos et al. [53] compared the efficacy and safety of Tetraspan® with conventional unbalanced HES in patients undergoing orthopedic surgery. There was less blood loss in the Tetraspan® group and a smaller amount of had to be fluid infused compared to non-balanced HES. The authors concluded that Tetraspan® provides excellent volemic filling and can be used throughout the perioperative period.

Key Concepts
- Physiopathology of hypotension during regional anesthesia
- Crystalloids/colloid in preventing hypotension in cesarean section
- Evaluation of fluid needs
- Invasive monitoring of cardiovascular parameters
- Optimized fluid therapy in the perioperative period improves patient outcome
- Liberal/restricted/GDT strategy

Key Words
- Spinal anesthesia
- Epidural anesthesia
- Hypotension
- Perioperative fluid management
- Crystalloids/colloids
- Balanced/Non-balanced solution

Focus on...
- Papakitsos G, Papakitsou T, Kapsali A (2010) A total balanced volume replacement strategy using a new balanced 6% hydroxyethyl starch preparation Tetraspan (HES 130/0.42) in patients undergoing major orthopaedic surgery: 6AP3-1. Eur J Anesthes 27:106
- Soni N (2009) British Consensus Guidelines on Intravenous Fluid Therapy for Adult Surgical Patients (GIFTASUP): Cassandra's view, Anaesthesia 64:235-238
- Holte K (2010) Pathophysiology and clinical implications of perioperative fluid management in elective surgery. Dan Med Bull 57: B4156

References

1. Hahn RG (1992) Haemoglobin dilution from epidural-induced hypotension with and without fluid loading, Acta Anaesthesiol Scand 36:241-244
2. Holte K, Foss NB, Svensén C, Lund C, Madsen JL, Kehlet H (2004) Epidural anesthesia, hypotension, and changes in intravascular volume. Anesthesiology 100:281-286
3. Ueyama H, He YL, Tanigami H, Mashimo T, Yoshiya I (1999) Effects of crystalloid and colloid preload on blood volume in the parturient undergoing spinal anesthesia for elective Cesarean section, Anesthesiology 91:1571-1576
4. Shin BS, Ko JS, Gwak MS, Yang M, Kim CS, Hahm TS, Lee SM, Cho HS, Kim ST, Kim JH, Kim GS (2008) The effects of prehydration on the properties of cerebrospinal fluid and the

spread of isobaric spinal anesthetic drug. Anesth Analg 106:1002-7
5. Coe AJ (1995) Haemodynamic effects of subarachnoid block in the elderly. Br J Anaesth 74:244
6. Pouta AM, Karinen J, Vuolteenaho OJ, Laatikainen TJ (1996) Effect of intravenous fluid pre-load on vasoactive peptide secretion during Caesarean section under spinal anaesthesia. Anaesthesia 51:128-132
7. Dyer RA, Farina Z, Joubert IA, Du Toit P, Meyer M, Torr G, Wells K, James MF (2004) Crys-talloid preload versus rapid crystalloid administration after induction of spinal anaesthesia (coload) for elective caesarean section. Anaesth Intensive Care 32:351-357
8. Teoh WH, Sia AT (2009) Colloid preload versus coload for spinal anesthesia for cesarean de-livery: the effects on maternal cardiac output. Anesth Analg 108:1592-1598
9. Ogata K, Fukusaki M, Miyako M, Tamura S, Kanaide M, Sumikawa K (2003) The effects of colloid preload on hemodynamics and plasma concentration of atrial natriuretic peptide dur-ing spinal anesthesia in elderly patients. Masui 52:20-25
10. Nishikawa K, Yokoyama N, Saito S, Goto F (2007) Comparison of effects of rapid colloid loading before and after spinal anesthesia on maternal hemodynamics and neonatal outcomes in cesarean section. J Clin Monit Comput 21:125-129
11. Tziavrangos E, Schug SA (2006) Regional anaesthesia and perioperative out come. Curr Opin Anaesthesiol 19:521-525
12. Price JD, Sear JW, Venn RM (2004) Perioperative fluid volume optimization following prox-imal femoral fracture. Cochrane Database Syst Rev CD003004
13. Cecconi M, Fasano N, Langiano N, Divella M, Costa MG, Rhodes A, Della Rocca G (2011) Goal-directed haemodynamic therapy during elective total hip arthroplasty under regional anaes-thesia. Crit Care 15:R132
14. Holte K, Sharrock NE, Kehlet H (2002) Pathophysiology and clinical implications of peri-operative fluid excess. Br J Anaesth 89:622-632
15. Siemionow K, Cywinski J, Kusza K, Lieberman I (2012) Intraoperative fluid therapy and pul-monary complications. Orthopedics 35:e184-e191
16. Järvelä K, Kööbi T, Kauppinen P, Kaukinen S (2001) Effects of hypertonic 75 mg/ml (7.5%) saline on extracellular water volume when used for preloading before spinal anaesthesia. Ac-ta Anaesthesiol Scand 45:776-781
17. Hamilton MA (2009) Perioperative fluid management: progress despite lingering controver-sies. Cleve Clin J Med 76 Suppl 4, S28-S31
18. Shoemaker WC, Appel PL, Kram HB, Waxman K, Lee TS (1988) Prospective trial of supra-normal values of survivors as therapeutic goals in high-risk surgical patients. Chest 94:1176-1186
19. Noblett SE, Snowden CP, Shenton BK, Horgan AF (2006) Randomized clinical trial assess-ing the effect of Doppler-optimized fluid management on outcome after elective colorectal resection. Br J Surg 93:1069-1076
20. Boyd AD, Tremblay RE, Spencer FC, Bahnson HT (1959) Estimation of cardiac output soon after intracardiac surgery with cardiopulmonary bypass. Ann Surg 150:613-626
21. Clowes GH, Del Guercio LR (1960) Circulatory response to trauma of surgical operations. Metabolism 9:67-81
22. Parker MJ, Griffiths R, Boyle A (2004) Preoperative saline versus gelatin for hip fracture pa-tients; a randomized trial of 396 patients. Br J Anaesth 92:67-70
23. Venn R, Steele A, Richardson P, Poloniecki J, Grounds M, Newman P (2002) Randomized controlled trial to investigate influence of the fluid challenge on duration of hospital stay and perioperative morbidity in patients with hip fractures. Br J Anaesth 88:65-71
24. Van De Water JM, Miller TW, Vogel RL, Mount BE, Dalton ML (2003) Impedance cardiog-raphy: the next vital sign technology? Chest 123:2028-2033
25. Bayram M, Yancy CW (2009) Transthoracic impedance cardiography: a noninvasive method of hemodynamic assessment. Heart Fail Clin 5:161-168
26. Summers RL, Shoemaker WC, Peacock WF, Ander DS, Coleman TG (2003) Bench to bed-side: electrophysiologic and clinical principles of noninvasive hemodynamic monitoring us-ing impedance cardiography. Acad Emerg Med 10:669-680

27. Michard F (2005) Changes in arterial pressure during mechanical ventilation. Anesthesiology 103:419-28; quiz 449-5
28. Pinsky MR (2006) Hemodynamic monitoring over the past 10 years. Crit Care 10:117
29. Holte K, Kehlet H (2002) Compensatory fluid administration for preoperative dehydration-does it improve outcome? Acta Anaesthesiol Scand 46:1089-1093
30. Ali SZ, Taguchi A, Holtmann B, Kurz A (2003) Effect of supplemental pre-operative fluid on postoperative nausea and vomiting. Anaesthesia 58:780-784
31. Maharaj CH, Kallam SR, Malik A, Hassett P, Grady D, Laffey JG (2005) Preoperative intravenous fluid therapy decreases postoperative nausea and pain in high risk patients. Anesth Analg 100:675-82
32. Brandstrup B, Tønnesen H, Beier-Holgersen R, Hjortsø E, Ørding H, Lindorff-Larsen K, Rasmussen MS, Lanng C, Wallin L, Iversen LH, Gramkow CS, Okholm M, Blemmer T, Svendsen PE, Rottensten HH, Thage B, Riis J, Jeppesen IS, Teilum D, Christensen AM, Graungaard B, Pott F, Danish Study Group on Perioperative Fluid Therapy (2003) Effects of intravenous fluid restriction on postoperative complications: comparison of two perioperative fluid regimens: a randomized assessor-blinded multicenter trial. Ann Surg 238:641-648
33. Nisanevich V, Felsenstein I, Almogy G, Weissman C, Einav S, Matot I (2005) Effect of intraoperative fluid management on outcome after intraabdominal surgery. Anesthesiology 103:25-32
34. Kabon B, Akça O, Taguchi A, Nagele A, Jebadurai R, Arkilic CF, Sharma N, Ahluwalia A, Galandiuk S, Fleshman J, Sessler DI, Kurz A (2005) Supplemental intravenous crystalloid administration does not reduce the risk of surgical wound infection. Anesth Analg 101:1546-1553
35. Holte K, Kristensen BB, Valentiner L, Foss NB, Husted H, Kehlet H (2007) Liberal versus restrictive fluid management in knee arthroplasty: a randomized, double-blind study. Anesth Analg 105:465-474
36. Holte K (2010) Pathophysiology and clinical implications of peroperative fluid management in elective surgery: Dan Med Bull 57, B4156
37. Gan TJ, Soppitt A, Maroof M, el-Moalem H, Robertson KM, Moretti E, Dwane P, Glass PS (2002) Goal-directed intraoperative fluid administration reduces length of hospital stay after major surgery. Anesthesiology 97:820-826
38. Wakeling HG, McFall MR. Jenkins CS, Woods WG, Miles WF, Barclay GR, Fleming SC (2005) Intraoperative oesophageal Doppler guided fluid management shortens postoperative hospital stay after major bowel surgery. Br J Anaesth 95:634-642
39. Singer M (2006) The FTc is not an accurate marker of left ventricular preload. Intensive Care Med 32:1089; author reply 1091
40. Soni N (2009) British Consensus Guidelines on Intravenous Fluid Therapy for Adult Surgical Patients (GIFTASUP): Cassandra's view. Anaesthesia 64:235-238
41. Verheij J, van Lingen A, Beishuizen A, Christiaans HM, de Jong JR, Girbes AR, Wisselink W, Rauwerda JA, Huybregts MA, Groeneveld AB (2006) Cardiac response is greater for colloid than saline fluid loading after cardiac or vascular surgery. Intensive Care Med 32:1030-1038
42. Chohan AS, Greene SA, Grubb TL, Keegan RD, Wills TB, Martinez SA (2011) Effects of 6% hetastarch (600/0.75) or lactated Ringer's solution on hemostatic variables and clinical bleeding in healthy dogs anesthetized for orthopedic surgery. Vet Anaesth Analg 38:94-105
43. Fries D, Innerhofer P, Klingler A, Berresheim U, Mittermay M, Calatzis A, Schobersberger W (2002) The effect of the combined administration of colloids and lactated Ringer's solution on the coagulation system: an in vitro study using thrombelastograph coagulation analysis (ROTEG, Anesth Analg 94, 1280-7, table of contents
44. Nielsen VG (2005) Colloids decrease clot propagation and strength: role of factor XIII-fibrin polymer and thrombin-fibrinogen interactions. Acta Anaesthesiol Scand 49:1163-1171
45. Mittermayr M, Streif W, Haas T, Fries D, Velik-Salchner C, Klingler A, Oswald E, Bach C, Schnapka-Koepf M, Innerhofer P (2007) Hemostatic changes after crystalloid or colloid fluid administration during major orthopedic surgery: the role of fibrinogen administration. Anesth Analg 105:905-17

46. Langeron O, Doelberg M, Ang ET, Bonnet F, Capdevila X, Coriat P (2001) Voluven, a lower substituted novel hydroxyethyl starch (HES 130/0.4), causes fewer effects on coagulation in major orthopedic surgery than HES 200/0.5. Anesth Analg 92:855-862

47. Kuitunen A, Hynynen M, Salmenperä M, Heinonen J, Vahtera E, Verkkala K, Myllylä G (1993) Hydroxyethyl starch as a prime for cardiopulmonary bypass: effects of two different solutions on haemostasis. Acta Anaesthesiol Scand 37:652-658

48. Huet, Siemons, Hagenaars, Van Oeveren (1998) Is hydroxyethyl starch 130/0.4 the optimal starch plasma substitute in adult cardiac surgery? Anesth Analg 90:274-279

49. Konrad CJ, Markl TJ, Schuepfer GK, Schmeck J, Gerber HR (2000) In vitro effects of different medium molecular hydroxyethyl starch solutions and lactated Ringer's solution on coagulation using SONOCLOT. Anesth Analg 90:274-279

50. Gandhi SD, Weiskopf RB, Jungheinrich C, Koorn R, Miller D, Shangraw RE, Prough DS, Baus D, Bepperling, F, Warltier DC (2007) Volume replacement therapy during major orthopedic surgery using Voluven (hydroxyethyl starch 130/0.4) or hetastarch. Anesthesiology 106:1120-1127

51. Felfernig M, Franz A, Bräunlich P, Fohringer C, Kozek-Langenecker SA (2003) The effects of hydroxyethyl starch solutions on thromboelastography in preoperative male patients. Acta Anaesthesiol Scand 47:70-73

52. Boldt J, Schöllhorn T, Münchbach J, Pabsdorf M (2007) A total balanced volume replacement strategy using a new balanced hydoxyethyl starch preparation (6% HES 130/0.42) in patients undergoing major abdominal surgery. Eur J Anaesthesiol 24:267-275

53. Papakitsos, Papakitsou, Kapsali (2010) A total balanced volume replacement strategy using a new balanced 6% hydroxyethyl starch preparation Tetraspan (HES 130/0.42) in patients undergoing major orthopaedic surgery: 6AP3-1. European Journal of Anesthesiology 27:106

Cardiac Surgery

9

Felice Eugenio Agrò, Dietmar Fries and Marialuisa Vennari

9.1 Pathophysiology

Adequate fluid replacement in cardiac patients is fundamental to successful surgery. In patients undergoing cardiac surgery, correct fluid management maintains an adequate circulatory volume and a proper electrolyte and acid-base balance, avoiding arrhythmic (i.e., atrial fibrillation) and hemodynamic (i.e., hypotension, pulmonary edema) complications.

In particular, hypovolemia is a frequent occurrence among cardiac surgical patients: fluid deficits are the result of fluid loss such as due to hemorrhage or mannitol-induced diuresis, often used during cardiopulmonary bypass (CPB). CPB patient may also present a Systemic Inflammatory Response Syndrome (SIRS) with a capillary leakage syndrome and a consequent shift of fluid from intravascular space (IVS) to interstitial space (ISS): hypovolemia develops in absence of obvious fluid loss.

Hypovolemia leads to a reduction in cardiac output (CO) and tissue perfusion, with a high risk of complications (organ failure), which in some cases may be fatal.

Another cause of concern is fluid overload, which may precipitate a worsening of cardiac function (especially in patients with impaired contractility), leading to acute pulmonary edema and cardiogenic shock. These events may complicate patient management (use of inotropes and other cardiovascular active drugs) during surgery (prior to CPB) and cause difficulties in weaning the patient from the CPB pump. Moreover, aggressive preoperative or intraoperative (prior to CPB) fluid administration may cause hemodilution, with an

M. Vennari (✉)
Postgraduate School of Anesthesia and Intensive Care, Anesthesia, Intensive Care and Pain Management Department, University School of Medicine Campus Bio-Medico of Rome, Rome, Italy
e-mail: m.vennari@unicampus.it

F. E. Agrò (ed.), *Body Fluid Management*,
DOI: 10.1007/978-88-470-2661-2_9 © Springer-Verlag Italia 2013

increased need for blood products, which is further augmented by CPB priming. Suboptimal Hb values may reduce O_2 delivery (DO_2) increasing transfusional need, especially in patients affected by coronary artery diseases [1].

In order to avoid either hypoperfusion, with major organ damage, or fluid overload, stabilization of the cardiovascular system through an adequate fluid therapy should take into account the type of surgery and the initial electrolyte balance of the patient [2, 3]. In this setting, Goal-Directed Therapy GDT) may be indicated to optimize the management of cardiac surgery patients. In fact, GDT can assure an adequate circulating volume, avoiding water overload and instead leading to an ideal perfusion condition (DO_2) for each patient.

9.2   Clinical Management of Fluid

In cardiac surgery, the debate regarding optimized fluid therapy concerns not only solutions given to patients during and after surgery but also those used in CPB priming. The treatment of hypovolemia using an appropriate intravascular volume means preventing organ dysfunction, without increasing cardiac work. However, the ideal approach to volume management is still debated in cardiac surgery patients. Recently, the historical debate crystalloid/colloid has enlarged to include colloid/colloid. Nonetheless, the physical and chemical properties of the various plasma substitutes determine the different therapeutic and adverse effects. Thus, any discussion of intravenous volume replacement should consider the potential side effects, involving the inflammatory response, endothelial integrity, coagulation, and organ function (e.g., the kidneys), and not only the effect of the chosen fluid on systemic hemodynamics.

9.2.1   Comparison Between Crystalloids and Colloids

In cardiac surgery, the use of crystalloids seems to be less appropriate for volume replacement than colloids. In fact, in the intravascular space (IVS), a major amount of crystalloids is needed to achieve the same volume replacement [4]. The distribution of crystalloids is mainly interstitial and the administration of a large dose may facilitate fluid overload and hemodilution. Moreover, a relationship between the administration of high fluid volumes and increased mortality has been reported [5]. According to the literature, the use of crystalloids for volume stabilization in patients with circulatory shock is related to a higher risk of altered lung function because of pulmonary edema (fluid overload, referred to as "Da Nang lung" based on the large number of cases in the Vietnam war) [6, 7]. In particular, the use of crystalloids seems to be less appropriate in patients with reduced myocardial function. Ley et al. compared fluid replacement with crystalloids or colloids in patients undergoing coronary artery bypass or valve substitution. In that study, patients treated with hydroxyethyl starches (HES) needed less time in the intensive care unit

Table 9.1 Comparison between crystalloids and colloids in cardiac surgery

Crystalloids	Colloids
Facilitate fluid overload	Less time in intensive care
Hemodilution	Less fluids after surgery
Pulmonary edema	Better hemodynamic performance
Fewer indications in patients with reduced myocardial function	Anaphylaxis reactions
Suggested for continuous loss	Coagulopathy
	Suggested for temporary loss

than patients treated with normal saline solution. In addition, they required fewer fluids after surgery and showed better hemodynamic performance than the crystalloids group [8]. On the other hand, colloids are associated with coagulopathy, and anaphylaxis, and may cause tubular damage (ATN) with renal dysfunction (Table 9.1).

The state of the art use of crystalloids is suggested for continuous losses (total body water loss, such as due to *perspiratio insensibilis* and urinary output) while colloids are suggested for temporary losses (IVS loss, such as due to hemorrhage).

9.2.1.1 Gelatins

Currently available gelatins come in cross-linked (e.g., Gelofundiol), urea-cross-linked (e.g., Haemacel), and succinylated (e.g., Gelofusine) forms and they have comparable volume-expanding power. All of them are safe enough with respect to coagulation and organ-function preservation but they are the second most frequent cause of anaphylactic shock in cardiac surgery, following antibiotics.

9.2.1.2 Hydroxyethyl Starches

In cardiac surgery patients, HES are widely used for correcting hypovolemia. The first- and second-generations HES demonstrated good hemodynamic effects but were the cause of important side effects involving renal function, coagulation, and tissue storage and frequently caused pruritus [9].

Second- and third-generation HES include HES 6% 550/0.75 and HES 6% 130/0.4, respectively. The first is exclusively used in USA, and the second widely in Europe. HES with a lower mean molecular weight (MMW) and a lower molar substitution rate (MSR) (third and fourth generations) are safer in terms of kidney injury, even at higher doses [10]. In fact, HES 6% 130/0.4 may confer protection in ischemic/toxic renal injury, at least compared to HES 6% 200/0.5. This is an important highlight considering that acute renal failure is a frequent complication in cardiac surgery patients, especially after CPB.

One concern regarding HES use in cardiac surgery is its association with coagulation disturbances and, consequently, a greater bleeding risk in patients receiving large amounts of blood or blood products. This is especially the case with first-generation HES preparations, which induce a fibrin polymerization disturbance, a type I von-Willebrand-like syndrome, decreased coagulation factor VIII levels, and alterations in platelet function. In a recent meta-analysis, the use of third- vs. second-generation HES was not related to clinical (and statistically significant) differences in patients with blood loss after surgery [11].

The effect of HES on platelet function during cardiac surgery is an additional concern of HES use. However, unlike HES 450/0.7, HES 200/0.6, and HES 70/0.5, HES 130/0.4 were not associated with negative effects on platelet function. The preservation of endothelial function and the maintenance of endothelial integrity using HES 6%130/0.4 was also reported [12].

HES solutions with a narrow range of MMW were shown to be effective in reducing capillary edema in an animal model [13]. Furthermore, an improvement in microcirculation and in tissue oxygenation secondary to HES infusion has been demonstrated [14]. One explanation for these results is a direct effect of HES on inflammation (e.g., via a reduction in NF-$\varkappa$B release) [15].

These observations point to potential beneficial effects of HES in reducing systemic stress and the inflammatory response due to surgery and CPB, which may cause a capillary leak syndrome, with vasodilatation, interstitial and pulmonary edema, increased O_2 consumption VO_2, and reduced O_2 delivery DO_2 and tissue diffusion. Thus, modern HES preparations can be expected to reduce cardiovascular changes that may alter or precipitate disturbances in the hemodynamic and metabolic equilibrium of these patients.

In recent years, the solution in which HES are diluted has also become a subject of interest [16]. Saline solutions, in which most colloids are dissolved, contain higher amounts of chloride than plasma and therefore may cause hyperchloremic acidosis and sodium overload, especially in the presence of clinical conditions such as renal dysfunction or heart failure. Accordingly, the latest-generation HES are dissolved in plasma-adapted solutions, with a composition very close to that of plasma.

9.2.1.3 Albumin

Albumin is generally considered the best volume-replacement solution for cardiac surgery patients, but it is very expensive and its use does not justify its cost.

A meta-analysis by Russell et al. showed that, compared to crystalloids, the use of albumin in cardiac surgery yields good results with respect to platelet count, as well as a positive influence on oncotic pressure and postoperative weight gain [17].

9.2.2 Comparison Between HES and Other Colloids

There is some evidence in cardiac surgery [18] that HES affect coagulation to a greater extent than gelatins. Specifically, there is greater blood loss and an

Table 9.2 Comparison between HES and gelatins in cardiac surgery

HES vs. gelatins
Decreased renal effects
Better oncotic characteristics
Maintenance of plasma oncotic pressure
Reduced plasma shift in the third space

Table 9.3 Comparison between HES and albumin in cardiac surgery

HES vs. albumin
Better effect on CO and DO_2
No acid-base alterations

increased need for allogenic blood products in patients treated with HES 200/0.5 [19].

In an isolated renal perfusion model in which tubular damage occurs, HES were shown to impair kidney function [20]. However, different results have emerged from studies on the latest-generation HES: compared to gelatins, third- and fourth-generation HES exhibit positive effects on both the inflammatory response [15] and endothelial integrity, with reduced renal effects and a decrease in the total volume of colloid required. Allison and colleagues [21] studied the influence of gelatin and HES 6% 200/0.5 on the renal excretion of albumin. Excretion was significantly higher in the gelatin group, consistent with a better integrity of vascular membranes in the HES-treated patients.

Ooi et al. [22] confirmed that HES 6% 130/0.4 maintains plasma oncotic pressure better than gelatins and that it is also capable of reducing third-space plasma shifts. They suggested the use of HES 6% 130/0.4 instead of gelatin solutions.

One of the most serious complications after cardiac surgery is renal dysfunction. Gelatins cause greater kidney damage than HES, especially when compared to third- and fourth-generation HES. However, in a study of CBP patients, HES use corresponded to a decrease in GFR and modest renal dysfunction. Based on these heterogeneous results, the role of HES in determining renal damage remains to be clarified [23] (Table 9.2).

The effect of albumin and modern HES on hemodynamic and acid-base equilibrium after cardiac surgery was evaluated by Niemi et al in a prospective randomized study [24] comparing volume replacement with HES 6% (130 kDa, n =15) to HES 6% (200 kDa, n =15) and 4% albumin (69 kDa, n =15) after CBP. In the early postoperative phase, the albumin group had a lower cardiac index and less O_2 delivery than either the HES 130 or HES 200 group. Moreover, HES 130 did not induce acid-base alterations, while albumin infusion had a negative base excess (Table 9.3).

9.2.3   Comparison Between Balanced and Unbalanced Solutions

When evaluating the effects of different volume replacement strategies, the electrolytic composition has to be taken into account. Hyperchloremia caused by non-balanced, nor non-plasma-adapted solutions can alter kidney sensitivity to vasoconstrictors, leading to increased vascular tone and a reduction in glomerular filtration. Balanced and plasma-adapted solutions avoid hyperchloremia, with a lower risk of kidney injury, even in cardiac surgery patients, as well as a reduced bleeding risk [9] and inflammatory response.

Clotting disturbances can be avoided or reduced by dissolving HES in balanced, plasma-adapted solutions. Furthermore, there is growing evidence that the use of balanced solutions reduces the need for blood products because of the improved coagulation status, even in the setting of CPB priming [25, 26].

Finally, balanced plasma-adapted solutions maintain acid-base balance, alterations of which may worsen the hemodynamic status of cardiac patients. In a prospective, randomized, double-blind study of cardiac surgery patients [27], a balanced HES 130/0.4 preparation was compared to an unbalanced HES 130/0.4. While the hemodynamic status did not differ between the two groups, the base excess at the end of surgery was significantly less negative in the balanced than in the unbalanced HES group.

9.2.4   Cardiopulmonary Bypass Priming

Priming consists in filling the tubes of extracorporeal circuits for CPB with a fluid, before CPB starts. CBP priming is still the subject of debate, as the ideal priming strategy has not been determined and there are no specific guidelines for the procedure. Nevertheless, CPB priming plays a central role in cardiac surgery, with the choice of the solution as one of the major factors influencing patient outcome.

The main goal of CBP priming is to avoid the drop in colloid-osmotic pressure (COP) that occurs during CBP, because of hemodilution. Several lines of evidence suggest that the use of crystalloids alone is not indicated for priming. In fact, they reduce the COP, increasing the risk of postoperative organ dysfunctions and pulmonary edema [28, 29].

A study comparing HES, albumin, and Ringer lactate solution as priming fluid for CBP showed that colloids are preferable to crystalloids. The study pointed out similar results for the HES and albumin groups, whereas fluid accumulation was demonstrated in the Ringer lactate group [30].

The more recent focus of the literature has been on the use of third- and fourth-generation HES for CBP priming. Some studies have reported fewer side effects with these solutions than with gelatin, especially regarding the effects on coagulation [31-33]. However, this conclusion was not supported by a recent study. Appelman et al. [34] did not find the expected preservation of clotting parameters in a comparison of a balanced HES priming solution with gelatin-based priming. Nonetheless, HES in balanced preparations are related to fewer post-operative alterations than either albumin or gelatin. However, there is still insufficient evidence supporting the "default" use of HES. Accordingly, these solutions should be used with caution in CBP priming, as is the case for all fluids. All CBP priming solutions should be considered as real drugs, i.e., with both beneficial effects but also negative side effects. The correct choice is based on literature evidence as well as on surgical experience and on the patient's risk factors for fluid therapy.

Key Concepts
- Comparison between crystalloids and colloids
- Different types of colloids
- Cardiopulmonary bypass priming

Key Words
- Hypovolemia
- Crystalloids
- Colloids
- Gelatins
- HES
- Albumin
- Priming

Focus on...
- Base EM, Standl T, Lassnigg A, Skhirtladze K, Jungheinrich C, Gayko D, Hiesmayr M (2011) Efficacy and safety of hydroxyethyl starch 6% 130/0.4 in a balanced electrolyte solution (Volulyte) during cardiac surgery. J Cardiothorac Vasc Anesth 25(3):407-14

References

1. Vretzakis G, Kleitsaki A, Aretha D, Karanikolas M (2011) Management of intraoperative fluid balance and blood conservation techniques in adult cardiac surgery. Heart Surg Forum 14:E28-39
2. Stephens R, Mythen M (2003) Optimizing intraoperative fluid therapy. Current Opinion in Anaesthesiology 16:385-392
3. Adams HA (2007) Volumen und Flüssigkeitsersatz – Physiologie, Pharmakologie und klinischer Einsatz. Anästh Intensivmed 48:448-60

4. Rackow EC, Falk JL, Fein IA, Siegel JS, Packman MI, Haupt MT, Kaufmann BS, Putnam D (1983) Fluid resuscitation in circulatory shock: a comparison of the cardio-respiratory effects of albumin, hetastarch, and saline solutions in patients with hypovolemic and septic shock. Crit Care Med 11:839-850
5. Pradeep A, Rajagopalam S, Kolli HK, Patel N, Venuto R, Lohr J, Nader ND (2010) High volumes of intravenous fluid during cardiac surgery are associated with increased mortality. HSR Proceedings in Intensive Care and Cardiovascular Anesthesia 2:287-296
6. Stein L, Berand J, Morisette M (1975) Pulmonary edema during volume infusion. Circulation 52:483-489
7. Rackow EC, Fein A, Leppo J et al (1977) Colloid osmotic pressure as a prognostic indicator of pulmonary edema and mortality in the critical ill. Chest 72:709-713
8. Ley SJ, Miller K, Skov P, Preig P (1990) Crystalloid versus colloid fluid therapy after cardiac surgery Heart Lung 19:31-40
9. Kozek-Langenecker SA (2005) Effects of hydroxyethyl starch solutionson hemostasis. Anesthesiology 103:654–60
10. Brunkhorst FM, Engel C, Bloos F et al (2008) German Competence Network Sepsis (Sep-Net). Intensive insulin therapy and pentastarch resuscitation in severe sepsis. N Engl J Med 358:125 –39
11. Raja SG, Akhtar S, Shahbaz Y, Masood A (2011) In cardiac surgery patients does Voluven® impair coagulation less than other colloids? Interact Cardiovasc Thorac Surg 12:1022-7
12. Dieterich HJ, Weissmuller T, Rosenberger P, Eltzschig HK (2006) Effect of hydroxyethyl starch on vascular leak syndrome and neutrophil accumulation during hypoxia. Crit Care Med 34:1775 –82
13. Traumer LD, Brazeal BA, Schmitz M et al (1992) Pentafraction reduces the lung lymph response after endotoxin administration in the ovine model. Circ Shock 36:93–6
14. Lang K, Boldt J, Suttner S, Haisch G (2001) Colloids versus crystalloids and tissue oxygen tension in patients undergoing major abdominal surgery. Anesth Analg 93:405–9
15. Tian J, Lin X, Guan R, Xu JG (2004) The effects of hydroxyethyl starch on lung capillary permeability in endotoxic rats and possible mechanisms. Anesth Analg 98:768–74
16. Gan TJ, Bennett-Guerrero E, Phillips-Bute BIH, Wakeling H, Moskowitz DM, Olufolabi Y, Konstadt SN, Bradford C, Glass PS, Machin SJ, Mythen MG (1999) Hextend, a physiologically balanced plasma expander for large volume use in major surgery: a randomized phase III clinical trial. Anesth Analg 88:992–8
17. Russell JA, Navickis RJ, Wilkes MM (2004) Albumin versus crystalloid for pump priming in cardiac surgery: meta-analysis of controlled trials. J Cardiothorac Vasc Anesth 18:429-37
18. Niemi TT, Suojaranta-Ylinen RT, Kukkonen SI, Kuitunen AH (2006) Gelatin and hydroxyethyl starch, but not albumin, impair hemostasis after cardiac surgery. Anesth Analg 102:998-1006
19. Van der Linden PJ, De Hert SG, Daper A, Trenchant A, Schmartz D, Defrance P, Kimbimbi P (2004) 3.5% urea-linked gelatin is as effective as 6% HES 200/0.5 for volume management in cardiac surgery patients. J Anaesth 51:236-41
20. Hüter L, Simon TP, Weinmann L, Schuerholz T, Reinhart K, Wolf G, Amann KU, Marx G (2009) Hydroxyethylstarch impairs renal function and induces interstitial proliferation, macrophage infiltration and tubular damage in an isolated renal perfusion model. Crit Care 13:R23. Epub Feb 25
21. Allison KP, Gosling P, Jones S, Pallister I, Porter KM (1999) Randomized trial of hydroxyethyl starch versus gelatin for trauma resuscitation. J Trauma 47:1114 –21
22. Ooi JS, Ramzisham AR, Zamrin MD (2009) Is 6% hydroxyethyl starch 130/0.4 safe in coronary artery bypass graft surgery? Asian Cardiovasc Thorac Ann 17(4):368-72
23. Winkelmayer WC, Glynn RJ, Levin R, Avorn J (2003) Hydroxyethyl starch and change in renal function in patients undergoing coronary arterybypass graft surgery. Kidney Int 64(3):1046
24. Niemi T, Schramko A, Kuitunen A, Kukkonen S, Suojaranta-Ylinen R (2008) Haemodynamics and acid-base equilibrium after cardiac surgery: comparison of rapidly degradable hydroxyethyl starch solutions and albumin. Scand J Surg 97(3):259-65

25. Roche AM, James MF, Grocott MP, Mythen MG (2002) Coagulation effects of in vitro serial haemodilution with a balanced electrolyte hetastarch solution compared with a saline-based hetastarch solution and lactated Ringer's solution. Anaesthesia 57:950 –5

26. Martin G et al (2002) A prospective, randomized comparison of thrombelastographic coagulation profile in patients receiving lactated Ringer's solution, 6% hetastarch in a balanced-saline vehicle, or 6% hydroxyethyl starch in saline during major surgery. J Cardiothorac Vasc Anesth 16:441– 6

27. Base EM, Standl T, Lassnigg A, Skhirtladze K, Jungheinrich C, Gayko D, Hiesmayr M (2011) Efficacy and safety of hydroxyethyl starch 6% 130/0.4 in a balanced electrolyte solution (Volulyte) during cardiac surgery J Cardiothorac Vasc Anesth 25(3):407-14

28. Foglia RP, Lazar HL, Steed DL et al (1978) Iatrogenic myocardial edema with crystalloid primes: effects on left ventricular compliance, performance and perfusion. Surg Forum 29:312-315

29. Hoeft A et al (1991) Priming of cardiopulmonary bypass with human albumin or Ringer's Lactate: effect on colloiosmotic pressure and extravascular lung water. Br J Anesth 66:73–80

30. RM Sade, MR Stroud, FA Crawford Jr, JM Kratz, JP Dearing and DM Bartles (1985) A prospective randomized study of hydroxyethyl starch, albumin, and lactated Ringer's solution as priming fluid for cardiopulmonary bypass. The Journal of Thoracic and Cardiovascular Surgery 89:713-722

31. Gallandat Huet RC, Siemons AW, Baus D, van-Rooyen-Butijn WT, Haagenaars JA, van Oeveren W, Bepperling F (2000) A novel hydroxyethyl starch (Voluven) for effective perioperative plasma volume substitution in cardiac surgery. Can J Anaesth 47:1207–1215

32. Haisch G, Boldt J, Krebs C, Suttner S, Lehmann A, Isgro F (2001) Influence of a new hydroxyethylstarch preparation (HES 130/0.4) on coagulation in cardiac surgical patients. J Cardiothorac Vasc Anesth 15:316–321

33. American Thoracic Society Consensus Statement (2004) Evidence-based colloid use in the critically ill. Am J Respir Crit Care Med 170:1247–1259

34. Appelman MH, van Barneveld LJ, Romijn JW, Vonk AB, Boer C (2011 May) The impact of balanced hydroxylethyl starch cardiopulmonary bypass priming solution on the fibrin part of clot formation: ex vivo rotation thromboelastometry. Perfusion 26(3):175-80

Sepsis and Septic Shock

10

Rita Cataldo, Marialuisa Vennari and Felice Eugenio Agrò

Sepsis and septic shock are major health issues involving millions of people worldwide each year.

10.1 Definitions

10.1.1 Systemic Inflammatory Response Syndrome (SIRS)

Systemic Inflammatory Response Syndrome (SIRS) is a condition often observed among critically ill patients. This syndrome is sustained by proinflammatory cytokines and factors that mediate endothelial activation and adhesion resulting in capillary leakage. Clinically, SIRS is diagnosed based on the presence of two or more of the following criteria:
- body temperature < 36°C or > 38°C [1];
- heart rate > 90 beats per minute;
- tachypnea (high respiratory rate), with > 20 breaths per minute or an arterial partial pressure of carbon dioxide < 4.3 kPa (32 mmHg);
- white blood cell count < 4000 cells/mm³ (4 × 109 cells/L) or > 12,000 cells/mm³ (12 × 109 cells/L), or the presence of > 10% immature neutrophils (band forms) [2, 3].

10.1.2 Capillary Leakage

Capillary leakage is a condition of increased capillary permeability to water, ions, and macromolecules. Generally, it is caused by an alteration of capillary per-

R. Cataldo (✉)
Director of the Anesthesia Department
University School of Medicine Campus Bio-Medico of Rome, Rome Italy
e-mail: r.cataldo@unicampus.it

F. E. Agrò (ed.), *Body Fluid Management*,
DOI: 10.1007/978-88-470-2661-2_10 © Springer-Verlag Italia 2013

meability due to an inflammatory response such as SIRS. The result is a loss of proteins (particularly albumin) from the plasma to the interstitial space (ISS), and a fluid shift from the intravascular space (IVS) to the ISS (third space syndrome), resulting in hypovolemia and interstitial edema (especially pulmonary edema).

10.1.3 Sepsis

Sepsis is a form of SIRS that is caused by an infection [4].

10.1.4 Severe Sepsis

Severe sepsis is defined as sepsis and sepsis-induced organ dysfunction or tissue hypoperfusion [4].

10.1.5 Sepsis-Induced Hypotension

Sepsis-induced hypotension is defined as [4]:
- a systolic blood pressure (SBP) < 90 mm Hg or
- mean arterial pressure < 70 mm Hg or
- a SBP decrease > 40 mm Hg or
- a SBP < 2 SD below normal for the patient's age in the absence of other causes of hypotension.

10.1.6 Sepsis-Induced Hypoperfusion

Sepsis-induced tissue hypoperfusion is defined as either [4]:
- septic shock;
- an increased lactate;
- oliguria.

10.1.7 Septic Shock

Septic shock is defined as hypotension induced by sepsis refractory to fluid-resuscitation.

10.2 Physiopathology

The physiopathological basis of sepsis is a redistribution of blood flow due to the migration of inflammatory cells into tissues, with increased vascular permeability and vasodilatation. The consequences of this mechanism are hypotension and hypoperfusion, with interstitial edema resulting in a stress-induced response that includes stimulation of the sympathoadrenergic and renin-angiotensin systems. Initially, the resulting increase in cardiac contractility helps to maintain an adequate cardiac output. Later, however, there is cardiac dysfunction: cardiac output decreases, tissue perfusion is inadequate, and the oxygen supply is dereased, which evolves into multi-organ failure (MOF) [5].

10.3   Clinical Management of Fluids

According to current published guidelines, fluid administration is the first therapeutic action that should be taken in order to guarantee adequate cardiac output and oxygen [6]. Fluid therapy should, ideally, improve tissue oxygenation and microcirculation, while preventing lung edema. The recent literature reports that extravascular lung water is an independent outcome indicator in septic patients [6].

Fluid management in patients with severe sepsis/septic shock is not easily managed. It is a severe condition that requires the administration of very large amounts of IV fluids over a short period of time. Accordingly, these patients require close clinical monitoring in which the hemodynamic response to fluid loading is evaluated and overload of the ISS is avoided. Due to vasodilatation and capillary leakage, most patients require a high volume fluid loading during the first 24 h [5].

10.3.1 Which Kind of Fluid?

An unresolved question of sepsis management is which kind of fluid to use? Are crystalloids better than colloids? To answer this question, the effects of crystalloids and colloids on septic patients have to be evaluated.

10.3.1.1 Crystalloids
Crystalloids are composed of water and electrolytes (or glucose) that diffuse easily through the endothelium into the ISS in amounts proportional to the extravascular water rate; specifically, the greatest amount of crystalloids localize into the ISS as it is more extensive than the IVS. In patients with sepsis, crystalloids have an increased distribution in the ISS (Fig. 10.1), resulting in a higher risk of tissue edema. Moreover these patients need higher-dose infusions (6–8 times normal) in order to obtain an effective volume expansion.

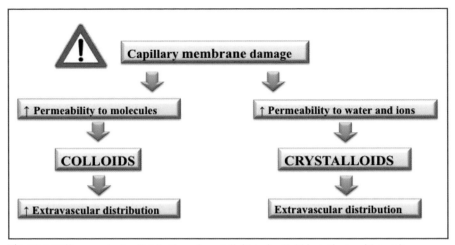

Fig. 10.1 Differences in the distribution of crystalloid and colloid in patients with sepsis

10.3.1.2 Colloids

Theoretically, colloids have a greater expanding power than crystalloids. In fact, colloids are composed of macromolecules that are unable to pass through semi-permeable biological membranes. In the presence of normal vascular permeability, colloids remain in the ISS, exerting a high colloid-osmotic pressure, which retains water in the ISS. If endothelial permeability increases, colloid macromolecules then shift from the IVS to the ISS [7] (Fig. 10.1). In particular, colloid molecules pass through the endothelium according to their molecular weight (MW): the lower the MW of the colloid (albumin, gelatins), the greater the membrane permeability. Thus, for higher MW colloids, such as hyydroxyethyl starches (HES), the membrane remains quite impermeable. The MW also determines the ability of the colloid to pass into the ISS, increasing its colloid-osmotic pressure and leading to water movement from the IVS to the ISS and thus to the formation of edema.

10.3.2   Comparison Between Crystalloids and Colloids in Balanced and Unbalanced Solutions

Different results are described in the literature regarding the hemodynamic effects of crystalloids and colloids [7-12]. If short-term effects (within 90 min from the beginning of fluid therapy) are considered, studies on small sample populations report a greater improvement of cardiovascular function in terms of volume expansion with colloids (4% gelatin, 6% albumin, 6% HES 200/0.5) [7, 8]. A non-randomized study on a large sample population (346 patients) reported mean arterial pressures of patients administered fluid therapy consisting of crystalloid or colloid (HES 130/0.4 or 4% gelatin) for a period of 2 weeks; the HES 130/0.4 group had higher mean arterial pressures [11].

A double-blind, randomized study on 475 patients reported that patients receiving crystalloids for primary resuscitation took longer to achieve initial cardiovascular stability than patients receiving colloids (6% HES 200/0.5 or dextran 70). However, this difference was not clinically important, as the degree of compromise during this period was generally not sufficient to require intervention with a rescue colloid. The same study reported that a reduction in hematocrit was greater in the colloid group 2 h after fluid therapy was initiated, but greater in the crystalloid group 6 h after fluid therapy was started [12] A randomized multi-center study on 537 patients reported that colloid (10% HES 200/0.5) therapy was associated with a more rapid achievement of the target central venous pressure and with a smaller total resuscitation fluid amount than achieved with crystalloid therapy, at least during the first 4 days of fluid therapy; however, the mean cardiovascular Sequential Organ Failure Assessment (SOFA) score of the entire fluid therapy period (21 days or one intensive care unit stay) was similar between the two groups [9]

Finally, a randomized, multi-center, double blind study on 1.218 patients found no difference in the mean cardiovascular SOFA score during one week in patients assigned to fluid resuscitation with either 4% albumin or crystalloids [10].

In a comparison of albumin or gelatin and crystalloids, albumin or gelatin resuscitation is associated with a greater hemodynamic improvement than crystalloids at least regarding short-term effects [7, 8]. If the longer-term actions of fluid therapy are considered, however, it seems that there are no significant differences in cardiovascular effects between crystalloids and albumin or gelatin [10, 11]. This may be due to the fact that over longer periods of time colloids are not as well retained in the IVS as crystalloids since sepsis increases endothelial permeability [11].

In evaluations of HES (200/0.5 or 130/0.4) and crystalloids, resuscitation with the former (in particular, HES 200/0.5, the most well-studied) is associated with a more rapid achievement of cardiovascular stability and a greater volume expansion, after both short and long-term fluid resuscitation [7-9, 11, 12]. It is unclear, however, whether the differences in hemodynamic effects are clinically significant [9, 12]. Only one study compared dextran 70 to crystalloids, concluding that dextran resuscitation is associated with a more rapid, but clinically not significant, achievement of cardiovascular stability [12].

10.3.3 Side Effects of Crystalloids and Colloids

10.3.3.1 Pulmonary Edema
The results of previously discussed studies provide support for the hypothesis that during severe sepsis/septic shock colloidal macromolecules diffuse across

the endothelial membrane due to the severely increased capillary membrane permeability. In the ISS, colloidal macromolecules exercise a colloid-osmotic pressure that tends to pull water into the extravascular space, potentially resulting in edema, including pulmonary edema. Studies comparing crystalloid and colloid resuscitation reported that the type of resuscitation fluid did not influence the incidence of pulmonary edema [8, 9, 19, 12].

10.3.3.2 Nephrotoxicity

Nephrotoxicity is a side effect associated with the use of some colloids. It is highly feared in septic patients because sepsis can cause renal failure and hemostatic disorders. In such cases, the rates of acute renal failure and renal-replacement therapy are higher following fluid resuscitation with HES 200/0.5, HES 130/0.4, or gelatin than with balanced crystalloids or saline [9, 11]. It seems that HES 200/0.5 but not HES 130/0.4 is more nephrotoxic than gelatin [11, 14]. The nephrotoxicity of HES 200/0.5 seems to be dose-dependent and occurs especially at doses > 20 mL/kg/die [9]. Interestingly, the administration of albumin vs. saline did not alter kidney function in septic patients [10].

10.3.3.3 Coagulation and Hemostasis

Coagulopathy [15] is another possible side effect of fluid administration. Normally, septic patients are at higher risk of clotting disorders (CID). The few studies on colloid-induced coagulopathy in septic patients yielded conflicting results [12, 16]. A randomized, double-blind study of a homogeneous population of 475 patients with septic shock reported similar bleeding manifestations and coagulation disorders for patients resuscitated with 6% dextran 70 and those resuscitated with 5–10 mL/kg of 6% HES 200/0.5; the patients were followed for 4 days after the beginning of fluid resuscitation [12]. However, these results should be considered with caution since they were obtained after a relatively short follow-up (4 days) and conflict with those of a large meta-analysis, on the hemostastic effects of colloids in a heterogeneous sample population, in which dextran and high-medium MW (kDa ≥ 200) HES was associated with a high risk of bleeding [15].

10.3.3.4 Inflammation

There is increasing evidence that some plasma substitutes possess additional effects besides volume replacement. These additional properties positively impact perfusion, microcirculation, tissue oxygenation, inflammation, endothelial activation, capillary leakage, and tissue edema [16, 17]. For example, Lang et al. [18] have shown that modern HES 130/0.4 is able to improve tissue oxygenation, increase microperfusion, and decrease endothelial inflammation; while crystalloids seem to mostly distribute into the ISS and reduce capillary perfusion. Neff et al. [19] suggested that a lower molar solubilization ratio (MSR) HES alters red blood cell aggregation, thus reducing blood viscosity. More studies are needed to confirm these findings.

10.3.4   Hypertonic Solutions

Hypertonic solutions allow an efficacious volume expansion using small fluid volumes. Studies performed mostly on animals have reported that volume replacement with hypertonic solutions not only results in hemodynamic improvements (by increasing preload, reducing afterload, and increasing inotropism) but also counters the formation of tissue edema and modulates the inflammatory response. These properties could be particularly useful in patients with severe sepsis/septic shock. Unfortunately, the findings in animals have yet to be confirmed in humans such that it is still not possible to recommend hypertonic solutions for fluid resuscitation in patients [20].

10.3.5   How Much Fluid?

According to the International Guidelines of the Surviving Sepsis Campaign (SSC), during the first 6 h, the goals of resuscitation from hypoperfusion induced by sepsis should include:

- central venous pressure (CVP) of 8–12 mmHg;
- mean arterial pressure ≥ 65 mmHg;
- urine output ≥ 0.5 mL/kg/h;
- central venous or mixed venous oxygen saturation ≥70% or ≥65%, respectively.

A high CVP target (12–15 mmHg), which means a high atrial filling pressure, should be considered for patients mechanically ventilated with diastolic dysfunction or high abdominal pressure, or those with pre-existing, clinically significant pulmonary artery hypertension. It must be remembered, however, that the CVP can be misleading regarding volume status as it depends not only on ventricular preload but also on ventricular compliance. More reliable measures are the volumetric parameters calculated, for example, by pulse contour continuous cardiac output (PiCCO); in fact, resuscitation directed toward hemodynamic goals in the first 6 h reduces mortality after 28 days of follow up [21].

Multiple studies have shown an improvement of mortality data when the goal-directed therapy was that indicated by the SSC guidelines [22-25]. For some patients, the administration of fluids can be dangerous, as acute right-ventricular failure, pulmonary or cerebral edema, and abdominal compartment syndrome may increase the damage caused by the fluid overload. Thus, it is important that clinicians identify those patients who will truly benefit from fluid therapy.

Depending on the available monitoring (arterial line, PAC, $ScvO_2$, echocardiography, Doppler ultrasound), a dynamic parameter is crucial to predict damage due to infusion therapy. Most often this will involve pulse pressure variation (PPV) (Fig. 10.2) [26].

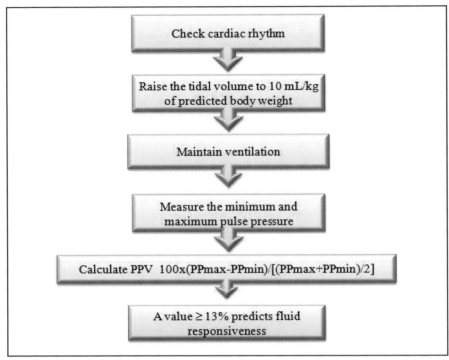

Fig. 10.2 How to measure pulse pressure variation (PPV)

10.4   Guidelines

The SCC guidelines recommend a goal-targeted fluid management with an initial target CVP ≥ 8 mmHg and the continuation of fluid therapy until the achievement of hemodynamic stability. The suggested fluids for resuscitation are crystalloids and natural/artificial colloids, but there is not enough evidence for the superiority of one particular fluid type over another [21]. A fluid challenge is recommended to calculate fluid responsiveness. It consists of either instantaneous infusion (within 10–15 min) of 250 ml of crystalloid or colloid, repeatable if indicated, with an increase of CVP ≥ 2 mmHg. Fluid responsiveness should bring an improvement in cardiac output and consequently an increase in tissue perfusion [27]. Fluid therapy must be started with 1 L of crystalloids or 300–500 mL of colloids over 30 min. Balanced solutions are reasonably preferable in patients with sepsis, in whom fluid resuscitation should be rapid and involve the use of large volumes. The rate of fluid administration must be decreased if the targeted CVP has not yet been achieved and when clinical signs of fluid overload arise (pulmonary edema, severe increase in CVP and wedge pressure) without any coexisting hemodynamic improvement [5, 21]. A meta-analysis on 1001 patients treated for sepsis reported a reduction in mortality in the group treated according to the SSC guidelines [28].

10.4.1 Current Results of Goal-Directed Therapy in Sepsis: a Systematic Review

An overview of the current results of hemodynamic monitoring and manipulation in sepsis was obtained by our group [29] in a systematic review and meta-analysis of randomized controlled trials comparing GDT with the standard of care. Studies were searched in MEDLINE, EMBASE, and Cochrane Library databases. The features of our review were as follows:

I. Randomized controlled trials (RCTs) were selected using the following inclusion criteria. RCTs on the effects of hemodynamic goal-directed therapy on mortality or morbidity in critically ill patients were the main research topic. Goal-directed therapy was defined as the monitoring and manipulation of hemodynamic parameters to reach normal or supranormal values by fluids and/or vasoactive therapy. Studies with no description of goal-directed therapy, no difference between groups in the optimization protocol, with therapy titrated to the same goal in both groups were excluded.

II. The presence of a control group with patients treated according to standard of care was required.

III. The study population consisted of critically ill, non-surgical patients, or postoperative patients with already established sepsis or organ failure. Studies involving mixed populations or surgical patients undergoing non-cardiac or cardiac surgery were excluded.

Among the 737 patients randomized in the four included studies, hospital mortality was recorded in 298 (40%). Of these, 179 patients had been assigned to the control group (47%), and 119 to the experimental group (32%). Table 10.1 shows the overall responses (ORs) and 95% confidence intervals (CIs) for the observed in-hospital mortality in each trial as well as the pooled estimate. The overall effect in the combined studies was a significant reduction in mortality for the experimental group [pooled OR of 0.50 (0.34–0.74); $P = 0.0006$] without a significant heterogeneity among studies ($P = 0.25$; $I^2 = 27\%$). Overall, the findings suggest that hemodynamic optimization can reduce mortality in sepsis.

10.5 Conclusions

According to the most recent clinical trials on fluid resuscitation of patients with severe sepsis/septic shock, a few hours after the beginning of fluid therapy, colloid resuscitation causes an improvement in cardiovascular function

Table 10.1 Effect of hemodynamic optimization on hospital mortality in patients with sepsis (experimental vs. control group)

Study	Experimental Group	Control Group	Weight	Odds Ratio (95%CI)
De Oliveira (2008)	8/51	21/51	5.3	0.27 [0.10, 0.68]
Lin (2006)	58/108	83/116	9.4	0.46 [0.27, 0.80]
Rivers (2001)	46/95	50/106	9.4	1.05 [0.60, 1.83]
Santhanam (2008)	13/74	13/73	6.0	0.98 [0.42, 2.30]
Overall	119/363	179/374	100	0.50 [0.34, 0.74]

Heterogeneity: $I^2 = 27\%$; $\chi^2 = 4$; $P = 0.25$; Overall effect: $Z = 3.44$; $P = 0.0006$

and plasma volume expansion that is greater than the recovery obtained with crystalloid resuscitation. The effects of fluid therapy are recordable after hours/days. The hemodynamic effects of albumin and gelatins are likely similar to those of crystalloids. HES, on the other hand, have a greater expanding power than crystalloids, even after hours or days and have been recommended for patients with sepsis. However, HES is associated with many side effects, some on which depend on MMW and MSR (i.e., nephrotoxicity, coagulopathy, risk of pulmonary edema) while others involve independent risk factors (i.e., allergic reactions and itching). Theoretically, patients with severe sepsis/septic shock are very susceptible to the development of colloid-induced kidney injury, coagulopathy, and pulmonary edema given that sepsis alone can already cause renal failure, hemostatic disorders, and pulmonary edema. There are several types of HES, which differ according to their MW and MSR. The side effects (nephrotoxicity, coagulopathy and risk of pulmonary edema) of medium-MW HES, especially HES 200/0.5, has been well studied. Compared to crystalloids, HES 200/0.5 therapy does not increase the risk of pulmonary edema but it is associated with a higher rate of acute kidney failure. Thus, comparatively speaking, low-MW HES (HES 130/0.4) poses less danger to the kidney and causes only minor changes in the clotting system. Nevertheless, current studies on the safety of HES 130/0.5 are of limited statistical power in addition to the fact that in septic patients this HES has been largely unexamined. A major ongoing study is aimed at assessing the safety and efficacy of HES 130/0.4 in patients with severe sepsis [30].

In conclusion, as HES have known side effects and their advantages compared to crystalloids in improving hemodynamic are still being evaluated, it seems rational that, at least for the time being, fluid resuscitation of patients with severe sepsis/septic shock should be mainly based on the use of crystalloids. This conclusion is in agreement with many recently published reviews on this topic [31, 32]. The use of HES should be limited to patients whose hemodynamic condition is particularly compromised. Low-MW HES, such as HES 130/0.4, are associated with less nephrotoxicity and coagulopathy than medium-MW HES, such as HES 130/0.5 (maximum daily dose of 50 mL/kg/die). As already recommended by guidelines on sepsis therapy, crystalloids and colloids in balanced solution should be preferred. Current studies on the safety of HES 130/0.4 in balanced solution may clarify whether this colloid can be considered the first-choice fluid for patients with severe sepsis or septic shock.

Key Concepts
- Definition of SIRS, sepsis, and septic shock
- Side effects of colloids and crystalloids

Key Words
- SIRS
- Sepsis
- Septic shock
- Side effects
- PPV

Focus on…
- Dellinger RP, Levy MM, Carlet JM et al (2008) Surviving Sepsis Campaign Guidelines Committee. Surviving Sepsis Campaign. International guidelines for management of severe sepsis and septic shock. Crit Care Med 34:17-60
- Scandinavian Critical Care Trials Group (2011) Comparing the effect of hydroxyethyl starch 130/0.4 with balanced crystalloid solution on mortality and kidney failure in patients with severe sepsis (6S-Scandinavian Starch for Severe Sepsis/Septic Shock trial): Study protocol, design and rationale for a double-blinded, randomized clinical trial. Trials 12:24
- Reinhart K, Perner A, Sprun CL et al (2012) Consensus statement of the ESICM task force on colloid volume therapy in critically ill patients. Intensive Care Med 38(3):368-83

References

1. American College of Chest Physicians/Society of Critical Care Medicine Consensus Conference: definitions for sepsis and organ failure and guidelines for the use of innovative therapies in sepsis (1992) Crit Care Med 20:864–74
2. Rippe JM, Irwin RS, Cerra FB (1999) Irwin and Rippe's intensive care medicine. Philadelphia, Lippincott-Raven
3. Tsiotou AG, Sakorafas GH, Anagnostopoulos G, Bramis J (March 2005) Septic shock; current pathogenetic concepts from a clinical perspective. Medical Science Monitor: International Medical Journal of Experimental and Clinical Research 11:RA76–85
4. Dellinger RP et al (2008) Surviving Sepsis Campaign: international guidelines for management of severe sepsis and septic shock. Crit Care Med 36:296-327
5. Dellinger RP, Levy MM, Carlet JM et al, for the International Surviving Sepsis Campaign Guidelines Committee (2008) Surviving Sepsis Campaign. International guidelines for management of severe sepsis and septic shock: 2008. Crit Care Med Vol. 36, No. 1
6. Rajnish KJ et al (2004) Albumin: an overview of its place in current clinical practice. J Indian An
7. Trof RJ, Sukul SP, Twisk JWR, Girbes ARJ, Groeneveld AB J (2010) Greater cardiac response of colloid than saline fluid loading in septic and non-septic critically ill patients with clinical hypovolaemia. Intensive Care Med 36:697–701
8. Van der Heijden M, Verheij J, van Nieuw Amerongen GP, Groeneveld AB (2009) Crystalloid or colloid fluid loading and pulmonary permeability, edema, and injury in septic and nonseptic critically ill patients with hypovolemia. Crit Care Med 37:1275–81
9. Brunkhorst FM, Englel C, Bloos F et al (2008) Intensive insulin therapy and pentastarch resuscitation in severe sepsis. N Engl J Med 358:125–39
10. The SAFE Study Investigators (2011) Impact of albumin compared to saline on organ function and mortality of patients with severe sepsis. Intensive Care Med 37:86–96
11. Bayer O, Reinhart K, Sakr Y et al (2011) Renal effects of synthetic colloids and crystalloids in patients with severe sepsis: A prospective sequential comparison. Crit Care Med Vol. 39, No. 6
12. Wills BA, Nguyen MD, Ha TL et al (2005) Comparison of three fluid solutions for resuscitation in dengue shock syndrome. N Engl J Med 353:877–89
13. Sakr Y et al (2007) Effects of hydroxyethyl starch administration on renal function in critically ill patients. Br J Anaesth 98:216–224
14. Schortgen F, Lacherade JC, Bruneel F, Cattaneo I, Hemery F, Lemaire F, Brochard L (2001) Effects of hydroxyethylstarch and gelatin on renal function in severe sepsis: a multicentre randomised study. Lancet 357:911-916
15. Blanloeil Y, Trossaërt M, Rigal JC, Rozec B (2002) Effects of plasma substitutes on hemostasis. Ann Fr Anesth Reanim 21:648-67
16. Wiedermann CJ (2008) Systematic review of randomized clinical trials on the use of hydroxyethyl starch for fluid management in sepsis. BMC Emerg Med 8:1–8
17. Mitra S, Khandelwal P (2009) Are all colloids same? How to select the right colloid? Indian Journal of Anaesthesia 53:592-607
18. Lang K, Boldt J, Suttner S, Haisch G (2001) Colloids versus crystalloids and tissue oxygen tension in patients undergoing major abdominal surgery. Anesth Analg 93:405–409
19. Neff TA, Fischler L, Mark M, Stocker R, Reinhart WH (2005) The influence of two different hydroxyethyl starch solutions (6% HES 130/0.4 and 200/0.5) on blood viscosity. Anesth Analg 100:1773–1780
20. Libert N, de Rudnicki S, Cirodde A, Thepenier C, Mion G (2010) Il y a-t-il une place pour le serum sale hypertonique dans les etats septiques graves? Annales Francaises d'Anesthesie et de Reanimation 29:25–35
21. Dellinger RP et al (2008) Surviving Sepsis Campaign: international guidelines for management of severe sepsis and septic shock: 2008. Crit Care Med 36:296-327

22. Gurnani PK et al (2010) Impact of the implementation of a sepsis protocol for the management of fluid-refractory septic shock: A single-center, before-and-after study. Clin Ther 32:1285-93
23. Micek ST et al (2006) Before-after study of a standardized hospital order set for the management of septic shock. Crit Care Med 34:2707–2713
24. Kortgen A et al (2006) Implementation of an evidence-based "standard operating procedure" and outcome in septic shock. Crit Care Med 34:943–949
25. Machado FR et al (2010) Improving mortality in sepsis: analysis of clinical trials. Shock 34 Suppl 1:54-8
26. Durairaj L et al (2008) Fluid therapy in resuscitated sepsis: less is more. Chest 133:252-63
27. Antonelli M et al (2007 Apr) Hemodynamic monitoring in shock and implications for management. International Consensus Conference, Paris, France, 27-28 April 2006. Intensive Care Med 33:575-90
28. Jones AE et al (2008) The effect of a quantitative resuscitation strategy on mortality in patients with sepsis: a meta-analysis. Crit Care Med 36:2734-9
29. Agrò FE, Benedetto U, Cocomello L, Benedetto M. A systematic review and meta-analysis of randomized controlled trials on the comparison between hemodynamic optimization versus standard care in non-surgical critically ill patients. Submitted
30. Perner A, Haase N, Wetterslev J et al, the Scandinavian Critical Care Trials Group (2011) Comparing the effect of hydroxyethyl starch 130/0.4 with balanced crystalloid solution on mortality and kidney failure in patients with severe sepsis (6S - Scandinavian Starch for Severe Sepsis/Septic Shock trial): Study protocol, design and rationale for a double-blinded, randomized clinical trial. Trials 12:24
31. Groeneveld ABJ, Navickis RJ, Wilkes MM (2011) Update on the Comparative Safety of Colloids: A Systematic Review of Clinical Studies. Ann Surg 253:470–483
32. Hartog CS, Bauer M, Reinhart K (2011) The Efficacy and Safety of Colloid Resuscitation in the Critically Ill. Anesth Analg 112:156–64

Fluid Management in Trauma Patients

11

Chiara Candela, Maria Benedetto and Felice Eugenio Agrò

11.1 Introduction

Trauma is a considerable health issue, given that each day 16 000 people die from trauma and several thousand are severely injured [1].

11.1.1 Chest Trauma

Chest trauma is the second most common cause of death after head trauma. Most cases of chest trauma are the consequence of motor vehicle accidents, which is the main cause of death [2].
Patients with chest trauma show several clinical manifestations: rib fractures, pneumothorax, hemothorax or both, lung contusion, cardiac contusion or laceration, blunt aortic injury, diaphragmatic injury, and lung laceration.

11.1.2 Hemothorax

Hemothorax is an intrapleural bleeding that results from injury to the chest wall, lung, or thoracic vessels. In massive hemothorax, the affected lung is collapsed, with right to left shunt and hypoxia. The blood loss leads to hemorrhagic shock and, potentially, circulatory failure. Hemothorax is very often accompanied by pneumothorax, a condition termed as hemopneumothorax.

C. Candela (✉)
Postgraduate School of Anesthesia and Intensive Care, Anesthesia, Intensive Care and Pain Management Department, University School of Medicine Campus Bio-Medico of Rome, Rome, Italy
e-mail: chiaracandela@yahoo.it

F. E. Agrò (ed.), *Body Fluid Management*,
DOI: 10.1007/978-88-470-2661-2_11 © Springer-Verlag Italia 2013

11.1.3   Cardiac Tamponade

Cardiac tamponade is a rare event in blunt chest trauma, mostly associated with penetrating trauma. It occurs when blood from an injured great vessel, cardiac chamber, or coronary or pericardial vessel accumulates in the pericardial space. The pericardium is poorly distensible and tamponade can occur with the accumulation of as few as 20 mL of blood. The heart is compressed, blocking the filling of the cardiac chambers and resulting in cardiac output reduction, hypotension and shock.

11.1.4   Flail Chest

Flail chest occurs when two or more adjacent rib fractures in two or more places interrupt the bony continuity of a segment of the chest wall with the rest of the thoracic cage, resulting in ventilatory mechanical failure. Flail chest is coupled with an underlying pulmonary contusion and very often with pneumothorax and/or hemothorax.

11.1.5   Pulmonary Contusion

Pulmonary contusions are injuries to the lung parenchyma that are caused by a high-energy blunt force to the thorax, with alveolar hemorrhage and edema. They are frequently associated with other chest injuries, such as rib fractures or flail chest but can also occur alone. This is especially the case in younger patients, whose thoracic cage is more elastic and flexible such that high-energy force is readily transmitted to the underlying lung without rib fractures. Hypoxia may develop according to the proportion of right to left shunt.

11.1.6   Aortic Injury

Aortic injury typically results from high-energy accidents, such as high-speed motor vehicle collisions or falls. It is fatal immediately at the scene of the accident in > 80% of the cases; patients who reach the hospital alive usually have a contained tear that most commonly involves the descending aorta below the origin of the left subclavian artery. If not rapidly diagnosed and treated, those patients are at very high risk of death shortly after their hospital admission.

11.1.7   Abdominal Trauma

Abdominal injuries are an important cause of death in trauma patients and should be evaluated very carefully based on the likelihood of occult bleeding, which may lead to catastrophic consequences if not promptly diagnosed and treated. Patients with abdominal trauma should be rapidly assessed and undergo early surgical consultation to avoid the misdiagnosis of abdominal injuries and preventable trauma-related death.

11.1.8 Pelvic Trauma

Fractures of the pelvis are associated with high rates of mortality and morbidity. Mortality is 30–50% for open pelvic fractures and 10–30% for closed injuries. Associated trauma to the abdominal and pelvic viscera, chest, spine, and musculoskeletal system is commonly seen.

Fractures of the pelvis usually involve the pelvic ring, iliac wings, and sacrum. Ligamentous disruption may lead to diastasis of the pubic symphysis and rupture of the sacroiliac joints.

Disruption of the pelvic bone, iliac arterial and venous vessels can lead to massive hemorrhage, 85% of which is venous or bony in origin. If not promptly and aggressively treated, those injuries lead to exsanguination and death.

11.2   Physiopathology

The first condition that should be suspected in cases of shock in the context of trauma, up to its exclusion, is hypovolemia due to hemorrhage. Indeed, absolute hypovolemia from blood loss is the main cause of shock in trauma patients, as well as the most frequent cause of death in the acute phase of trauma. It is responsible for a large majority of the deaths occurring within the first hours of hospital admission.

However, hypovolemia in trauma patients is also caused by hemorrhages, internal organ damage, capillary leakage, systemic inflammatory response syndrome (SIRS) and third-space syndrome. Hypotension may have three sequential components: hypovolemia, vasodilatation, and cardiac failure, leading to multiple organ failure (MOF).

Considering these observations, it is evident that the earliest goals in the management of trauma patients are the control of bleeding and hemodynamic stabilization.

11.3   Clinical Management of Fluids

According to WHO guidelines, trauma care with fluid resuscitation depends on the type of fluids, the ability to administer them and to monitor the hemodynamic response and the treatment of complications. One of the most important complications in trauma patients is blood loss, which may cause hemodynam-

Table 11.1 Clinical manifestations of blood loss

Blood losses	Clinical manifestations
Over 40% of blood volume	Most patients die quickly.
30–40% of total blood volume	Hemorrhagic shock: hypotension, mental impairment, high respiratory rate, heart rate over 100 bpm, oliguria.
15–30% of total blood volume	High heart rate, high respiratory rate, cold extremities, decreased urine output, increased diastolic pressure.
0–15% of total blood volume	No hemodynamic alteration, urine output slightly decreased, mild anxiety.

ic instability. The clinical manifestations of hemorrhage depend on the amount of blood loss (Table 11.1).

Blood losses up to 15% of blood volume are compensated by hormonal and autonomic responses to hypovolemia, with minor clinical manifestations. Consequently, they must not necessarily be treated with IV fluid and can optionally be replaced with crystalloid. Blood loss > 15% (750 mL) should be treated with colloid infusion solutions; while major blood loss (> 30%) must be replaced with colloids [3,4]. The limitation of any volume replacement is hemodilution, because a reduction in the hematocrit leads to a decrease in tissue oxygen delivery. The critical level of the Hb concentration in patients with no apparent heart or pulmonary diseases is approximately 7 g/dL.

Early deaths within the first 24 h after injury, are typically due to massive uncontrolled hemorrhage in about 50% of patients and fatal traumatic brain injury in the remainder. In addition, 56% of hemorrhagic deaths take place in the pre-hospital setting [5].

11.3.1 Which Kind of Fluid?

Data on the ideal first-line fluid for trauma resuscitation are unclear. The type of fluid and the timing of its administration remain poorly standardized. Although pre-hospital fluid administration does not show any significant benefit with respect to clinical outcomes, it is currently routinely performed.

11.3.1.1 Crystalloids
According to the eighth edition of Advanced Trauma Life Support, fluid resuscitation in trauma starts with warm isotonic crystalloids (Ringer lactate or saline), as they provisionally allow expansion of the intravascular space (IVS). More recently, a more restrained and prudent use of crystalloids in the pre-hospital setting was recommended.

11.3.1.2 Colloids

Colloids (mainly HES), administered in bolus form, are suggested when hemodynamic instability or cognitive deterioration occurs [6]. However, capillary leakage is an important consideration in patients receiving colloids, as it may cause a worsening of pre-existing edema and impairment of tissue oxygenation due to the shift of colloid into the interstitial space (ISS). Furthermore, several side effects (kidney injury, clotting disorders, and anaphylaxis) have been reported, especially after the infusion of older-generation colloids. Colloids have not been shown to be superior to crystalloids in the treatment of hypovolemia in critically ill patients [7].

11.3.1.3 Hypertonic Solutions

Hypertonic solutions are alternative fluids in the early stages of trauma. They are especially useful in patients with brain injury as they have been shown to decrease the intracranial pressure [8] with a better efficacy than mannitol [6]. Another possible benefit of hypertonic solutions is a rapid increase in the mean arterial pressure by using small volumes and a consequent reduction of lung edema in the days following resuscitation [9]. However, there are no convincing data on better survival [10-12], as discussed elsewhere in this volume.

11.3.2   How Much Fluid?

A bolus of fluid is recommended for patients with isolated injuries involving the extremities and isolated brain injury. Patients at high risk of internal hemorrhage, however, should be managed with a deliberate hypotensive approach until the achievement of complete hemostasis [13].

According to the Eastern Association for the Surgery of Trauma [6]:
- in case of superficial wounds, intravenous access is not necessary;
- if the patient is conscious and a radial pulse is present, the pre-hospital personnel may place a venous access but fluids should be withheld;
- venous access should be achieved and fluid infusion started (500 mL of HES in bolus) if there is no radial pulse or the patient's mental status is confused;
- fluid infusion should be stopped if the pulse and mental status improve;
- if the patient is refractory to fluids, a bolus of 500 mL HES should be repeated.

The Tactical Combat Casualty Care Guidelines (TCCC) guidelines recommend [14]:
a. Trauma without shock:
   - IV fluids are not required;
   - per os fluids are allowed if the patient is conscious and able to swallow.
b. Trauma with shock:

- an IV bolus of 500 mL HES should be administered;
- if the patient remains in shock, an additional bolus should be repeated after 30 min;
- no more than 1000 mL of HES in an IV bolus should be administered.

c. Trauma with persistent hemodynamic instability:
   - fluid resuscitation with Ringer lactate, HES, and blood are appropriate.

d. Brain trauma in unconscious patients with weak or absent peripheral pulse:
   - resuscitation should be performed until a systolic blood pressure $\geq$ 90 mmHg is achieved.

Fluid resuscitation should be rationally delayed, i.e., until definitive hemorrhage control is achieved. This is especially important in out-of hospital settings, where transport times are short [15].

11.3.3 The Risk of Fluid Overload

Excessive fluid infusion in the acute trauma setting is often associated with complications that can lead to MOF and increased mortality. The administration of excessive fluids in a patient with uncontrolled hemorrhage could lead to a dilution of coagulation factors and platelets, thus worsening the bleeding. A large amount of crystalloids or colloids may promote interstitial and pulmonary edema.

In the presence of SIRS and MOF, fluid overload may reduce organ perfusion and lead to abdominal compartment syndrome. A retrospective study conducted on 3137 trauma patients showed increased mortality following the administration of > 1.5 L of fluids; this was especially pronounced in elderly patients (> 70 years) [16].

11.3.4 Current results of Goal-Directed Therapy in Trauma. Systematic Review

An overview of current results of hemodynamic monitoring and manipulation in critically ill patients has been carried out by our group [17]. It is a systematic review and meta-analysis of randomized controlled trials comparing GDT versus standard of care. Studies were searched in MEDLINE, EMBASE and Cochrane Library databases.

I. Randomized controlled trials (RCTs) were selected using the following inclusion criteria. RCTs on the effects of hemodynamic goal-directed therapy on mortality or morbidity in critically ill patients as main research topic. Goal-directed therapy was defined as monitoring and manipulation of hemodynamic parameters to reach normal or supranormal values by fluids and/or vasoactive therapy. Studies with no description of goal-directed therapy, no difference between groups in the optimization protocol, with therapy titrated to the same goal in both groups were excluded.

Table 11.2 Effect of hemodynamic optimization in the experimental group versus control on hospital mortality in trauma patients

| Study or subgroup | Experimental Group | | Control Group | | | Odds Ratio |
	Events	Total	Events	Total	Weight M-H	Random, 95% CI
Bishop et al. (1995)	9	50	24	65	5.7%	0.38 [0.16,0.90]
Citra et al. (2007)	13	80	18	82	6.5%	0.69 [0.31,1.52]
Fleming et al. (1992)	8	33	15	34	4.5%	0.41 [0.14,1.15]
Velmahos et al. (2000)	6	40	4	35	3.0%	1.37 [0.35,5.30]
Subtotal (95% CI)		203		216	19.8%	0.56 [0.34,0.92]
Total events	26		61			

II. Presence of a control group with patients treated according to the standard of care.

III. Study population consisted of critically ill, non-surgical patients, or postoperative patients with already established sepsis or organ failure. Studies involving mixed population or surgical patients undergoing non-cardiac or cardiac surgery were excluded.

The overall effect when combining the studies was a significant reduction in mortality for the experimental group without a significant heterogeneity among studies (Table 11.2).

From the study emerged that hemodynamic optimization can reduce mortality in non-surgical critically ill patients with relevant benefits for trauma patients.

Key Concepts
- Hypovolemia due to hemorrhage in trauma patients
- The management of fluid administration in trauma patients
- Risk of fluid overload

Key Words
- Blood loss
- Hemorrhagic shock
- Crystalloids
- Colloids
- Hypertonic solutions

Focus on...
- Van den Elsen MJ, Leenen LPH, Kesecioglu J (2010) Hemodynamic support of the trauma patient. Curr Opin Anaesthesiol 23(2):269-75
- Roppolo LP, Wigginton JG, Pepe P (2010) Intravenous fluid resuscitation for the trauma patient. Curr Opin Crit Care 16(4):283-8
- Ertmer C, Kampmeier T, Rheberg S, Lange M (2011) Fluid resuscitation in multiple trauma patients. Curr Opin Anaesthesiol 24(2):202-8
- Reinhart K, Perner A, Sprun CL et al (2012) Intensive Care Med 38(3):368-8

References

1. WHO (2004) Guidelines for essential trauma care
2. Hanafi M, Al-Sarraf N, Sharaf H, Abdelaziz A (2011) Pattern and presentation of blunt chest trauma among different age groups. Asian Cardiovasc Thorac Ann 19:48-51
3. Garrioch MA (2004) The body's response to blood loss. Vox Sanguinis 87 (Suppl. 1)S74–S76
4. Riddez L, Hahn RG, Brismar B et al (1997) Central and regional hemodynamics during acute hypovolemia and volume substitution in volunteers. Crit Care Med 25:635-640
5. Kauvar DS et al (2006) Impact of hemorrhage on trauma outcome: an overview of epidemiology, clinical presentations, and therapeutic considerations. J Trauma 60(suppl):S3-11
6. Cotton BA et al (2009) Guidelines for prehospital fluid resuscitation in the injured patient. J Trauma Aug 67:389-402
7. Van den Elsen MJ et al (2010) Hemodynamic support of the trauma patient. Curr Opin Anaesthesiol 23:269-75
8. Bratton SL et al (2007) Guidelines for the management of severe traumatic brain injury. II. Hyperosmolar therapy. J Neurotrauma 24(suppl1):S14-20
9. Patanwala AE et al (2010) Use of hypertonic saline injection in trauma. Am J Health Syst Pharm 67:1920-8
10. Kortbeek JB et al (2008) Advanced trauma life support, 8th edition, the evidence for change. J Trauma 64:1638-50
11. Hashiguchi N et al (2007) Hypertonic saline resuscitation: efficacy may require early treatment in severely injured patients. J Trauma 62:299–306
12. Pinto FC et al (2006) Volume replacement with lactated Ringer's or 3% hypertonic saline solution during combined experimental hemorrhagic shock and traumatic brain injury. J Trauma 60:758–763
13. Roppolo LP et al (2010) Intravenous fluid resuscitation for the trauma patient. Curr Opin Crit Care 16:283-8
14. Tactical Combat Casualty Care Guidelines 18 August 2010
15. Ertmer C et al (2011) Fluid resuscitation in multiple trauma patients. Curr Opin Anaesthesiol 24:202-8
16. Arlati S et al (2007) Decreased fluid volume to reduce organ damage: a new approach to burn shock resuscitation? A preliminary study. Resuscitation 72:371–378
17. Agrò FE, Benedetto U, Cocomello L, Benedetto M. A systematic review and meta-analysis of randomized controlled trials on the comparison between hemodynamic optimization versus standard care in non-surgical critically ill patients. Submitted

Fluid Management in Burn Patients

12

Felice Eugenio Agrò, Hans Anton Adams
and Annalaura Di Pumpo

12.1 Physiopathology

Severe burns result in a combination of hypovolemic and redistribution shock, manifested by a decreased intravascular volume, a low occlusion pressure in the pulmonary artery, a high systemic vascular resistance, and a reduced cardiac index [1]. The balance of water, plasma protein (albumin), and inorganic solute between the intravascular and interstitial spaces (IVS and ISS, respectively) is modified by the alteration of capillary permeability, resulting in hypovolemia.

12.2 Clinical Management of Fluids

The basis of fluid management in burn patients is to prevent shock. A delay of 2 h in fluid administration complicates resuscitation and increases mortality [2].

The total amount of fluid infusion mainly depends on the severity of the burn(s) and the extent of the body surface involved, but cannot be calculated exactly. At best, a rough estimation is possible.

12.2.1 Which Kind of Fluid?

12.2.1.1 Crystalloids
Currently, crystalloids are widely used for fluid resuscitation in burn patients,

A. Di Pumpo (✉)
Postgraduate School of Anesthesia and Intensive Care, Anesthesia, Intensive Care and Pain Management Department, University School of Medicine Campus Bio-Medico of Rome, Rome, Italy
e-mail: annalaurad.p@live.it

F. E. Agrò (ed.), *Body Fluid Management*,
DOI: 10.1007/978-88-470-2661-2_12 © Springer-Verlag Italia 2013

even if the infusion of large volumes reduces plasma protein concentrations and produces tissue edema. While Ringer's lactate is widely used, a balanced solution with acetate or malate is preferred due to the reduced degree of oxygen consumption during its metabolism.

12.2.1.2 Colloids

According to the American Burn Association guidelines, colloids can be used 12 to 24 h from the injury, when the integrity of the capillary membrane has been restored. The use of colloids results in a reduction of tissue edema and of the overall fluid requirement [1, 3]. The literature is significantly focused on the use of albumin in treating hypovolemia in burn patients. However, data on mortality following the use of albumin in burn patients are still contradictory [4]. In some burn centers, gelatin solutions are preferred based on cost reduction, whereas hydroxyethyl starch solutions are avoided due to probable renal impairment.

12.2.1.3 Hypertonic Solutions

Hypertonic saline solutions need to be used with caution because of possible hypernatremia, hyperchloremia, and renal failure [1, 2].

12.2.2 How Much Fluid?

12.2.2.1 The Role of Total Burned Surface Area (TBSA)

According to the American Burn Association guidelines, patients with burns involving > 20 % of the total body surface area (TBSA) must receive fluid replacement using the total burned area estimation (Fig. 12.1). A need for crystalloids at 2–4 mL/kg/% TBSA in the first 24 h has been estimated (Parkland formula according to Baxter). A half volume should be administered during the first 8 h and the remaining part in the following 16 h [1].

Children need higher infusion amounts than adults. The typical fluid requirement is 6 mL/kg/% TBSA. They also may need the addition of dextrose in the first 24 h to maintain glucose homeostasis [1]. Patients with deep lesions and inhalation trauma also need larger volumes of fluid [5].

Fluid resuscitation should be carried out to maintain a urine output > 0.5 mL/kg/h in adults and > 1.0 mL/kg/h in children [1, 6]. However diuresis is not recognized in the literature as the unique parameter to evaluate the efficacy of fluid resuscitation [7]. The crucial goal of fluid administration should be to ensure an adequate blood perfusion to major organs rather than to normalize hemodynamic parameters [7]. Consequently, goal-directed fluid therapy has been recommended for burn patients as well [7].

12.2.2.2 The Risk of Fluid Overload

Burn patients are high-fluid-need patients but this does not mean an indiscriminate and never-ending use of fluids. Indeed, fluid overload may worsen inter-

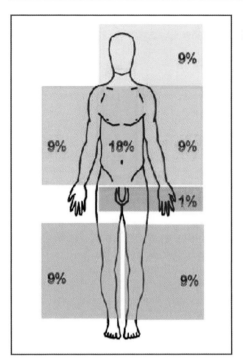

Fig. 12.1 Rule of nines to rapidly assess the percentage of body surface involved by burns

stitial edema, leading to complications such as intra-abdominal hypertension, abdominal compartment syndrome, as well as ocular compartment syndrome [8]. Accordingly, current guidelines require the use of advanced invasive or minimally invasive hemodynamic monitoring, especially in patients with refractory shock or with poor cardiopulmonary reserve [1].

The first step in burn patients: infuse fluids at calculated rates, as ordered by the treating physician. To avoid the inappropriate use of fluid therapy, vital signs and urine output should be measured.

The main goals of a fluid regimen in the first phase are:
- no increase in the hemoglobin concentration or the hematocrit;
- mean arterial pressure at least 65 mmHg;
- urine output at least 0.5 mL/kg/h;
- central venous pressure 10–15 mmHg, if necessary 20 mmHg;
- central venous oxygen saturation > 70%;
  Step one should be repeated every hour.
- If urine output is less than 15 mL/h (Table 12.1) for longer than 2 h, despite an increase in the fluid administration rate, urinary catheter and vital signs should be checked. Furthermore, gelatin should be considered in the treatment protocol.

Table 12.1 Fluid management in burn patients with stable vital signs

Urine output < 15 mL	Urine output between 15 and 30 mL	Urine output between 30 and 50 mL	Urine output between 50 and 200 mL	Urine output > 200 mL
Increase the IV rate of fluid by 20% or 200 mL/h	Increase the IV rate of fluid by 10% or 100 mL/h	Left IV as it is	Decrease the IV rate of fluid by 10% or 100 mL/h	Decrease the IV rate of fluid by 10% or 100 mL/h every 30 and the in minutes meanwhile blood sugar, lactate and hemoglobin should be checked

- If the calculated maintenance rate is achieved and held for 2 h and the patient is at least 24 h post-burn, fluid resuscitation should be considered complete and maintenance IV treatment should then be instituted. Attention must be paid to an eventual new onset of oliguria. In this case, crystalloids or even gelatin should be administered again at the current rate. If the patient requires an overly large volume of crystalloids (> 2× the normal amount) at the current calculated rate for ≥ 2 h, colloid resuscitation with gelatin should be considered.

Key Concepts
- Physiopathology of burns
- The role of total burned surface area
- Risk of fluid overload

Key Words
- Hypovolemic shock
- Crystalloids
- Colloids
- TBSA
- Fluid overload

Focus on...
- Pham TN, Cancio LC, Gibran NS (2008) American Burn Association practice guidelines burn shock resuscitation. J Burn Care Res 29(1):257-66

References

1. Pham TN, Cancio LC, Gibran NS (2008) American Burn Association practice guidelines burn shock resuscitation. J Burn Care Res 29:257-66
2. Latenser BA (2009) Critical care of the burn patient: the first 48 hours. Crit Care Med 37:2819-26
3. Vlachou E et al (2010) Hydroxyethylstarch supplementation in burn resuscitation—a prospective randomised controlled trial. Burns 36:984-91
4. Cochran A et al (2007) Burn patient characteristics and outcomes following resuscitation with albumin. Burns 33:25–30
5. Csontos C et al (2007) Factors affecting fluid requirement on the first day after severe burn trauma. ANZ J Surg 77:745–748
6. Rogers AD et al (2010). Fluid creep in major pediatric burns. Eur J Pediatr Surg 20:133-8
7. Wang GY et al (2008) Esophageal echo-Doppler monitoring in burn shock resuscitation: are hemodynamic variables the critical standard guiding fluid therapy? J Trauma 65:1396-401
8. Klein MB et al (2007) The association between fluid administration and outcome following major burn: a multicenter study. Ann Surg 245:622–8

Fluid Management in Pediatric Patients

13

Robert Sümpelmann, Marialuisa Vennari
and Felice Eugenio Agrò

13.1 Physiology

13.1.1 Body Fluid Distribution

The total body water (TBW) consists of intracellular (ICF) and extracellular fluid (ECF) and represents up to 90% of the body weight in neonates. TBW decreases significantly during the first six months of life and reaches adult levels of about 60% after one year of age. The extracellular fluid (ECF) represents the main part of TBW and decreases in parallel from 40% in term neonates to adult levels of 20–25% after one year of age. The ICF does not vary much during infancy, from 30% at birth to 40% in adults [1]. The composition of the ECF or plasma is similar in neonates, children, and adults, but dehydration occurs more rapidly in children because they need more fluids.

13.1.2 Renal Function

Renal function is related to the maturation and size of the nephrons, which have the ability to filter the blood and to collect the filtrate. At birth, the kidneys are still undeveloped and the reabsorptive areas of the tubular cells are small. Thus, neonates cannot concentrate urine as effectively as adults, and they are unable to excrete large salt loads. After one month, the kidneys reach about 60% of their maturation but the reabsorptive areas of the tubular cells are still small and the capacity, e.g., for glucose reabsorption or potassium

M. Vennari (✉)
Postgraduate School of Anesthesia and Intensive Care, Anesthesia, Intensive Care and Pain Management Department, University School of Medicine Campus Bio-Medico of Rome, Rome, Italy
e-mail: m.vennari@unicampus.it

F. E. Agrò (ed.), *Body Fluid Management*,
DOI: 10.1007/978-88-470-2661-2_13 © Springer-Verlag Italia 2013

excretion is lower than in adults. In the first two years, the maturity and function of the kidneys increase greatly and reach adult levels [2].

13.1.3 Cardiovascular System

The newborn heart has a lower density of contractile elements and therefore less reserve such that it does not respond to stress as well as the adult heart. A higher percentage of non-contractile elements results in decreased ventricular compliance and less responsiveness to changes in vascular tone and preload. Cardiac output is tightly coupled with oxygen consumption, which is several times higher in neonates and infants than in adults. The stroke volume of the small heart is limited; consequently, a high cardiac output strongly depends on a high heart rate. Normally, the heart pumps all of the venous return (VR) it receives, and under most conditions VR is the main determinant of cardiac output in all age groups. Since VR depends strongly on the intravascular volume, the maintenance of normovolemia is of paramount importance in young age groups in order to maintain circulatory function and to stabilize the high tissue perfusion needed [3].

13.2 Concerns Regarding Crystalloids

For half a century, maintenance fluid therapy in children has been based on Holliday and Segar's recommendation, i.e., the administration of hypotonic fluids with 5% glucose added. Recently, however, many authors have found that the wide use of such fluids may cause serious complications, such as hyponatremia or hyperglycemia, and, more rarely, may result in permanent neurological consequences or even death [4-9]. Perioperative hyponatremia develops in response to two main factors: (1) the stress-induced secretion of ADH, which decrease the body's ability to excrete free water and (2) the use of hypotonic solutions as a source of free water [10-12].

Severe hyponatremia is a very dangerous condition, leading to a shift of water from the interstitial space (ISS) into neuronal cells. This process increases brain volume, inducing cerebral edema, brainstem herniation, and death. Infants are particularly susceptible to hyponatremia-related complications. In fact, they have a reduced Na-K-ATPase activity compared to adults and their brain size/cranial vault ratio is higher [13]. It was also found that the use of high volumes of normal saline may cause bicarbonate dilution and hyperchloremic acidosis, with renal vasoconstriction and impaired renal function. All of these sequelae can be avoided by the use of balanced electrolyte solutions containing both a physiological osmolarity and electrolyte composition and metabolic anions (acetate, lactate, or malate) as bicarbonate precursors for acid-base stabilization [14]. Generally, the intravascular volume effect of crystalloids depends on the ratio between the intravascular (IVFV) and the extracellular fluid volume (ECFV). The ECFV of neonates and infants is larger than that of adults [1], and the intravascular volume effect of crystalloids is therefore, in theory, lower in the younger age groups.

Infants have higher metabolic requirements than adults, potentially leading to perioperative lipolysis and hypoglycemia. Hypoglycemia can result in cerebral metabolism and blood flow alterations [15], and subsequently to long-lasting neurodevelopmental impairment, if unrecognized or undertreated. It can be prevented by administering 5% dextrose solutions in the perioperative period, although these solutions often cause hyperglycemia because of stress-induced insulin resistance [16]. The brain is also vulnerable to damage by hyperglycemia, in which intracellular acidosis (due to increased lactate levels) compromises cellular functions [17]. Lastly, the administration of glucose-free solutions increases the risk of lipolysis, with the release of ketone bodies and free fatty acids [18,19].

The literature suggests the intraoperative use of isotonic solutions with a reduced dextrose (i.e., 1–2.5%) concentration to avoid the above-mentioned consequences of hypoglycemia/lipolysis and hyperglycemia in children (Table 13.1) [20-22].

13.3   Concerns Regarding Colloids

13.3.1   Types of Colloids

Among colloids, human albumin (HA) was often used in children because it is well tolerated [23]. Recently gelatin and hydroxyethyl starch solutions (HES) are becoming more widely adopted as they have been shown to be equally effective and safe but less costly than HA (review in [24]). In adults, anaphylactoid reactions occurred more frequently after gelatin than in response to HES, whereas the risk of severe reactions seems to be lower in younger age groups.

While the use of older-generation HES (MW > 450 kDa or 200 kDa) in children is not recommended because of the negative side effects involving coagulation, organ function, and accumulation, latest-generation HES 130/0.42 have been reported to be safe and effective for volume replacement. Accordingly, they should be preferred in perioperative volume replacement management (review in [25]).

Interstitial fluid edema is a direct consequence of the administration of high volumes of crystalloids to replace significant acute blood losses. Since interstitial fluid overload may be related to postoperative complications [26], crystalloids should be used for cutaneous, enteral or renal fluid loss (= fluid replacement), and colloids for the substitution of significant blood loss or when the patient's circulation is in urgent need of additional volume (= volume replacement).

In perioperative fluid management, care must be taken to avoid hypervolemic iatrogenic peaks, which can cause endothelial damage [27].

Table 13.1 Composition (in mmol/L) of extracellular fluid (ECF) and various intravenous fluids for use in children

	Cations					Anions				Theoretical osmolarity[4]
	K+	Na+	Mg^{2+}	Ca^{2+}	HCO$_3^-$	Cl$^-$	Acetate	Lactate	Glucose	
ECF	4.5	142	1.25	2.5	24	103	-	1.5	2.78-5	291
Normal saline	-	154	-	-	-	154	-	-	-	308
BEL[1] w/ 1% glucose	4	140	2	2	-	118	30	-	55.5	296
RL[2]	5	130	1	1	-	112	-	27	-	276
2/3 ESG[3]	18	100	3	2	-	90	38	-	277.5	251
1/2 ESG[3]	2	70	0.5	1.25	-	55	22.5	-	277.5	151
1/3 ESG[3]	25	45	2.5	-	-	45	20	-	277.5	148

[1]Balanced electrolyte solution.
[2]Ringer's lactate.
[3]Hypotonic electrolyte solutions with 5% glucose.
[4]Σ (cations+anions).

13.3.2 Side Effects

Possible adverse drug reactions to artificial colloids include anaphylactoid reactions, coagulation disorders, renal function impairment, and tissue accumulation. Animal experiments and clinical studies in pediatric patients have shown minor changes in clotting parameters after moderate doses (10–20 mL/kg) of gelatin or HES but significant impairment of the coagulation system after hemodilution > 50% of the estimated blood volume [28, 29]. In a recent observational study in 1,130 children, HES 130 was found to be safe even in small infants and newborns [30]. Moreover, acid-base balance was found more stable when HES were used in a balanced solution rather than in normal saline. Since HES-related side effects are dose-dependent, moderate doses of 10–20 mL/kg are very safe whereas doses close to the maximum daily dose of 50 mL/kg should be used with caution because they may lead to critical hemodilution, dilutional coagulopathy, or iatrogenic hypervolemia.

13.4 Clinical Concerns in Surgical Pediatric Patients

The objective of perioperative fluid therapy is to maintain circulatory function and to stabilize the water-acid-base-electrolyte balance. In line with current recommendations, children should be allowed to drink clear fluids until 2 h before the induction of anesthesia, unless other considerations mandate otherwise. Balanced Electrolyte Solutions (BES) are recommended for intraoperative fluid replacement therapy in all age groups in order to avoid hyponatremia and hyperchloremic acidosis. For preterm infants, neonates and toddlers, it is always advisable to at least compensate the deficit caused by preoperative fasting and the intraoperative maintenance requirements, using BES with 1–2% glucose. Since these solutions are currently not available commercially in many countries, they need to be prepared extemporaneously in the hospital pharmacy or by the treating physician (e.g., by adding 6–12 mL of glucose 40% to 250 mL of IV fluid) [31, 32]. To compensate for preoperative deficits (e.g., from fasting), the overall infusion rate in the first hour may be 10–20 mL/kg/h. As blood glucose concentrations increase, glucose-containing IV fluids should be reduced or stopped, correspondingly infusing more glucose-free BES. Older toddlers and school-age children may also be given glucose-free BES within the recommended fasting periods. In cases of clinical evidence of hypovolemia, 10 mL/kg of BES or 5 mL/kg of artificial colloid solution may additionally be administered as required. Postoperatively, children should be allowed oral fluids as soon as possible, unless other considerations mandate otherwise (Table 13.2) [33].

Table 13.2 Suggested perioperative intravenous fluid therapy for neonates, infants, and toddlers [33]

Before surgery	Minimize fasting periods (clear fluids up to 2 h preop)
Minor procedures	Background infusion of 10-20 mL/Kg/h of a balanced electrolyte solution with 1-2% glucose (add 6-12 mL of glucose 40% to 250 mL of balanced electrolyte solution); older toddlers and school-age children may also be given glucose-free balanced electrolyte solutions
Larger procedures	Reduce glucose-containing background infusion to maintenance requirements after one hour, use balanced electrolyte solution for correction requirements; consider artificial colloids in case of hypovolemia – the objective is to achieve normovolemia and hemodynamic stability
Major procedures	Same as larger procedures; administer blood products in case of critical hemodilution
After surgery	Permit oral fluid soon after surgery

13.4.1 Monitoring Perioperative Intravenous Fluid Therapy

Conscious children, especially neonates and small infants, are able to maintain blood pressure for long periods of time through vasoconstriction in the presence of larger fluid deficits, even if a shock situation has already occurred. In deeply anesthetized children, however, some or all of the regulatory mechanisms are suppressed so that hypotension is more likely to occur in the presence of reduced blood volume. Shallow anesthesia, on the other hand, may mask hypovolemia. Therefore, apart from the standard parameters of heart rate and arterial blood pressure, other parameters must be used to estimate a child's volume status [34]. An abnormal respiratory-synchronous invasive blood pressure curve or pulse oximetry signal variations (i.e., perfusion or pleth variability index) and low central venous pressure may be signs of low filling pressures even in young children. Perioperative metabolic acidosis and increasing lactate concentrations typically arise from hypovolemia with reduced oxygen delivery. Major surgical procedures should therefore be accompanied by routine blood gas analyses (e.g., at hourly intervals), with central venous oxygen saturation ($ScvO_2$) as a particularly rapid indicator of peripheral organ and tissue utilization of oxygen delivery. Other important parameters for estimating volume status include urine output, refilling time, and skin temperature.

13.5 Clinical Concerns in Septic Pediatric Patients

Severe sepsis in children is much less frequent than in adults, and pediatric mortality caused by sepsis is estimated to be 10% in the USA [35]. For sepsis treatment, an initial resuscitation volume of 40–60 mL/kg is recommended but can be as much as 200 mL/kg. Subsequent therapy should be guided by invasive hemodynamic monitoring. In fact, the filling pressure and blood-gas monitoring, including ScvO$_2$, can provide important information during fluid therapy, suggesting that the venous system needs more fluid or that it is overloaded [36]. Given that venous access in pediatric patients is more difficult to obtain, the American Heart Association and the American Academy of Pediatrics have developed guidelines that encourage the use of an intraosseous access in emergent cases. Brierley suggested decreasing the rate of fluid administration if clinical signs of cardiac filling are identified but there is no hemodynamic improvement [37]. However, the wide use of fluids for acute hemodynamic stabilization in children has not been shown to increase the incidence of cerebral edema or acute respiratory distress syndrome. Increased fluid requirements may be evident for several days secondary to fluid loss from the intravascular compartment when there is profound capillary leak. As there is currently no evidence on the choice of fluids in children with sepsis, the routine fluid and volume replacement therapy may include isotonic crystalloids, colloids, and blood products.

Key Concepts
- Recommendations for fluid and volume replacement in pediatrics
- Safety of balanced electrolyte solutions and HES in small infants

Key Words
- Hyponatremia
- Hyperchloremia
- Acidosis

Focus on…
- Saudan S (2010) Is the use of colloids for fluid replacement harmless in children? Curr Opin Anaesthesiol 23(3):363-7
- Bailey AG, McNaull PP, Jooste E, Tuchman JB (2010) Perioperative crystalloid and colloid fluid management in children: where are we and how did we get here? Anesth Analg 110:375-390

References

1. Fris-Hansen B (1961) Body water compartments in children: changes during growth and related changes in body composition. Pediatrics 28:169-81
2. Bissonnette B (2011) Pediatric Anesthesia. People's Medical Publishing House- USA, Shelton, Connecticut
3. Nichols DG, Ungerleider RM, Spevak PJ et al (2006) Critical heart disease in infants and children. Mosby Elsevier, Philadelphia
4. Choong K, Kho ME, Menon K, Bohn D (2006) Hypotonic versus isotonic saline in hospitalised children: a systematic review. Arch Dis Child 91:828-835
5. Duke T, Molyneux EM (2003) Intravenous fluids for seriously ill children: time to reconsider. Lancet 362:1320-1323
6. Hoorn EJ, Geary D, Robb M, Halperin ML, Bohn D (2004) Acute hyponatremia related to intravenous fluid administration in hospitalized children: an observational study. Pediatrics 113:1279-1284
7. Moritz ML, Ayus JC (2003) Prevention of hospital-acquired hyponatremia: a case for using isotonic saline. Pediatrics 111:227-230
8. Moritz ML, Ayus JC (2004) Hospital-acquired hyponatremia: why are there still deaths? Pediatrics 113:1395-1396
9. Moritz ML, Ayus JC (2005) Preventing neurological complications from dysnatremias in children. Pediatr Nephrol 20:1687-1700
10. Fraser CL, Arieff AI (1997) Epidemiology, pathophysiology, and management of hyponatremic encephalopathy. Am J Med 102:67-77
11. Arieff AI, Ayus JC, Fraser CL (1992) Hyponatraemia and death or permanent brain damage in healthy children. BMJ 304:1218-1222
12. Arieff AI (1998) Postoperative hyponatraemic encephalopathy following elective surgery in children. Paediatr Anaesth 8:1-4
13. Ayus JC, Achinger SG, Arieff A (2008) Brain cell volume regulation in hyponatremia: role of sex, age, vasopressin, and hypoxia. Am J Physiol Renal Physiol 295:F619-624
14. Witt L, Osthaus WA, Bünte C et al (2010) A novel isotonic- balanced solution with 1% glucose for perioperative fluid management in children- an animal experimental study. Pediatr Anesth 20:734
15. Sieber FE, Traystman RJ (1992) Special issues: glucose and the brain. Crit Care Med 20:104-114
16. Welborn LG, McGill WA, Hannallah RS, Nisselson CL, Ruttimann UE, Hicks JM (1986) Perioperative blood glucose concentrations in pediatric outpatients. Anesthesiology 65:543-547
17. Bailey AG, McNaull PP, Jooste E, Tuchman JB (2010) Perioperative crystalloid and colloid fluid management in children: where are we and how did we get here? Anesth Analg 110:375-390
18. Mikawa K, Maekawa N, Goto R, Tanaka O, Yaku H, Obara H (1991) Effects of exogenous intravenous glucose on plasma glucose and lipid homeostasis in anesthetized children. Anesthesiology 74:1017-1022
19. Nishina K, Mikawa K, Maekawa N, Asano M, Obara H (1995) Effects of exogenous intravenous glucose on plasma glucose and lipid homeostasis in anesthetized infants. Anesthesiology 83:258-263
20. Dubois MC GL, Murat I et al (1992) Lactated Ringer with 1% dextrose: an appropriate solution for peri-operative fluid therapy in children. Paed Anaesth 2:99-104
21. Berleur MP, Dahan A, Murat I, Hazebroucq G (2003) Perioperative infusions in paediatric patients: rationale for using Ringer-lactate solution with low dextrose concentration. J Clin Pharm Ther 28:31-40
22. Sümpelmann R, Becke K, Crean P et al (2011) European consensus statement for intraoperative fluid therapy in children. Eur J Anaesthesiol 28:637–639

23. Söderlind M, Salvignol G, Izard P, Lönnqvist PA (2001) Use of albumin, blood transfusion and intraoperative glucose by APA and ADARPEF members: a postal survey. Paediatr Anaesth 11:685-9
24. Saudan S (2010) Is the use of colloids for fluid replacement harmless in children? Curr Opin Anaesthesiol 23:363-7
25. Westphal M, James MF, Kozek-Langenecker S, Stocker R, Guidet B, Van Aken H (2009) Hydroxyethyl starches: different products—different effects. Anesthesiology 111:187-202
26. Arikan AA, Zappitelli M, Goldstein SL, Naipaul A, Jefferson LS, Loftis LL (2011) Fluid overload is associated with impaired oxygenation and morbidity in critically ill children. Pediatr Crit Care Med: epub
27. Chappell D, Jacob M, Hofmann-Kiefer K, Conzen P, Rehm M (2008) A rational approach to perioperative fluid management. Anesthesiology 109:723-40
28. Witt L, Osthaus WA, Jahn W, Rahe-Meyer N, Hanke A, Schmidt F, Boehne M, Sümpelmann R (2012) Isovolaemic hemodilution with gelatin and hydroxyethyl starch 130/0.42: effects on hemostasis in piglets. Pediatr Anesth 22:379
29. Osthaus WA, Witt L, Johanning K, Boethig D, Winterhalter M, Huber D, Heimbucher C, Sümpelmann R (2009) Equal effects of gelatin and hydroxyethyl starch (6% HES 130/0.42) on modified thrombelastography in children. Acta Anaesthesiol Scand 53:305-10
30. Sümpelmann R, Kretz FJ, Luntzer R, de Leeuw TG, Mixa V, Gäbler R, Eich C, Hollmann MW, Osthaus WA (2011) Hydroxyethyl starch 130/0.42/6:1 for perioperative plasma volume replacement in 1130 children: results of an European prospective multicenter observational postauthorization safety study (PASS). Pediatr Anesth: epub
31. Sümpelmann R, Mader T, Dennhardt N, Witt L, Eich C, Osthaus WA (2011) A novel isotonic balanced electrolyte solution with 1% glucose for intraoperative fluid therapy in neonates: results of a prospective multicentre observational postauthorisation safety study (PASS). Paediatr Anaesth 21:1114-8
32. Sümpelmann R, Mader T, Eich C, Witt L, Osthaus WA (2010) A novel isotonic-balanced electrolyte solution with 1% glucose for intraoperative fluid therapy in children: results of a prospective multicentre observational post-authorization safety study (PASS). Paediatr Anaesth 20:977-81
33. Sümpelmann R, Hollnberger H, Schmidt J, Strauss JM (2006) Recommendations for perioperative intravenous fluid therapy for neonates, infants, and toddlers. Anästh Intensivmed 47:616-619
34. Osthaus WA, Huber D, Beck C, Roehler A, Marx G, Hecker H, Sümpelmann R (2006) Correlation of oxygen delivery with central venous oxygen saturation, mean arterial pressure and heart rate in piglets. Paediatr Anaesth 16:944-7
35. Carcillo JA, Linde-Zwirble WT et al (2003) The epidemiology of severe sepsis in children in the United States. Am J Respir Crit Care Med 167:695-701
36. Carcillo JA, Fields Al (2002) Clinical practice parameters for hemodynamic support of pediatric and neonatal patients in septic shock. Crit Care Med 30:1365-78
37. Brierley J, Carcillo JA, Choong K et al (2009) Clinical practice parameters for hemodynamic support of pediatric and neonatal septic shock: 2007 update from the American College of Critical Care Medicine. Crit Care Med 37:666-88

Fluid Management in Neurosurgery

14

Pietro Martorano, Chiara Candela, Roberta Colonna
and Felice Eugenio Agrò

14.1 Physiopathology

The brain and spinal cord are isolated from other tissues by the blood-brain barrier (BBB): a uniquely composed, strictly controlled, extracellular environment surrounding the central nervous system (CNS), i.e., neurons, astrocytes, and pericytes. Anatomically, the walls of the BBB differ from the peripheral capillaries as a continuous and not fenestrated endothelium, which blocks the free diffusion of interstitial fluid solutes [1].

In order to protect the CNS from the influx of any toxic or pathogenic agents, all molecules with a radius of $> 7-9\text{Å}$ are blocked [2]; the BBB, in contrast, is freely crossed by H_2O, O_2, and CO_2, while glucose passes through by facilitated diffusion. The reduced size of the pores of the BBB prevents the passage of plasma proteins and electrolytes (Na+, Cl-, K+). It also determines a unique phenomenon in the body: the movement of water through the BBB is driven only by the osmotic gradient between plasma and extracellular fluids. This is in contrast to the peripheral tissues, where the movement of fluids between the various compartments is regulated by oncotic pressure. Hence the statement, "brain parenchyma acts as an osmometer rather than an oncometer"; in case of an intact BBB, indeed, plasma osmolarity is the only determining factor in fluid movement between the CNS and the intravascular space [3].

An analysis of the pathophysiological mechanisms regulating intracranial pressure (ICP) can better explain the significance of this phenomenon. Monroe-Kellie's law states that, since the skull is considered a rigid recipient, relationships between the volumes of intracranial components is a constant

C. Candela (✉)
Postgraduate School of Anesthesia and Intensive Care, Anesthesia, Intensive Care and Pain Management Department, University School of Medicine Campus Bio-Medico of Rome, Rome, Italy
e-mail: chiaracandela@yahoo.it

F. E. Agrò (ed.), *Body Fluid Management*,
DOI: 10.1007/978-88-470-2661-2_14 © Springer-Verlag Italia 2013

(K = total intracranial volume = V (brain 85–90%) + V (cerebrospinal fluid 3%) + V (blood 10%) [4, 5]. According to this law, to guarantee a constant ICP, any increase in one of the three components has to be coupled with a compensatory reduction in one of the other factors [6,7].

During pathological conditions (e.g., the development of an intracranial hematoma), there is progressive utilization of these compensatory mechanisms; when they are exhausted, even slight increases of volume suffice to cause a potentially harmful increase in the ICP [8, 9].

Conversely, an overload in the infusion of solutions could lead to an increase of the parenchymal component of the intracranial contents, thereby also increasing the ICP [10]. With an undamaged BBB, the intravenous administration of hypertonic solutions, through a rapid increase of plasma osmolality, creates an osmotic gradient between the CNS and the intravascular compartment, leading to a reduction in brain volume and ICP.

When a brain injury occurs, whether of ischemic or traumatic nature, this fine regulation could become weak—due to possible losses of BBB integrity—with increased permeability of the brain capillaries and the subsequent extravasation of plasma proteins [11-13].

14.2   Fluid Management

In the past, fluid management in neurosurgical or brain-injured patients mainly focused on a reduction of infusions (hypovolemic hemoconcentration), with the aim of preventing the development of brain edema [14]. However, further studies established the catastrophic impact of water restriction on brain trauma [15], pointing to hypovolemia as one of the most negative factors determining the outcome of these patients.

Clifton et al. confirmed these results in a retrospective study (2002) performed on 392 patients with brain trauma. The results evidence the critical involvement of ICP, mean arterial pressure (MAP), cerebral perfusion pressure (CPP) derangements leading to a poor prognosis, and water unbalance and hypotension [16]. Consequently, while the development of cerebral edema and intracranial hypertension still represents the most feared complication of brain damage, the risks due to hypovolemia and hypotension must be underlined, too [17]. Currently, the strategy for volume replacement in these patients aims at keeping the volume within normal levels (CVP $\approx$ 8 cm H_2O) setting the arterial pressure such that it guarantees adequate cerebral blood flow (CBF), and CPP, avoiding brain ischemia [17].

It should be considered that hypoperfusion may represent an independent risk factor for the development of coagulopathy in patients with head trauma [18]. A high incidence (> 40%) of this complication has been detected and investigated, including in children whereas a close correlation with the severity of the brain damage; low Glasgow coma scale, increasing age, Injury Severity Score (ISS) $\geq$ 16 and intraparenchymal lesions were found to be independently associated [19]. Conversely, it must be considered that an overestimated fluid administration, leading to hemodilution, could cause an imbalance of the hemoglobin/hematocrit ratio [20,21]. Hemodilution for hematocrit values under 27%, could increase the ICP, with a reduction in CPP. In vitro studies have shown that the highest oxygen supply to tissues is coupled with hematocrit values of about 30% while the supply of oxygen to the tissues is compromised at a hematocrit < 25%, with a risk of hypoxia in damaged brain tissues. Conversely, unwarranted hemodilution in patients with a hematocrit < 30% should be avoided [22].

14.3   Which Kind of Fluid?

Optimized fluid management plays an essential role during the perioperative period: an adequate handling of fluid must maintain good cardiovascular stability, allows an efficient organ perfusion, and improves patient recovery after surgery.

Patients undergoing neurosurgery often have important and rapid hemodynamic imbalances due to the combination of factors such as prolonged surgery, bleedings, prolonged fluid restriction, and diabetes insipidus. Thus, the choice of the type and dose of liquid administered must be carefully targeted to maintain adequate values of perfusion pressure and blood volume.

14.3.1   Crystalloids

14.3.1.1 Saline Solution (NaCl 0.9%)
Most often, crystalloids in neurosurgical patients are iso-osmolar, such as normal saline solutions, due to their lack of action on plasma osmolality and therefore the absence of water accumulation in the brain. Administration is keyed to balancing the patient's urine output and transepidermal water losses (30–35 mL/kg/day), keeping in mind that the amounts can vary in critically ill patients, related to various factors such as fever and mechanical ventilation. Moreover, a correct fluid replacement should be aimed at maintaining an adequate cardiac output, avoiding excessive fluid replacement.

As previously stated, inadequate fluid infusions with a "dry patient" can lead to harmful scenarios, especially in cases of marked hypovolemia [15-17].

All glucose-containing solutions should be avoided, as well as all hypotonic solutions, due to their ability to lower plasma osmolality and, conversely, to increase the amount of incoming free water into the brain parenchyma, with an accompanying worsening of cerebral edema [23, 24]. Moreover, glucosate solutions, by increasing the amount of lactate in ischemic areas of the brain (injured by the use of retractors during surgery or pathological situations), could worsen outcome.

14.3.1.2 Mannitol

Mannitol is the most commonly infused hyperosmolar solution in neuro-surgery. It is administered for a broad range of purposes: for intracranial hypertension therapy in neurotrauma, to obtain a "relaxed brain" during neurosurgical procedures, with the aim of reducing both the pressure exerted by surgical retractors on the brain parenchyma and to increase tumor definition during surgery.

Mannitol is available in several different concentrations, usually administered by intravenous infusion (15–20 min) at a dose of 0.25–1 g/kg. Due to its high osmolality (1000–1300), mannitol is able to decrease ICP by establishing (in an undamaged BBB) a high intravascular osmotic gradient with the movement of free water from the brain parenchyma into the intravascular space.

The sudden increase in plasma osmolality could induce a transient increase in ICP, probably due to an improved volume in the cerebral vessels [25-27], as well as a transient increase in Na^+ and a decrease in K^+. In the latter case, high doses of mannitol (2 mg/kg) can lead to the onset of transient hyperkalemia, probably due to solvents in the formulations or to red cells lysis at the infusion site in response to the high concentration of mannitol; this can cause the onset of specific electrocardiographic alterations [28].

14.3.1.3 Hypertonic Saline

In analogy with mannitol, hypertonic saline administration acts, by smaller volumes, to increase plasma osmolality, with the swift passage of water from the interstitial and intracellular compartments to the intravascular one. This approach has favorable effects in patients with intracranial hypertension [29, 30].

Hypertonic saline is able to reduce the water content also in extracerebral organs, especially when serum osmolality is > 350 mOsm/l. Here, potential therapeutic effects are achieved in the perioperative management of fluids in brain-injured patients [31]. Recent studies seem to confirm this approach; Hauer et al. found that the early and continuous infusion of hypertonic saline in patients with severe brain damage and signs of intracranial hypertension was safe and helpful in reducing the frequency of seizures and intracranial hypertension and thus in lowering mortality; the incidence of adverse events in that study was comparable to that of the control group [32]. Although these solutions are commercially available in different concentrations, clinical studies seem to show that concentration does not play a substantial role in changing serum osmolarity [33].

Both mannitol and hypertonic saline solutions exert beneficial effects on ICP but through different features. Francony et al., comparing the effect of equiosmolar doses of mannitol and hypertonic saline ranging from 20% to 7.5%, concluded that mannitol is as effective as hypertonic saline in decreasing ICP in patients with brain injuries, but differs with respect to additional effects on cerebral circulation by improving the rheology of the blood [34].

In contrast, a recent meta-analysis suggested that hypertonic saline solution is more effective than mannitol for high-grade intracranial hypertension treat-

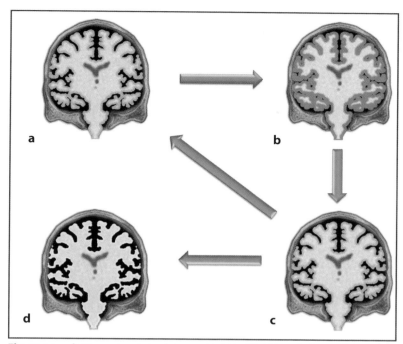

Fig. 14.1 a → **b** Hyponatremia leads to a rapid shift of fluid into the intracellular compartment, producing cerebral edema. **b** → **c** The brain adapts to the decreased osmolality by removing cell electrolytes (rapid adaptation) and subsequently organic osmolytes (slow adaptation). **c** → **a** A slow and controlled correction of hyponatremia allows a return to the normal condition. **c** → **d** If correction of hyponatremia is too fast, it can cause serious and irreversible consequences such as pontine myelinolysis

ment [35]. In a study conducted in children with intracranial hypertension unresponsive to other therapies, Khanna et al. evaluated the effects of 3% saline continuous infusion for a mean of 7.6 days. They observed that the increase in serum sodium correlated with a decrease in ICP and an increase of CBF [36].

Hypertonic saline may also be used to correct hyponatremia, especially when the patient is already symptomatic. In this case, a slow and controlled administration of hypertonic saline, usually associated with furosemide to control iatrogenic expansion of extracellular fluid, allows for an effective correction of hyponatremia, avoiding serious sequelae such as myelinolysis (Fig. 14.1).

Despite the demonstrated efficacy of hypertonic saline therapy in intractable intracranial hypertension, it should be borne in mind that its use may result in the onset of secondary hypernatremia, even in response to small amounts of infusion [37-39]. To counteract this risk, it may be safer to use a 3% hypertonic saline solution as it has been shown, compared to 7.5% saline, to exert similar effects on hemodynamics and ICP, with less of an impact on Na+ concentration and the same increase in cerebral dehydration [40].

The administration of furosemide in combination with hypertonic solutions, in order to enhance the osmotic effects, is widespread in common clinical practice. This strategy has yielded favorable and seems to be slightly more effective when hypertonic saline rather than mannitol is administered [41, 42].

It is worth emphasizing that the use of hypertonic solutions requires an uncompromised renal function, as intravascular volume expansion leads to an increase in diuresis and natriuresis (in the case of hypertonic saline) in order to maintain water and electrolyte homeostasis. Many studies have shown that hyperosmolar solutions can produce several degrees of renal injury coupled with arteriolar spasm and osmotic diuresis [43]. In vitro and in vivo studies of hypertonic saline and mannitol have found direct damage to kidney cells with a consequent reduction in renal blood flow and glomerular fraction rate.

Osmotic nephrosis is the mechanism leading to nephrotoxicity following high doses of mannitol, immunoglobulins, dextrans, and hetastarch. It is characterized by swelling and the vacuolar degeneration of epithelial cells of the proximal convoluted tubules following development of an oncotic gradient induced in the tubular cells by administered and non-metabolizable substances. Hyperosmolality seems to act through different mechanisms, such as activation of tubulo-glomerular feedback, or simply as a function of intravascular volume depletion as a result of osmotic diuresis [44]. Moreover, mannitol augmentation drives an increase in plasma oncotic pressure higher than the glomerular filtration ability, resulting in intense renal artery vasoconstriction and reductions in the glomerular filtration rate [45]. The quick regression of renal failure observed after the removal of mannitol by peritoneal dialysis seems to confirm this hypothesis. Renal toxicity induced by the administration of hetastarch has been linked to a pro-inflammatory effect, as shown by the detection of macrophage interstitial infiltration and proliferation as well as tubular damage [46].

14.3.2 Colloids

14.3.2.1 Hetastarches (HES)

Although HES have a remarkable effect on volume filling, their use is negligible due to their negative effects on coagulation and hemostasis. These adverse effects, though slighter than older generation HES, seem to apply to the latest-generation HES as well [47, 48]. Thus, their use is still debated in neuroanesthesia and in patients suffering from coagulopathies.

Dextrans are not available either in Europe or in the USA, since their use is tempered by several adverse effects, involving not only alterations in hemostasis, but also the triggering of severe allergic reactions, such as bronchospasm, and heart failure.

14.3.2.2 Albumin

Albumin is the main plasma-derived protein. Its high costs, due to the complicated and rigorous procedures necessary for its production, strongly limit its use. The benefits of albumin in the field of neurosurgery and neuroanesthesia are still not clear. The University Health System Consortium fully acknowledges the use of other colloids but does not confirm the usefulness of albumin in this particular setting [50].

14.3.3 Hypertonic/Hyperosmotic Solutions

The recent introduction of hypertonic/hyperosmotic solutions has generated wide clinical and scientific interest, as confirmed by the large amount of literature investigating their effectiveness and superiority over other currently available solutions. A comparative study performed in animals demonstrated that the administration of small volumes of hypertonic/hyperoncotic solutions afford both a stable systemic-splanchnic hemodynamic level, (by increasing blood flow and O_2 delivery, to reduce secondary hemodilution), without any increase of pulmonary arterial pressure, a common event after saline 0.9% and dextran infusion [51]. Improvement of hemodynamic status in humans was confirmed in a randomized single-blind study, underlining the capability of these particular solutions to significantly reduce the ICP and increase cardiac index [52].

Compared to hypertonic solutions, hypertonic hyperosmotic solutions may exert, in addition to a faster onset of volume refilling, more favorable effects on brain tissue damage and cerebral edema, with no increase in ICP [53]. In particular, at equimolar doses, these solutions reduce ICP more effectively compared than mannitol, and are longer lasting [54].

14.4   Conclusions

The main goals of peri-operative fluid management are to ensure adequate tissue oxygenation and to prevent oxygen debt following an increase in the cerebral metabolic rate of oxygen ($CMRO_2$) during surgery. In uneventful patients, fluid therapy is directed at achieving balanced urinary and transepidermal water losses. In neurosurgical patients with brain tumor, hematoma, or head injury an increased ICP may be due to mass effect and perilesional edema. Conversely, in this particular class of patients, hemodynamic stability represents a necessary but insufficient target to ensure a favorable outcome.

Consequently, fluid therapy, in addition to the above objectives (standard intravascular volume, CBF and $CMRO_2$, regardless of intracranial pathology [16, 17]), should be adjusted to prevent/counteract the increase in ICP. Therefore, in neurosurgical patients, an isovolemic state should be achieved by the infusion of iso-osmolar crystalloid, of approximately 300 mOsm (0.9%

saline solution), in order to avoid alterations in plasma osmolality, the main determinant of fluid balance in the brain, thereby avoiding water accumulation in the brain parenchyma.

Hyperosmotic solutions, such as mannitol and hypertonic saline, should be used in patients with intracranial hypertension, reserving the use of hypertonic saline to those with intracranial hypertension refractory to conventional therapy (hyperventilation, mannitol, diuretics). Hypertonic solutions might be necessary even in the course of neurosurgical operations, e.g., in which brain debulking could facilitate the exposure and subsequent excision of a brain tumor. In these case, mannitol is the first option, followed, if necessary, by the infusion of hypertonic saline coupled or not with a loop diuretic in order to obtain a synergistic effect.

Key Concepts
- Water movement through the blood-brain barrier
- Liberal/restrictive fluid strategy
- Peri-operative fluid management

Key Words
- Cerebral edema
- Hypovolemia
- Crystalloids
- Colloids
- Hypertonic/hyperosmotic solutions

Focus on...
- Tommasino C (2002) Fluids and the neurosurgical patient. Anesth Clin N Am 20:329-346
- Hauer EM, Stark D, Staykov D et al (2011) Early continous hypertonic saline infusion in patients with severe cerebrovascular disease. Crit Care Med 39:1766-1772 (Abstract)
- Talving P, Lustenberger T, Lam L et al (2011) Coagulopathy after isolated severe traumatic brain injury in children. J Trauma 71:1205-1210 (Abstract)

References

1. Begley DJ (2004) Delivery of therapeutic agents to the central nervous system: the problems and the possibilities. Pharmacol Ther 104:29-45
2. Fenstermacher JD, Johnson JA (1966) Filtration and reflection coefficient the rabbit blood-brain barrier. Am J Phisiol 211:341-346
3. Zornow MH, Todd MM, More SS (1987) The acute cerebral effects of changes in plasma osmolality and oncotic pressure. Anesthesiology 67:936-941
4. Avezaat JH, Van Eijndhoven JH, Wyper DJ (1979) Cerebrospinal fluid pulse pressure and intracranial volume-pressure relationships. J Neurol Neurosurg Psychiatry 42:687-700
5. Bouma GJ, Muizelaar JP, Bandoh K et al (1992) Blood pressure and intracranial pressure-volume dynamics in severe head injury: relationship with cerebral flow. J Neurosurg 77:15-19
6. Paulson OB, Strandgaard S, Edvinsson L (1990) Cerebral autoregulation. Cerebrovasc Brain Metab Rev 2:161-192
7. Tans JT, Poortvliet DC (1989) Relationship between compliance and resistance to outflow of CSF in adult hydrocephalus. J Neurosurg 71:59-62
8. Langfitt TW, Weistein JD, Kassel NF (1965) Cerebral vasomotor paralysis produced by intracranial hypertension. Neurology (Minneap.) 15:622-641
9. Langfitt TW (1969) Increased intracranial pressure. Clinical Neurosurgery 16:436-471
10. Dodge PR, Crawford JD, Probst JH (1960) Studies in experimental water intoxication. Arch Neurol 5:513-529
11. Zornow MH, Scheller MS, Todd MM et al (1988) Acute cerebral effects of isotonic crystalloid and colloid solutions following cryogenic brain injury in the rabbit. Anesthesiology 69:180-184
12. Kaieda R, Todd MM, Warner DS (1989) Prolonged reduction in colloid oncotic pressure does not increase brain edema following cryogenic injury in rabbits. Anesthesiology 71:554-560
13. Tommasino C, Picozzi V (2007) Volume and electrolyte management. Best Pract Res Clin Anaesthesiol 21:497-516
14. Shenkin HA, Benzier HO, Bouzarth W (1976) Restricted fluid intake: rational management of the neurosurgical patient. J Neurosurg 45:432-6
15. Chestnut RM, Marshall LF, Klauber MR et al (1993) The role of secondary brain injury in determining outcome from severe head injury. J Trauma 34:216-22
16. Clifton GL, Miller ER, Choi SC, Levin HS. (2002) Fluid thresholdsand outcome from severe brain injury. Critical Care Medicine 30:739-745
17. Andrews BT (1993) The intensive care management of patients with head injury. In: Andrews BT (ed) Neurosurgical Intensive Care. New York, McGraw-Hill, pp 227-242
18. Lustenberger T, Talving P, Kobayashi L, Barmparas G et al (2010) Early coagulopathy after isolated severe traumatic brain injury: relationship with hypoperfusion challenged. Journal of Trauma-Injury Infection & Critical Care 69:1410-1414
19. Talving P, Lustenberger T, Lam L et al (2011) Coagulopathy after isolated severe traumatic brain injury in children. Journal of Trauma-Injury Infection & Critical Care 71:1205-1210. Abstract.
20. Harrison MJG (1989) Influence of haematocrit in the cerebral circulation. Cerebrovasc Brain Metabol Rev 1:55-67
21. Hudak ML, Koehler RC, Rosenberg AA et al (1986) Effect of hematocrit on cerebral blood flow. Am J Phisiol 251:H63-70
22. Tango HK, Schmidt AP, Mizumoto N, Lacava M, Auler JOC Jr (1986) Low Hematocrit levels increase intracranial pressure in an animal model of cryogenic brain injury. Journal of Trauma-injury Infection & critical Care 66:720-726
23. Tommasino C, More S, Todd MM (1988) Cerebral effects of isovolemic hemodilution with crystalloid or colloid solutions in normal rabbits. Crit Care Med 16:862-8
24. Tommasino C (2002) Fluid and neurosurgical patient. Anesthesiology Clin N Am 20:329-346

25. Shenkin HA, Goluboff B, Haft H (1964) Further observations on the effects of abruptly increased osmotic pressure of plasma on cerebrospinal pressure in man. J neurosurg 22:563-568

26. Ravussin P, Archer DP,Meyer E et al (1985) The effects of rapid infusions of saline and mannitol on cerebral blood volume and intracranial pressure in dogs. Can Anaesth Soc J 32:506-15

27. Kassell NF, Baumann KW, Hitchon PW et al (1982) The effects of high dose mannitol on cerebral blood flow in dogs with normal intracranial pressure. Stroke 13:59-61

28. Moreno M, Murphy C, Goldsmith C (1969) Increase in serum potassium resulting from the administration of hypertonic mannitol and other solutions. J Lab Clin Med 73:291-298

29. Worthley LIG, Cooper DJ, Jones N (1988) Treatment of resistant intracranial hypertension with hypertonic saline. J Neurosurg 68:478-481

30. Suarez JI, Qureshi AI, Bhardwaj A et al (1998) Treatment of refractory intracranial hypertension with 23,4% saline. Crit Care Med 26:1118-1122

31. Toung TJK, Chen CH, Lin C, Bhardwaj A (2007) Osmotherapy with hypertonic saline attenuates water content in brain and extracerebral organs. Critical Care Medicine 35:526-531 (Abstract)

32. Hauer EM, Stark D, Staykov D et al (2011) Early continous hypertonic saline infusion in patients with severe cerebrovascular disease. Crit Care Med 39:1766-1772 (Abstract)

33. Toung TJ, Nyquist P, Mirski MA (2008) Effect of hypertonic saline concentration on cerebral and visceral organ water in an uninjuredrodent model. Crit Care Med 36:256-261(Abstract)

34. Francony G, Fauvage B, Falcon D et al (2008) Equimolar doses of mannitol and hypertonic saline in the treatment of increate intracranial pressure. Crit Care Med 36:795-800 (Abstract)

35. Kamel H, Navi BB, Nakagawa K et al (2011) Hypertonic saline versus mannitol for the treatment of elevated intracranial pressure: A meta-analysis of randomized clinical trials. Crit Care Med 39:554-559 (Abstract)

36. Khanna S, Davis D, Peterson B et al (2000) Use of hypertonic saline in the treatment of severe refractory posttraumatic intracranial hypertension in pediatric traumatic brain injury. Crit Care Med 28:1144-1151 (Abstract)

37. Froelich M, Ni Q, Wess C et al (2009) Continous hypertonic saline therapy and the occurrence of complications in neurocritically ill patients. Crit Care Med 37:14331441 (Abstract)

38. Shackford SR, Fortlage DA, Peters RM et al (1987) Serum osmolar and electrolyte changes associated with large infusions of hypertonic sodium lactate for intravascular volume expansion of patients undergoing aortic reconstruction. Surg Gynecol Obstet 164:127-136

39. Shackford SR, Sise MJ, Fridlund PH et al (1983) Hypertonic sodium lactate versus lactated ringer's solution for intravenous fluid terapy in operations on the abdominal aorta. Surgery 94:41-51

40. Sheikh AA, Matsuoka T, Wisner DH (1996) Cerebral effects of resuscitation with hypertonic saline and a new low-sodium hypertonic fluid in hemorrhagic shock and head injury. Critical Care Medicine 24:1226-1232 (Abstract)

41. Mayzler O, Leon A, Eilig I et al (2006) The effect of hypertonic (3%) saline with and without furosemide on plasma osmolality, sodium concentration, and brain water content after closed head trauma in rats. J Neurosurg Anesth 18:24-31

42. Todd MM, Cutkomp J, Brian JE (2006) Influence of mannitol and furosemide, alone and in combination, on brain water content after fluid percussion injury. Anesthesiology 105:1176-1181

43. Rudnick MR, Goldfarb S (2003) Pathogenesis of contrasted-induced nephropathy: Experimentaland clinical observations with an emphasis on the role of osmolality. Rev Cardvasc Med 4(Suppl 5):s28-33

44. Visweswaran P, Massin EK, Dubose TD (1997) Mannitol-induced acute renal failure. J Am Soc Nephrol 8:1028-1033

45. Moran M, Kapsner C (1987) Acute renal failure associated with elevated plasma oncotic pressure. N Eng J Med 317:150-153

46. Hüter L, Simon TP, Weinmann L et al (2009) Hydroxyethylstarch impairs renal function and induces interstitial proliferation, macrophage infiltration and tubular damage in an isolated renal perfusion model. Critical Care 13:R23

47. Treib J, Haass A, Pindur G (1997) Coagulation disorders caused by hydroxyethyl starch. Thromb Haemost 78:974-983

48. Franz A, Bräunlich P, Gamsjäger T, Felfernig M et al (2001) The effects of hydroxyethyl starches of varying molecular weights on platelet function. Anesth Analg 92:1402-1407

49. Varney KL, Young B, Hatton J (2003) Albumin use in Neurosurgical Critical Care. Pharmacotherapy 23:88-92

50. University Health System Consortium (2000) Technology assessment: albumin, non protein colloid, and crystalloid solutions. Oak Brook IL: University Health System Consortium, 25

51. Chiara O, Pelosi P, Brazzi L et al (2003) Resuscitation from hemorrhagic shock: Experimental model comparing normal saline, dextran, and hypertonic saline solutions. Critical Care Medicine 31:1915-1922 (Abstract)

52. Bentsen G, Breivic H, Lundar T et al (2006) Hypertonic saline (7,2%) in 6% hydroxyethyl starch reduces intracranial pressure and improves hemodynamics in a placebo-controlled study involving stable patients with subarachnoid hemorrhage. Critical Care Medicine 34:2912-2917 (Abstract)

53. Elliott MB, Jallo JJ, Gaughan JP, Tuma RF (2007) Effects of crystalloid-colloid solutions on traumatic brain injury. J Neurotrauma 24:195-202

54. Battison C, Andrews PJD, Graham C, Petty T (2005) Randomized, controlled trial on the effect of a 20% mannitol solution and a 7,5% saline/6%dextran solution on increased intracranial pressure after brain injury. Critical Care Medicine 33:196-202 (Abstract)

Fluid Management in Obstetric Patients

15

Maria Grazia Frigo, Annalaura Di Pumpo
and Felice Eugenio Agrò

15.1 Physiopathology

In pregnancy, hemodynamic and cardiovascular changes occur that prevent blood loss during delivery. In fact, there is an increase in blood volume, during the first trimester [1]. The volume of blood continues to expand rapidly in the second trimester before reaching a plateau in the last trimester. At the same time, the increase in Red Blood Cell (RBC) mass occurs more slowly, leading to a relative anemia and hemodilution [2], with the latter peaking by 30–32 weeks of gestation. Dilutional anemia is therefore common, especially between 28 and 34 weeks gestation, when hemoglobin concentrations are lowest. The accretion in RBC mass results in an 18–25% increase in the first months of pregnancy, followed by a drop after childbirth due to hemorrhage [3-5]. The increase in red cell volume provides for the extra oxygen demands of the mother and fetus. The lower end of the normal range for hemoglobin in pregnancy is 11–12 g/dL. These physiological responses have considerable advantages during pregnancy: improved placental perfusion, decreased risk of thrombosis and an adequate blood supply despite the bleeding that occurs with childbirth [6-8].

The White Blood Cell (WBC) count increases in pregnancy beginning in the first trimester, as a result of selective marrow erythropoiesis. This causes a left shift, with granulocytosis and more immature white cells in the circulation. The normal WBC count for pregnancy is 5000–12,000 WBC/mm^3, although values as high as 15,000 WBC/mm^3 are not uncommon [9].

A. Di Pumpo (✉)
Postgraduate School of Anesthesia and Intensive Care, Anesthesia, Intensive Care and Pain Management Department, University School of Medicine Campus Bio-Medico of Rome, Rome, Italy
e-mail: annalaurad.p@live.it

F. E. Agrò (ed.), *Body Fluid Management*,
DOI: 10.1007/978-88-470-2661-2_15 © Springer-Verlag Italia 2013

In pregnancy, there is a decrease in the platelet count, perhaps due to hemodilution and endothelial activation; the latter causes an increase in platelet consumption. In response, there is an increase in immature platelets [10-12].

Mild thrombocytopenia ($100,000–150,000/mm^3$), which is not particularly significant, is present in approximately 8% of pregnant women and has been termed "gestational thrombocytopenia" [13].

Pregnancy causes alterations of coagulation and fibrinolysis. These changes promote clotting, which acts as a defense mechanism against hemorrhage during childbirth [14]. Circulating levels of factors VII, VIII, IX, X, and XII, fibrinogen and von Willibrand factor increase, factor XI decreases, and prothrombin and factor V remain unchanged. The natural anticoagulants antithrombin III and protein C levels are unchanged or increase, and protein S levels fall [15]. There is a reduction in fibrinolytic activity that is mainly due to the marked increase in the plasminogen activator inhibitors PAI-I and PAI-2. Together, these changes increase the risk of thrombosis during pregnancy and during the postpartum period.

A variety of physiological changes occurs during pregnancy. In the early months, the retention of about 500 up to 900 mEq of sodium [16-18] generates an increase in total body water from 6 to 8 L. Resistance to the pressor effects of angiotensin II develops along with a rise in all components of the renin-angiotensin system. This results in a large increase in the volume of extracellular water (by 4–7 L) and in the retention of sodium and water, which acts to maintain normal blood pressure [19-20]. Stroke volume and heart rate increase. Cardiac output rises in the first trimester and then peaks by the end of the second trimester, having reached approximately 30–50% of the non-pregnant values (3.5–6.0L/min). The increase in cardiac output occurs rapidly beginning at the fifth week of gestation (4.88 L/min) and continuing until the 32nd week. After birth, cardiac output decreases and is restored to normal levels at 24 weeks postpartum. Between 8 and 16–20 weeks of gestation, stroke volume increases [21-24].

Colloid osmotic pressure (COP) may also undergo changes that can affect the well-being of the mother during pregnancy. For example, a decrease in the plasma COP from 25 mmHg to 18–20 mmHg may cause edema.

All of these factors must be taken into account in the fluid management of complicated obstetric patients.

15.2   Hemorrhage

Bleeding is a major cause of maternal mortality and of complications associated with childbirth [25]. In fact, a blood transfusion is required in 1–2% of pregnancies [26-27]. In most women, however, the loss of blood is tolerated due to the physiological changes that occur during pregnancy, as discussed above.

Bleeding may develop before or after childbirth. The causes include: uterine atony, placenta previa and placental abruption [28]. Other causes of postpartum hemorrhage are a retained placenta, uterine inversion, placenta accreta, uterine rupture, and trauma involving the genital tract [29, 30]. The risk factors for postpartum hemorrhage include pre-existing anemia, obesity, chorioamnionitis, fetal macrosomia, prior caesarean section, and multiple gestations [31].

The objectives of the management of obstetric hemorrhage are control of the source of blood loss and the maintenance of tissue perfusion [31, 38]. Decreased cardiac output, hypotension, and vasoconstriction may result in the decreased end-organ perfusion of vital organs, including the kidneys, heart, and brain [36]. In order to restore the oxygen carrying capacity and maintain adequate tissue perfusion, fluid resuscitation should begin with volume expansion using crystalloid, at a volume approximately three times that of the estimated blood loss. This should be followed immediately with red cell replacement using packed RBCs to restore the oxygen carrying capacity, with the goal of maintaining hemoglobin at 7–10 g/dL. Lastly, clotting factors and platelets should be replaced in order to prevent or correct coagulopathy [32, 33]. This replacement should begin with fresh, frozen plasma and be followed by cryoprecipitate and platelets. In cases in which coagulopathy does not respond to these measures, the administration of recombinant activated factor VII can be considered [37]. Since these products are not always available, some authors recommend massive transfusion [38].

Often, however, transfusion is delayed due to an underestimation by physicians of the amount of hemorrhage. While waiting for blood products, perfusion pressure and blood volume are initially maintained with crystalloids or colloids. The optimal fluid type in hypovolemic patients has been the subject of much debate; most studies have concentrated on traumatic hemorrhage. Nonetheless, peripartum hemorrhage is a condition in which a lack of treatment contributes to morbidity and mortality. Two difficulties arise in the pregnant woman compared with other patient groups. First, hypovolemia is much more difficult to recognize, owing to the physiological changes that occur during pregnancy. Second, when the volume of blood decreases, the oxygen supply is insufficient but the use of crystalloids and colloids contributes to the hemodilution. Thus, some colloids should be avoided because they negatively affect hemostasis [39]. In addition, according to Van der Linden and Ickx, there is no advantage in using albumin rather than saline solution in terms of morbidity and mortality [40]. Yet in other studies the administration of saline solution 0.9% was not recommended because it causes hyperchloremic acidosis. Instead, there is an argument for balanced fluid resuscitation using fluid (crystalloids and colloids) containing a physiological balance of electrolytes [41]. The use of hypertonic saline has been suggested in cases of hemorrhagic shock, but there are no studies demonstrating the effectiveness of this approach [42]. The presence of relative anemia requires the limited administration of clear liquids, with the amounts adapted to intravascular volume to ensure perfusion [43].

15.3   Pregnancy-Induced Hypertension

For the patient with pregnancy-induced hypertension (PIH), in particular those with pre-eclampsia, fluid management is a very important challenge because in many cases neither the physiology nor the cause of the PIH is known. PIH is characterized by the combination of intravascular volume depletion and an increase in the extracellular volume, which makes fluid management difficult. Some authors [44-45] advocate volume replacement to compensate the loss of intravascular volume, while others [46-47] recommend diuretics or volume limits because of the excess extracellular fluid. In simple PIH, crystalloid infusion at a rate of 75–125 mL/h in childbirth and the postpartum period is decisive [48-49]. In complicated cases of PIH or if there are other therapeutic interventions, intravascular volume becomes an important factor to consider in fluid management.

In the presence of oliguria, an infusion of 500-1000 mL of crystalloids is appropriate [50]. If the condition persists, then the oxygenation state must be taken into account because an excess of fluid can lead to pulmonary or cerebral edema. Clark and colleagues [50] showed that in patients with oliguria who fail to respond to the infusion of crystalloids, alternative treatment strategies may be required, depending on the cause. In the case of intravascular volume depletion, there is a need for the further infusion of crystalloid, but if, instead, the oliguria is due to the renal artery, vasospasm is required, i.e., by the administration of dopamine, without an infusion of fluids. In patients requiring volume expansion, due to a postpartum decrease in COP, then colloids are the first choice [51] (Fig. 15.1).

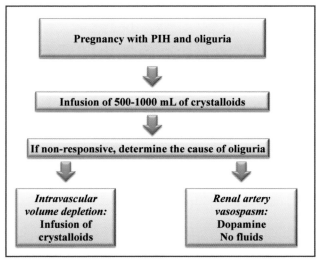

Fig. 15.1 Therapeutic approach in PIH complicated by oliguria

Another aspect to be considered in patients with PIH is regional anesthesia. The intravascular volume depletion, present in PIH, may exacerbate the sympathetic block, leading to vasodilatation and thus a decrease in blood pressure. Without adequate rehydration, the patient may experience hypotension, which may adversely affect fetal well-being. However, the excessive infusion of fluids can lead to overhydration, with the development of edema to the extent that early studies [52, 53] advised against the use of regional anesthesia in women with pre-eclampsia. This is no longer the accepted position as regional anesthesia cannot be implicated [54]. Indeed, recent studies [55] have shown that spinal anesthesia may cause less hypotension in patients with PIH than in healthy ones. In the former, to give crystalloids a few minutes before spinal anesthesia induction may prevent an increase in CVP [56]. In hypotensive patients, vasopressors should be used, not fluids.

In general, in pregnant patients with PIH, fluid management is complex and must be adapted to each case, considering the potential for complications and the other therapeutic interventions that the patient may require.

Key Concepts
- Causes and treatment of hemorrhage in pregnancy
- Factors that influence the treatment of PIH

Key Words
- Hypertension
- Hemorrhage
- Spinal anesthesia
- Oliguria

Focus on...
- Dahlgren G, Granath F, Pregner K et al (2005) Colloid vs. crystalloid preloading to prevent maternal hypotension during spinal anaesthesia for elective cesarean section. Acta Anaesthesiol Scand 49:1200–1206
- Watson J (2011) The effect of intrapartum intravenous fluid management on breastfed newborn weight loss J Obstet Gynecol Neonatal Nurs 40;S97

References

1. Ickx BE (2010) Fluid and blood transfusion management in obstetrics. European Journal of Anaesthesiology 27:1031-5
2. Bernstein IM, Ziegler W, Badger GJ (2001) Plasma volume expansion in early pregnancy. Obstet Gynecol 97:669
3. Hytten F (1985) Blood volume changes in normal pregnancy. In: Letsky EA (ed) Haematological Disorders in Pregnancy. London, W.B. Saunders, pp 601–612
4. Harstad TW, Mason RA, Cox SM (1992) Serum erythropoietin quantitation in pregnancy using an enzyme-linked immunoassay. Am J Perinatol 9:233–235
5. De Leeuw NK, Lowenstein L, Tucker EC et al (1968) Correlation of red cell loss at delivery with changes in red cell mass. Am J Obstet Gynecol 100:1092–1101
6. Cavill I (1995) Iron and erythropoiesis in normal subjects and in pregnancy. J Perinat Med 23:47–50
7. Koller O (1982) The clinical significante of hemodilution during pregnancy. Obstet Gynecol Surv 37:649–652
8. Clapp JF III, Little KD, Widness JA (2003) Effect of maternal exercise and fetoplacental growth rate on serum erythropoietin concentrations. Am J Obstet Gynecol 188:1021
9. Peck TM, Arias F (1979) Hematologic changes associated with pregnancy. Clin Obstet Gynecol 22:785–798
10. Sejeny SA, Eastham RD, Baker SR (1975) Platelet counts during normal pregnancy. J Clin Pathol 28:812–813
11. O'Brien JR (1976) Letter: platelet counts in normal pregnancy. J Clin Pathol 29:174
12. Rakoczi I, Tallian F, Bagdany S et al (1979) Platelet life-span in normal pregnancy and preeclampsia asdetermined by a non-radioisotope technique. Thromb Res 15:553–556
13. Burrows RF, Kelton JG (1990) Thrombocytopenia at delivery: a prospective survey of 6715 deliveries. Am J Obstet Gynecol 162: 731–734
14. Hellgren M (1996) Hemostasis during pregnancy and puerperium. Haemostasis 26(Suppl 4):244–247
15. Davis GL (2000) Hemostatic changes associated with normal and abnormal pregnancies. Clin Lab Sci 13:223–228
16. Seitchik J (1967) Total body water and total body density of pregnant women. Obstet Gynecol 29:155
17. Theunissen IM, Parer JT (1994) Fluid and electrolytes in pregnancy. Clin Obstet Gynecol 37:3
18. Lindheimer MD, Katz AI (1973) Sodium and diuretics in pregnancy. N Engl J Med 288:891
19. Lindheimer M, Barron WM (1998) Renal function and volume homeostasis. In: Gleicher N, Buttino L, Elkayam U (eds) Principles and Practice of Medical Therapy in Pregnancy. 3 edn. Stanford, CT, Appleton and Lange, pp 1043–1052
20. Davison JM, Vallotton MB, Lindheimer MD (1981) Plasma osmolality and urinary concentration and dilution during and after pregnancy: evidence that lateral recumbency inhibits maximal urinary concentrating ability. Br J Obstet Gynaecol 88:472–479
21. Bader RA, Bader MG & Rose DG (1955) Hemodynamics at rest and during exercise in pregnancy as studied by cardiac catherization. J Clin Invest 34:1524
22. Clark SL, Cotton DB, Wetal L (1989) Central hemodynamic assessment of normal term pregnancy. Am J Obstet Gynecol 161:1439–1442
23. Easterling TR, Watts DH, Schmucker BC et al (1987) Measurement of cardiac output during pregnancy: validation of Doppler technique and clinical observations in preeclampsia. Obstet Gynecol 69:845–850
24. Katz R, Karliner JS, Resnik R (1978) Effects of a natural volume overload state (pregnancy) on left ventricular performance in normal human subjects. Circulation 58:434–441
25. Atrash HK, Koonin LM, Lawson HW et al (1990) Maternal mortality in the United States, 1979 - 1986. Obstet Gynecol 76:1055
26. Kamani AA, McMorland GH, Wadsworth LD (1988) Utilization of red blood cell transfusion

in an obstetric setting. Am J Obstet Gynecol 159:1177

27. Kapholz H (1990) Blood transfusion in contemporary obstetric practice. Obstet Gynecol 75:940

28. Tsu VD, Langer A, Aldrich T (2004) Postpartum hemorrhage in developing countries: is the public health community using the right tools? Int J Gynaecol Obstet 85(Suppl 1):S42–S51

29. Doumouchtsis SK, Papageorghiou AT, Arulkumaran S (2007) Systematic review of conservative management of postpartum hemorrhage: what to do when medical treatment fails. Obstet Gynecol Surv 62:540–547

30. Chichakli LO, Atrash HK, Mackay AP et al (1999) Pregnancy-related mortality in the United States due to hemorrhage: 1979–1992. Obstet Gynecol 94:721–725

31. Cohen WR (2006) Hemorrhagic shock in obstetrics. J Perinat Med 34:263–271

32. Chong Y-S, Su L-L, Arulkumaran S (2004) Current strategies for the prevention of postpartum haemorrhage in the third stage of labour. Curr Opin Obstet Gynecol 16:143–150

33. Letsky EA (2001) Disseminated intravascular coagulation. Best Pract Res Clin Obstet Gynaecol 15:623–644

34. Bick RL (2002) Disseminated intravascular coagulation: a review of etiology, pathophysiology, diagnosis, and management: guidelines for care. Clin Appl Thromb Hemost 8:1–31

35. Djelmis J, Ivanisevic M, Kurjak A et al (2001) Hemostatic problems before, during and after delivery. J Perinat Med 29:241–246

36. Kobayashi T, Terao T, Maki M et al (2001) Diagnosis and management of acute obstetrical DIC. Semin Thrombosis Hemostasis 27:161–167

37. DeLoughery TG (2005) Critical care clotting catastrophies. Crit Care Clin 21:531–562

38. Pepas LP, Arif-Adib M, Kadir RA (2006) Factor VIIa in puerperal hemorrhage with disseminated intravascular coagulation. Obstet Gynecol 108:757–761

39. Burtelow M, Riley E, Druzin M et al (2007) How we treat: management of life-threatening primary postpartum hemorrhage with a standardized massive transfusion protocol. Transfusion 47:1564–1572

40. Van der Linden P, Ickx BE (2006) The effects of colloid solutions on hemostasis. Can J Anaesth 53(6 Suppl):S30–S39

41. Finfer S, Bellomo R, Boyce N et al (2004) A comparison of albumin and saline for fluid resuscitation in the intensive care unit. N Engl J Med 350:2247–2256

42. Boldt J (2007) The balanced concept of fluid resuscitation. Br J Anaesth 99:312–315

43. Mion G, Rüttimann M (1997) Loading with hypertonic saline solution during pregnancy toxemia. Ann Fr Anesth Reanim 16:1046–1047

44. American Society of Anesthesiologists Task Force on Perioperative Blood Transfusion and Adjuvant Therapies (2006) Practice guidelines for perioperative blood transfusion and adjuvant therapies. Anesthesiology 105:198–208

45. Cotton DB, Longmire S, Jones MM et al (1986) Cardiovascular alterations in severe pregnancy-induced hypertension: Effects of intravenous nitroglycerin coupled with blood volume expansion. Am J Obstet Gynecol 154:1053-9

46. Wasserstrum N (1992) Issues in fluid management during labor: Maternal plasma volume status and volume loading. Clin Obstet Gynecol 35:514-26

47. Hankins SDV, Wendel GD, Cunningham FG et al (1984) Longitudinal evaluation of hemodynamic changes in eclampsia. Am J Obstet Gynecol 150:506-12

48. Pearson JF (1992) Fluid balance in severe pre-eclampsia. Br J Hosp Med 48:47-51

49. Jones MM, Longmire S, Cotton DB et al (1986) Influence of crystalloid versus colloid infusion on peripartum colloid osmotic pressure changes. Obstet Gynecol 68:659-61

50. Kirshon B, Moise JK Jr, Cotton DB et al (1988): Role of volume expansion in severe preeclampsia. Surg Gynecol Obstet 167:367-71

51. Clark SL, Greenspoon JS, Aldahl D et al (1986) Severe preeclampsia with persistent oliguria: Management of hemodynamic subsets. Am J Obstet Gynecol 154:490-4

52. Kapholz H (1990) Blood transfusion in contemporary obstetric practice. Obstet Gynecol 75:940-3

53. Pritchard JA, MacDonald PC, Leveno KJ et al (1985) Hypertensive disorders in pregnancy. In: Pritchard JA, MacDonald PC, Leveno KJ et al (eds) Williams Obstetrics, 17 edn. Connecticut, Appleton-Century-Crofts, p 551
54. Lindheimer MD, Katz AI (1985) Current concepts: Hypertension in pregnancy. N Engl J Med 313:675
55. Dyer RA, Piercy JL, Reed AR (2007) The role of the anaesthetist in the management of the pre-eclamptic patient. Curr Opin Anaesthesiol 20:168–174
56. Aya AG, Mangin R, Vialles N et al (2003) Patients with severe preeclampsia experience less hypotension during spinal anesthesia for elective cesarean delivery than healthy parturients: a prospective cohort comparison. Anesth Analg; 97:867–872

Fluid Management in Palliative Care

16

Massimiliano Carassiti, Annalaura Di Pumpo
and Felice Eugenio Agrò

16.1   Palliative Sedation

Palliative sedation is a medical procedure in which consciousness is reduced or abolished, as the only therapeutic resource to relieve refractory symptoms that are intolerable for the patient. It is carried out through gradual titration of a sedative accompanied by periodic monitoring of the patient's vital signs, level of sedation, and degree of symptom relief. A team of experts in palliative care must perform this procedure, taking into account the indication and timing and the complete history of the patient. Ethical principles of proportionality, beneficence, and non-malfeasance, as well as the principle of patient autonomy are important considerations.

Refractory symptoms are those in which interventions do not bring any benefit to the patient, produce intolerable side effects, and/or do not provide relief within a reasonable amount of time. Palliative sedation is based on the following conditions [1]:
- the life expectancy of the patient is judged to be hours or days;
- the presence of intense pain;
- a sign that the suffering is refractory;
- the patient's consent.

Life expectancy is measured in palliative care using prognostic factors and prognostic indices, most commonly, the Palliative Prognostic Score [2] (Table 16.1) and the Palliative Prognostic Index [3].

Palliative sedation is indicated for the following refractory symptoms: dyspnea, delirium, pain, massive bleeding, and asphyxiation. The etiology of

M. Carassiti (✉)
Intensive Care Department, University School of Medicine Campus Bio-Medico of Rome,
Rome, Italy
e-mail: m.carassiti@unicampus.it

F. E. Agrò (ed.), *Body Fluid Management*,
DOI: 10.1007/978-88-470-2661-2_16 © Springer-Verlag Italia 2013

Table 16.1 Palliative Prognostic Score

Cryterion	Assessment	Partial Score
Anorexia	No	0
	Yes	1.5
Karnofsky Performance Scale	> 30	0
	10-20	2.5
Dyspnea	No	0
	Yes	1
Total WBC (x 10^9/L)	< 8.5	0
	8.6-11	0.5
	> 11	2.5
Lynphocyte percentage	20-40%	0
	12-19.9%	1
	< 12%	2.5
Clinical prediction of survival	> 12	0
	11-12	2
	7-10	2.5
	5-6	4.5
	3-4	6
	1-2	8.5
RISK GROUP	**30-DAY SURVIVAL**	**TOTAL SCORE**
A	> 70%	0-5.5
B	30-70%	5.6-11
C	< 30%	11.1-17.5

the various symptoms is important to understand the cause(s) of their possible irreversibility and refractoriness [4].

Palliative sedation follows not only clinical but also ethical principles, including the following [4-7]:

- the principle of double effect [5]: An intervention that is motivated by a good end is considered to be legitimate even though it may produce further effects that are negative but were neither sought nor desired;
- the principle of proportionality;
- the principle of beneficence;
- the principle of autonomy is respected when the patient, properly informed and competent, decides to accept or to refuse palliative sedation.

Some studies have shown that palliative sedation does not reduce the patient's life span [8-13]; rather, this can happen in a small proportion of patients because of the onset of respiratory depression, aspiration, and/or hemodynamic instability, as reported by Morita et al. [14].

In palliative care, nutrition and hydration play important roles in the terminally ill patient.

Palliative sedation follows a decision algorithm, most commonly, Portnoy's algorithm, which can be integrated as shown in Fig. 16.1.

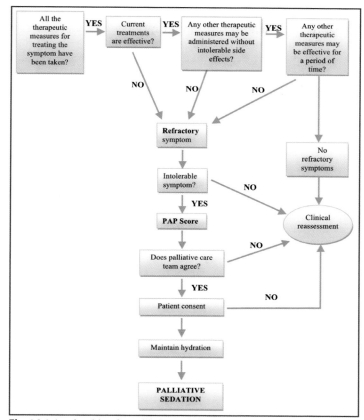

Fig. 16.1 An algorithm for palliative sedation

16.2   Hydration in Palliative Sedation

Dying patients, for example, those with advanced cancer, gradually stop eating and drinking. Hypercalcemia may occur and lead to a state of dehydration, thereby worsening the patient's condition [15].

Some studies [16] have shown that, for a terminally ill patient, less fluid is needed than in a patient undergoing surgery. The terminally ill patient, however, is more susceptible to fluid deficit. In addition, the majority of patients are elderly and their renal function is less effective in maintaining water balance and a state of hydration [17-21]. The reduced water demand is due to a number of factors: age, body weight, and the clearance of free water. Oskvig found that the loss of fluid occurs mainly in the intracellular rather than in the extracellular space [22].

A lack of fluids can cause symptoms such as cognitive impairment, altered behavior, confusion, delirium, fainting, or syncope, which may lead to a further fluid reductions [23] and thus a rapid deterioration of the patient, until death.

16.3   Advantages and Disadvantages of Hydration

The aim of hydration is to prevent or correct the symptoms that may occur with dehydration, especially delirium and opioid neurotoxicity. Numerous studies have shown that in terminally ill cancer patients hydration can prevent the onset of delirium [20, 24, 25]; in a Canadian study, vigorous hydration resulted in a lower incidence of delirium among patients in a palliative care unit [24] (Table 16.2).

Hydration is not only able to prevent delirium but it can also correct it. Several studies [26-30] have shown that the administration of fluids can permanently correct or is able to improve delirium arising after dehydration. In addition, delirium may indicate an accumulation of opioids and their metabolites, since terminally ill patients undergo a progressive deterioration of renal and hepatic function. The administration of fluids can reverse this accumulation [31], thus preventing the onset of delirium.

The level of hydration, however, does not act on symptoms of thirst and dry mouth [32]. This assertion is supported by several studies. Bourge [33] showed that there was no significant correlation between markers of hydration status in terminally ill patients and thirst. We therefore hypothesized that the homeostatic mechanisms controlling liquid and water balance are altered in dying patients. The study of Waller confirmed this hypothesis [34]. Therefore, hydration is not required, and may indeed be useless, to relieve the symptom of thirst [32].

Some authors have related certain side effects to hydration, i.e., vomiting, nausea, increased secretions, edema, ascites, urinary tract infections (due to increased use of urethral catheters in hydrated patients), airway secretions

Table 16.2 Advantages and disadvantages of hydration

Advantages	Disavantages
To prevent symptoms: confusion, agitation, and neuromuscular irritability	Painful and invasive therapy
To prevent complications	Nausea, vomiting
To relieve thirst	Increased secretions
To provide standard care	Edema
	Ascites

[35], and feelings of discomfort [36]. However, Dalal and Bruera [23] found no concrete evidence for these effects but did acknowledge that side effects can arise with excessive fluid administration.

In terminally ill patients, hypoalbuminemia may occur [32], which can lead to pulmonary or peripheral edema and ascites, if crystalloids are administered. If serum albumin is less than 26 g/L, Dunlop et al. [15] advised against the administration of fluids, whether intravenously or subcutaneously, to avoid adverse effects. Instead, intravenous colloids were recommended.

16.4   Method of Administration

Fluids can be administered via several different routes, as discussed in the following.

16.4.1   Intravenous Route

Traditionally, the administration of fluids intravenously is carried out at the peripheral level. However, in some cases, placement of a central venous access device may be required, The various devices differ from each other in terms of where and how they are positioned and the length of time they can remain in place. Peripherally inserted central catheters (PICCs) are suitable for patients who require prolonged intravenous therapy.

Importantly, intravenous therapy is not without risks, as infection and occlusion of the catheter [37] may occur. Furthermore, in the case of a central catheter, there may be complications related to the positioning procedure: arterial puncture, arrhythmias, cardiopulmonary arrest, pneumothorax, and incorrect location of the catheter tip have been reported [23].

16.4.2   Subcutaneous Route

Hypodermoclysis is the administration of fluid subcutaneously and is relevant in geriatric and palliative care [23]. Hypodermoclysis eliminates the disadvantages of intravenous therapy even if it cannot be used in emergency situations. It also should not be applied in patients with generalized edema and bleeding disorders.

Fluids that can be administered subcutaneously include electrolytic solutions (saline 0.9% and 0.45%), dextrose-saline, and saline-glucose [38-41]. Non-electrolytic solutions are not suitable because they can accumulate in the interstitial spaces and can lead to tissue desquamation. Colloids and hyperosmolar solutions cannot be administered by hypodermoclysis [23].

16.4.3 Enteral Route

The enteral route is indicated in malnourished patients because of their inability to ingest substances orally. It is chosen based on duration and in accordance with the patient's anatomy and physiology. Enteral nutrition is indicated in patients with cancer of the head and neck causing dysphagia and in those with esophageal obstruction, gastric outlet obstruction, or a prolonged critical illness requiring mechanical ventilation.

16.4.4 Proctoclysis

Proctoclysis is the administration of fluids through the rectum. It is indicated in patients in whom the enteral route is not an option. It cannot be used in patients with colon cancer or generalized edema.

This procedure was only recently considered as a viable alternative for hydration, although it was evaluated in several earlier studies [42, 43]. The side effects of proctoclysis are fluid loss, pain during the infusion, and catheter insertion. Proctoclysis offers a valid alternative also based on its low cost, ease of administration, and low maintenance.

The hydration of a terminally ill patient is not an act of "charity", but a medical gesture. Indeed, to ensure proper hydration does not mean extending the life of the patient but simply to prevent complications that arise due to sedation, such as electrolyte disorders.

Key Concepts
- Palliative sedation
- Complications of dehydration
- Methods of fluid administration in palliative sedation

Key Words
- Palliative sedation
- Hydration
- Opioids
- Delirium
- Intravenous route
- Hypodermoclysis
- Enteral route
- Proctoclysis

Focus on...
- Juth N (2010) European Association for Palliative Care (EAPC). Framework for palliative sedation: an ethical discussion. BMC Palliative Care 9:20
- Dalal S, Bruera E (2004) Dehydration in Cancer Patients: To Treat or Not To Treat. J Support Oncol 2:467–487

References

1. Nathan I Cherny, Lukas Radbruch and The Board of the European Association for Palliative Care European Association for Palliative Care (EAPC) (2009) recommended framework for the use of sedation in palliative care. Palliat Med 23:581
2. Maltoni M (1999) Successful validation of the palliative prognostic score (Pap Score) in terminally ill cancer patients. J pain symptom manage 17:240-247
3. Morita T (1999) The palliative prognostic index: a scoring system for survival prediction of terminally ill cancer patients. Support care cancer 7:128-133
4. Morita T (2005) Ethical validity of palliative sedation therapy: a multicenter, prospective, observational study conducted on specialized palliative care units in Japan. Journal of Pain and Symptom Management 30:308-319
5. Boyle J (2004) Medical ethics and double effect: the case of terminal sedation. Theoretical Medicine 25:51–60
6. Juth N (2010) European Association for Palliative Care (EAPC) framework for palliative sedation: an ethical discussion. BMC Palliative Care 9:20
7. Olsen ML (2010) Ethical decision making with end-of-life care: palliative sedation and withholding or withdrawing life-sustaining treatments. Mayo Clin Proc 85(10):949-954

8.   Claessens P, Menten J, Schotsmans P, Broeckaert B (2008) Palliative sedation: a review of the research literature. J Pain Symptom Manage 36:310–333

9.   Rietjens JA (2008) Palliative sedation in a specialized unit for acute palliative care in a cancer hospital: comparing patients dying with and without palliative sedation. J Pain Symptom Manage 36:228–234

10. Stone P, Phillips C, Spruyt O, Waight C (1997) A comparison of the use of sedatives in a hospital support team and in a hospice. Palliat Med 11:140–4

11. Chiu TY, Hu WY, Lue BH, Cheng SY, Chen CY (2001) Sedation for refractory symptoms of terminal cancer patients in Taiwan. J Pain Symptom Manage 21:467–472

12. Sykes N, Thorns A (2003) Sedative use in the last week of life and the implications for end-of-life decision making. Arch Intern Med 163:341–344

13. Maltoni M, Pittureri C, Scarpi E et al (2009) Palliative sedation therapy does not hasten death: results from a prospective multicentre study. Ann Oncol 20:1163–1169

14. Morita T, Chinone Y, Ikenaga M et al (2005) Efficacy and safety of palliative sedation therapy: a multicenter, prospective, observational study conducted on specialized palliative care units in Japan. J Pain Symptom Manage 30:320–328

15. Dunlop RJ, Ellershaw JE, Baines MJ, Sykes N, Saunders CM (1995) On withholding nutrition and hydration in the terminally ill: has palliative medicine gone too far? A reply. Journal of medical ethics 21:141-143

16. Bruera E, Belzile M, Watanabe S, Fainsinger RL (1996) Volume of hydration in terminal cancer patients. Support Care Cancer 4:147–150

17. Ciccone A, Allegra JR, Cochrane DG, Cody RP, Roche LM (1998) Age related differences in diagnoses within the elderly population. Am J Emerg Med 16:43–48

18. Hoffman NB (1991) Dehydration in the elderly: insidious and manageable. Geriatrics 46:35–38

19. Lavizzo-Mourey R, Johnson J, Stolley P (1988) Risk factors for dehydration among elderly nursing home residents. J Am Geriatr Soc 36:213–218

20. Seymour DG, Henschke PJ, Cape RD, Campbell AJ (1980) Acute confusional states and dementia in the elderly: the roles of dehydration/volume depletion, physical illness and age. Age Ageing 9:137–146

21. Warren JL, Bacon WE, Harris T et al (1994) The burden and outcomes associated with dehydration among US elderly, 1991. Am J Public Health 84:1265–1269

22. Oskvig RM (1999) Special problems in the elderly: the aging kidney and liver. Chest 115(5 suppl):158S–164S

23. Dalal S, Bruera E (2004) Dehydration in cancer patients: to treat or not to treat. J Support Oncol 2:467–487

24. Bruera E, Franco JJ, Maltoni M, Watanabe S, Suarez-Almazor M (1995) Changing patterns of agitated impaired mental status in patients with advanced cancer: association with cognitive monitoring, hydration, and opioid rotation. J Pain Symptom Manage 10:287–291

25. Inouye SK, Bogardus ST Jr, Charpentier PA et al (1999) A multicomponent intervention to prevent delirium in hospitalized older patients. N Engl J Med 340:669–676

26. Agostini JV, Leo-Summers LS, Inouye SK (2001) Cognitive and other adverse effects of diphenhy- dramine use in hospitalized older patients. Arch Intern Med 161:2091–2097

27. Gagnon P, Allard P, Mâsse B, DeSerres M (2000) Delirium in terminal cancer: a prospective study using daily screening, early diagnosis, and continuous monitoring. J Pain Symptom Manage 19:412–426

28. Maddocks I, Somogyi A, Abbott F, Hayball P, Parker D (1996) Attenuation of morphine-induced delirium in palliative care by substitution with infusion of oxycodone. J Pain Symptom Manage 12:182–189

29. Tuma R, DeAngelis LM (2000) Altered mental status in patients with cancer. Arch Neurol 57:1727–1731

30. Breitbart W, Gibson C, Tremblay A (2002) The delirium experience: delirium recall and delirium-related distress in hospitalized patients with cancer, their spouses/caregivers, and their nurses. Psychosomatics 43:183–194

31. Fainsinger RL, Bruera E (1997) When to treat dehydration in a terminally ill patient. Support Care 5:205–11
32. Ellershaw J E, Sutcliffe J M, Saunders CM (1995) Dehydration and the dying patient. Journal of pain and symptom management 10:192–197
33. Burge FI (1993) Dehydration symptoms of palliative care cancer patients. Journal of pain and symptom management 8:454-464
34. Waller A, Adunski A, Hershkowitz M (1991) Terminal dehydration and intravenous fluids. Lancet 337:745
35. Wildiers H, Menten J (2002) Death rattle: prevalence, prevention and treatment. J Pain Symptom Manage 23:310–7
36. Fainsinger R (2006) Non-oral hydration in palliative care #133. J Palliat Med 9:206–7
37. Krzywda EA (1999) Predisposing factors, prevention, and management of central venous catheter occlusions. J Intraven Nurs 22(6 suppl):S11–S17
38. Slesak G, Schnurle JW, Kinzel E, Jakob J, Dietz PK (2003) Comparison of subcutaneous and intravenous rehydration in geriatric patients: a randomized trial. J Am Geriatr Soc 51:155–160
39. Schen RJ, Singer-Edelstein M (1981) Subcutaneous infusions in the elderly. J Am Geriatr Soc 29:583–585
40. O'Keeffe ST, Lavan JN (1996) Subcutaneous fluids in elderly hospital patients with cognitive impairment. Gerontology 42:36–39
41. Bruera E, Brenneis C, Michaud M et al (1988) Use of the subcutaneous route for the administration of narcotics in patients with cancer pain. Cancer 62:407–411
42. Fainsinger RL, Bruera E (1991) Hypodermoclysis (HDC) for symptom control versus the Edmonton Injector (EI). J Palliat Care 7:5–8
43. Bruera E, Schoeller T, Pruvost M (1994) Proctoclysis for hydration of terminal cancer patients. Lancet 344:1699

Infusion-Related Complications

17

Annalaura Di Pumpo, Maria Benedetto
and Felice Eugenio Agrò

17.1 Phlebitis

Infusion therapy requires the use of a peripheral venous catheter (PVC),
whose position can be complicated by phlebitis, defined as an inflammation
of the tunica intima of a vein. Inflammation, in turn, may have mechanical,
chemical, or bacterial origins [1].
- Mechanical phlebitis occurs when the cannula generates friction with the
  wall of the vein, leading to inflammation.
- Chemical phlebitis is due to the infusion of fluids and medications, according to their osmolarity or pH [2].
- Bacterial phlebitis is due to the presence of infectious bacteria. The main
  risk factors are: a high number of administrations, inadequate practices
  during infusion, or a lack of cleanliness of the skin before the cannula is
  inserted [3, 4].

17.1.1 Signs and Symptoms

The three types of phlebitis share several signs and symptoms:
- erythema;
- swelling;
- warm skin at the cannula insertion;
- pain during fluid infusion.
  Other signs and symptoms that may indicate phlebitis are: difficulty of

M. Benedetto (✉)
Postgraduate School of Anesthesia and Intensive Care, Anesthesia, Intensive Care and Pain
Management Department, University School of Medicine Campus Bio-Medico of Rome,
Rome, Italy
e-mail: m.benedetto@unicampus.it

F. E. Agrò (ed.), *Body Fluid Management*,
DOI: 10.1007/978-88-470-2661-2_17 © Springer-Verlag Italia 2013

Table 17.1 Phlebitis grading system

Phlebitis Grading
Grade 0: No symptoms
Grade 1: Erythema and pain
Grade 2: Pain, erythema and edema
Grade 3: Pain, erythema, edema, streak formation, palpable venous cord
Grade 4: Pain, erythema, edema, streak formation, palpable venous cord and purulent drainage

infusion, the presence of a transudate, and fever of unknown origin. The presence of such events is the basis for the recognition of five degrees of phlebitis [5] (Table 17.1).

17.1.2 Treatment and Complications

The treatment of phlebitis varies depending on the clinical severity. Mild phlebitis (grades 0 and 1) reverts without treatment. More severe phlebitis mandates that the infusion be stopped and the cannula removed [6]. An anti-inflammatory cream should then be applied to the affected areas.

When phlebitis is not treated, patients may experience further complications, such as infection, thrombosis, superficial thrombophlebitis [7], and septic thrombophlebitis (a rare but very serious complication) [8].

17.2 Infiltration

Infiltration is defined as a loss of intravenous fluid into the surrounding tissue, mainly due to displacement of the catheter tip. Elderly patients are particularly vulnerable because their veins are fragile and thin.

17.2.1 Signs and Symptoms

Several signs and symptoms characterize fluid infiltration: skin swelling, discomfort, burning, tightness, and blanching. Accordingly, various degrees of infiltration are distinguished [9] (Table 17.2).

17.2.2 Prevention and Treatment

The prevention of infiltration is mainly related to clinical practice; it is based on the chosen veins and on the site of catheter placement. As an example, areas of flexion or fragile veins should be avoided.

Table 17.2 Infiltration scale

Infiltration scale
Grade 0: No symptoms
Grade 1: Edema < 2,5 cm, cold and pale skin, pain
Grade 2: Edema 2,5 to 15 cm, cold and pale skin, pain
Grade 3: Edema > 15 cm, mild pain, cold skin, numbness
Grade 4: Pale translucent, swollen, bruised tight skin, edema > 15 cm, moderate or severe pain, infiltration of any amount of blood product, irritant, or vesicant

The treatment consists of small clinical procedures:
1. Stoppage of the infusion.
2. Removal of the catheter.
3. Application of cold packs.

In addition, it is necessary to check the patient's pulse and to monitor the potential development of blisters, necessitating surgical consultation.

17.3 Extravasation

Extravasation is defined as the leakage of medications or fluids into the tissues close to the site of intravenous infusion.

Two types of extravasation are recognized:
- irritating, accompanied by inflammatory reactions;
- vesicant, with serious consequences.

17.3.1 Signs and Symptoms

Based on the amount of liquid, type, and position of the extravasation, the consequences will differ, ranging from irritation to tissue necrosis. The main symptoms are: swelling, pain, redness, and heating.

17.3.2 Prevention and Treatment

The best treatment for extravasation is prevention, which requires the placement of the cannula in large and intact veins. The veins of the hands and wrists should be avoided because they are areas rich in nerves and tendons, which can be easily damaged.

If extravasation is already present, the infusion must be stopped and the catheter removed. The extravasation is then aspirated from the subcutaneous tissue in order to prevent an inflammatory reaction. If a drug is instilled, as in the case of antineoplastic or vasopressors, an antidote should be administered.

17.4   Hematoma

Hematoma is a pool of blood organized external to a blood vessel (artery, vein or capillary). It occurs after damage to the blood vessel wall, which allows leakage of blood into the surrounding tissues. Hematoma differs from ecchymosis which is an expansion of blood located at skin level or in a mucous membrane in a thin layer.

Several factors are related to the accumulation of blood under the skin. For example, patients under anti-coagulant drugs tend to develop large hematomas. Consequently, the detection of a hematoma must be evaluated with respect to the basic health status of the patient [10].

The most common complication of hematomas is bacterial infection of the extravasated blood. There are different kinds of hematomas and both their symptoms and their clinical management will be influenced by their site, size, and the possible inflammation of nearby structures.

17.4.1   Signs and Symptoms

Blood is a strong tissue irritant and thus may induce inflammation and irritation, together with pain, redness, and swelling.

17.4.2   Prevention and Treatment

Hematoma should be managed following the R.I.C.E protocol: rest, ice, compression, elevation. The pain associated with hematoma is caused by inflammation and can be treated with anti-inflammatory drugs, taking into account the patient's health status.

Hematomas caused by infusion can be prevented by applying a compressive dressing at the vein insertion site. Patient cooperation can be useful in preventing hematoma, since if the arm is moved within a short period following venous puncture, the risk of bleeding will increase.

17.5   Hemorrhage/Thrombosis

These disorders are characterize by the onset of bleeding and the formation of intravascular thrombi. Bleeding disorders can be due to a dilution of clotting factors in the bloodstream or to the interaction of colloid molecules with platelet adhesion or with clot formation.

17.5.1 About Crystalloids and Colloids

In general, crystalloids are less likely than colloids to cause coagulation disorders. However, dilution with crystalloids seems to induce a significant hypercoagulability status because of the reduction in serum antithrombin III levels [11].

By contrast, albumin may impact coagulation and hemostasis by enhancing antithrombin III activity and inhibiting platelet function [12, 13]. Albumin may also be associated with hypocoagulability. Dietrich et al. showed an increased bleeding time in vitro [14], suggesting an increased risk of hemorrhage in patients.

Dextrans have been shown to decrease factor VIII levels, increase fibrinolysis, and alter platelet function, with a significant risk of bleeding especially after their high-dose administration [15, 16].

Gelatins were classically thought not to significantly impair coagulation, although recently evidence was presented for their causing platelet dysfunction and clotting disorders [17].

Regarding hydroxyethyl starches (HES), previous literature showed a severe increase of bleeding risk with those of high molecular weight. This is due to a von-Willebrand-like syndrome, with decreased factor VIII activity as well as reductions in von Willebrand factor antigen and factor VIII-related ristocetin cofactor [18-21]. However, fewer effects on the clotting system have been reported for the latest-generation HES.

An impairment of platelet function is another unwanted activity of HES. This effect is more significant in high molecular weight HES (e.g., HES 450/0.7 or HES 200/0.62) than in lower molecular weight preparations [22-24]. Modern HES, when diluted in balanced plasma-adapted solutions, seem to have no negative effects on platelets. In fact, reports have confirmed the importance of the solution in which the HES molecules are dispersed [25].

17.6 Bloodstream Infections

Bloodstream infections are severe infections that can increase patient morbidity and mortality. They are frequently related to the use of intravenous devices and can result in serious complications.

17.6.1 Causes and Risk Factors

The incidence of bloodstream infections related to CVP placement is quite low, even if serious infective complications from peripheral catheter placement may increase the morbidity and length of hospital stay.

Table 17.3 Risk factors of bloodstream infection

Risk factors of bloodstream infection
Central venous catheter
Comorbidity
Compromised immune status
Pathogen virulence
Device material
Non-sterility

The most common cause of bloodstream infections is related to the use of central venous catheters (CVC), particularly in intensive care unit (ICU) patients, with an estimated rate of 5.3 per 1,000 catheter days in the ICU [26]. This reflects the fact that ICU patients often have several comorbidities, including nosocomial infections.

In addition, a CVC may have been inserted under emergency conditions in which a sterile procedure may not have been possible.

The development of bloodstream infections depends on various factors. Pathogens enter the body usually through the skin, eventually colonizing the catheter tip and creating a focus of infection. Nevertheless, this is not enough for the development of a bloodstream infection. Other factors must be present, such as a virulent pathogen with a large adhesive capacity. Also, bloodstream infections often occur in patients with other comorbidities or with a compromised immune status, which may facilitate the infective colonization. Moreover, many intravascular devices are made of materials that favor colonization and the adhesion of microorganisms [27, 28] (Table 17.3).

17.6.2 Prevention

Infusion therapy should include measures that minimize the infection risk associated with intravenous therapy. These measures have an important impact not only on patient outcome but also on management costs. The most generic prevention measures concern hygienic requirements for the operator, antisepsis of the environment and of the instrumentation, and skin disinfection. In addition, catheters and cuffs can be coated or impregnated with antimicrobial or antiseptic agents. There are also materials that hinder the development of infections by preventing the adhesion of microorganisms.

Even the site of catheter insertion may predispose the patient to the development of infections, according to the density of the skin flora at the involved site. Many authors have argued that femoral and jugular catheters are more frequently associated with the risk of infection than subclavian catheters [29-32].

17.7   Venous Air Embolism

Venous air embolism is a possible side effect of fluid therapy that impacts morbidity and mortality. It is the result of a communication between the venous system and an air source. The positive pressure gradient allows the passage of air from the outside (atmospheric pressure) into the vessels (sub-atmospheric pressure) [33].

Generally, when a very small amount of air enters the venous system, it is rapidly reabsorbed without complications. In other cases, it may cause arrhythmias or lead to severe inflammatory disorders in the pulmonary vessels, such as direct endothelial damage and the accumulation of platelets, fibrin, neutrophils, and lipid droplets [34].

17.7.1 Prevention

Measures for the prevention of air embolism must be practiced during both catheter insertion and removal.

During CVC insertion, Trendelenburg position is needed for optimal CVC placement. Catheter removal should take place during a Valsalva maneuver, with the patient either supine or in the Trendelemburg position [35, 36].

Key Concepts
- Recognizing and treating phlebitis
- Treatment of extravasation
- Differences between colloids and crystalloids with respect to hemorrhage and thrombosis
- Risk factors of bloodstream infections
- Definition of venous air embolism

Key Words
- Phlebitis
- Infiltration
- Extravasation
- Hematoma
- Hemorrhage
- Bloodstream infection
- Venous air embolism

Focus on...
- Webster J et al (2010) Clinically-indicated replacement versus routine replacement of peripheral venous catheters. Cochrane Database of Systematic Reviews; Issue 3, Art No: CD007798.DOI: 10.1002/14651858. CD007798.pub2

References

1. Higginson R, Parry A (2011) Phlebitis: treatment, care and prevention. Nursing Times 107:18-21
2. Kohno E et al (2009) Effects of corticosteroids on phlebitis induced by Intravenous infusion of antineoplastic agents in rabbits. International Journal of Medical Sciences 6:218-223
3. Uslusoy E, Mete S (2008) Predisposing factors to phlebitis in patients with peripheral intravenous catheter: a descriptive study. Journal of the American Academy of Nurse Practitioners 20:172-180
4. Malach T et al (2006) Prospective surveillance of phlebitis associated with peripheral intravenous catheters. American Journal of Infection Control 34:308-312
5. Infusion Nurses Society (2006) Infusion Nursing Standards of Practice. Hagerstown, MD JP Lippincott
6. Webster J et al (2010) Clinically-indicated replacement versus routine replacement of peripheral venous catheters. Cochrane Database of Systematic Reviews; Issue 3, Art No: CD007798. DOI: 10.1002/14651858.CD007798.pub2
7. Loewenstein R (2011) Treatment of superficial thrombophlebitis. New England Journal of Medicine 364:380

8. Mermel LA et al (2009) Clinical practice guidelines for the diagnosis and management of intravascular catheter-related infection: update by the Infectious Diseases Society of America. Clinical Infectious Diseases 49:1-45

9. Infusion Nurses Society (2006) Infusion nursing standards of practice. Journal of Infusion Nursing 29(1S):S1-S92

10. Scales K (2008) Vascular access in the acute care setting. In: Dougherty L, Lamb J (eds) Intravenous therapy in nursing practice, 2 edn. Oxford, Blackwell Publishing (III)

11. Ruttmann TG, James MFM, Finlayson J et al (2002) Effects on coagulation of intravenous crystalloid or colloid in patients undergoing peripheral vascular surgery. Br J Anaesth 89:226-307

12. Rajnish KJ et al (2004) Albumin: an overview of its place in current clinical practice. J Indian An

13. Jorgensen KA, Stofferson E (1979) Heparin-like activity of albumin. Thrombos Res 16:573-578

14. Tobias MD, Wambold D, Pilla MA, Greer F (1998) Differential effects of serial hemodilution with hydroxyethyl starch, albumin, and 0.9% saline on whole blood coagulation. J Clin Anesth 8:366-71

15. Moran M, Kapsner C (1987) Acute renal failure associated with elevated plasma oncotic pressure. N Engl J Med 317:150-3

16. Linder P, Ickx B (2006) The effects of colloid solutions on haemostasis. Can J Anesth 53:s30–39

17. Gines A, Fernandez-Esparrach G, Monescillo A et al (1996) Randomized trial comparing albumin, dextran-70 and polygeline in cirrhotic patients with ascites treated by paracentesis. Gastroenterology 111:1002-10

18. DeJonge E, Levi M (2001) Effects of different plasma substitutes on blood coagulation: a comparative review. Crit Care Med 29:1261–7

19. Sanfelippo MJ, Suberviola PD, Geimer NF (1987) Development of a von Willebrand-like syndrome after prolonged use of hydroxyethyl starch. Am J Clin Pharmacol 88:653–5

20. Treib J, Baron JF, Grauer MT, Strauss RG (1999) An international view of hydroxyethyl starches. Intensive Care Med 25:258–68

21. Madjdpour C, Dettori N, Frascarolo P, Burki M, Boll M, Fisch A, Bombeli T, Spahn DR (2005) Molecular weight of hydroxyethyl starch: is there an effect on blood coagulation and pharmacokinetics? Br J Anaesth 94:569–76

22. Kozek-Langenecker SA (2005) Effects of hydroxyethyl starch solutions on hemostasis. Anesthesiology 103:654–60

23. Strauss RG, Pennell BJ, Stump DC (2002) A randomized, blinded trial comparing the hemostatic effects of pentastarch versus hetastarch. Transfusion 42:27–36

24. Haynes GH, Havidich JE, Payne KJ (2004) Why the Food and Drug Administration changed the warning label for hetastarch. Anesthesiology 101:560 –1

25. Treib J, Haass A, Pindur G (1997) Coagulation disorders caused by hydroxyethyl starch. Thromb Haemost 78:974–83

26. CDC. National Nosocomial Infections Surveillance (NNIS) (1998) System report, data summary from October 1986-April 1998. Am J Infect Control 26:522—33

27. Sheth NK, Franson TR, Rose HD, Buckmire FL, Cooper JA, Sohnle PG (1983) Colonization of bacteria on polyvinyl chloride and Teflon intravascular catheters in hospitalized patients. J Clin Microbiol 18:1061-3

28. Ashkenazi S, Weiss E, Drucker MM, Bodey GP (1986) Bacterial adherence to intravenous catheters and needles and its influence by cannula type and bacterial surface hydrophobicity. J Lab Clin Med 107:136-40

29. Heard SO, Wagle M, Vijayakumar E et al (1998) Influence of triple-lumen central venous catheters coated with chlorhexidine and silver sulfadiazine on the incidence of catheter-related bacteremia. Arch Intern Med 158:81-7

30. Goetz AM, Wagener MM, Miller JM, Muder RR (1998) Risk of infection due to central venous catheters: effect of site of placement and catheter type. Infect Control Hosp Epidemiol 19:842-5

31. Durbec O, Viviand X, Potie F, Vialet R, Albanese J, Martin C (1997) A prospective evaluation of the use of femoral venous catheters in critically ill adults. Crit Care Med 25:1986-9
32. Merrer J, De Jonghe B, Golliot F et al (2001) Complications of femoral and subclavian venous catheterization in critically ill patients: a randomized controlled trial. JAMA 286:700-7
33. Van Hulst RA, Klein J, Lachmann B (2003) Gas embolism: pathophysiology and treatment. Clin Physiol Funct Imaging 23:237-46
34. Mirski MA, Lele AV, Fitzsimmons L, Toung TJ (2007) Diagnosis and treatment of vascular air embolism. Anesthesiology 106:164-77
35. Scales K (2008) A practical guide to venepuncture and blood sampling, Nursing Standard 22:29-36
36. Bodenham AR, Simcock L (2009) Complications of central venous access. In: Hamilton H, Bodenham AR (eds) Central venous catheters. Oxford, Wiley Blackwell Publishing, pp 175-205 (III)

Commercially Available Crystalloids and Colloids

18

Marialuisa Vennari, Maria Benedetto and Felice Eugenio Agrò

18.1 Crystalloids on the Market

In this chapter, the main commercially available crystalloids and colloids are reviewed.

The characteristics of each product are described according to pharmaceutical company indications.

18.1.1 Sodium Chloride Injection, Solution (B Braun)

Composition

The properties of a 0.9% sodium chloride injection USP (per mL) are as follows:
- sodium chloride USP 9 mg;
- water for injection USP qs;
- pH adjusted to 5.5 (4.5–7.0) with hydrochloric acid NF;
- pH: 5.5 (4.5–7.0);
- calculated osmolarity: 310 mOsmol/L;
  The electrolytes concentration (mEq/100 mL) is:
- sodium 15.4 ;
- chloride 15.4.

Indications

This intravenous solution is indicated for use in adults and pediatric patients as a source of electrolytes and water for hydration. It is used as a diluent and as a

M.Vennari (✉)
Postgraduate School of Anesthesia and Intensive Care, Anesthesia, Intensive Care and Pain Management Department, University School of Medicine Campus Bio-Medico of Rome, Rome, Italy
e-mail: m.vennari@unicampus.it

F. E. Agrò (ed.), *Body Fluid Management*,
DOI: 10.1007/978-88-470-2661-2_18 © Springer-Verlag Italia 2013

delivery system for the intermittent intravenous administration of compatible drug additives. The prescribing information should be consulted regarding the indications and instructions for drug additives to be administered in this manner.

Contraindications
This solution is contraindicated when the administration of sodium or chloride could be clinically detrimental.

Adverse Reactions
Reactions may occur because of the solution itself or the technique of its administration. Among the reported reactions are: febrile response, infection at the injection site, venous thrombosis or phlebitis extending from the injection site, extravasation, and hypervolemia.

The physician should also be alert to the possibility of adverse reactions to drug additives diluted and administered from the plastic partial-fill container. Prescribing information for drug additives to be administered in this manner should be consulted.

Symptoms may result from an excess or deficit of one or more of the ions present in the solution; therefore, frequent monitoring of electrolyte levels is essential.

Hypernatremia may be associated with edema and an exacerbation of congestive heart failure due to the retention of water, resulting in an expanded extracellular fluid volume.

If an adverse reaction does occur, discontinue the infusion, evaluate the patient, institute appropriate therapeutic countermeasures, and save the remainder of the fluid for examination if deemed necessary [1].

18.1.2   Ringer's (B Braun) (Fig. 18.1)

Composition
One liter of Ringer's solution contains:
- sodium chloride 8.60 g;
- potassium chloride 0.30 g;
- calcium chloride $2H_2O$ 0.33 g;
- water for injection;
  The electrolytes concentration (mmol/L) is:
- sodium 147.20;
- potassium 4.02;
- calcium 2.24;
- chloride 155.70.

Indications
- Irrigation and cleaning during surgical intervention;
- irrigation of wounds and burns;

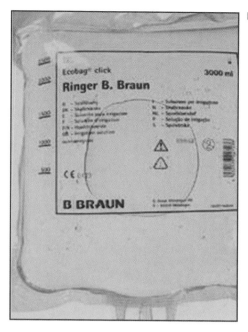

Fig. 18.1 Ringer's

- irrigation during endoscopic examinations of body cavities;
- intra-operative irrigation during arthroscopy with a mechanical instrumentarium;
- postoperative irrigation.

Adverse Side Effects
None are known.

Warning
Do not use for infusion. Only use the solution if the seal of the container is undamaged and the solution is clear. Opened containers must not be saved; quantities left over must be discarded. Store out of reach of children [2].

18.1.3   Ringer Lactate (B Braun) (Fig. 18.2)

Composition
One liter of Ringer's lactate contains:
- sodium chloride 6.00 g;
- potassium chloride 0.30 g;
- calcium chloride $2H_2O$ 0.20 g;
- magnesium chloride $6H_2O$ 0.20 g;

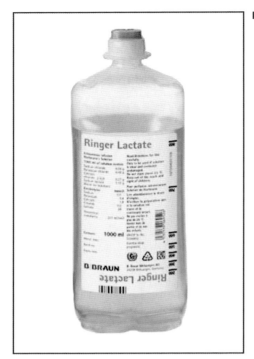

Fig. 18.2 Ringer Lactate

- sodium lactate 3.1 g;
- water for injection;
  The electrolytes concentration (mmol/L) is:
- sodium 130.00;
- potassium 4.00;
- calcium 1.40;
- magnesium 1.00;
- chloride 111.00;
- lactate 28.00.

Indications
- Irrigation and cleaning during surgical intervention;
- irrigation of wounds and burns;
- irrigation during endoscopic examinations of body cavities;
- intra-operative irrigation during arthroscopy with a mechanical instrumentarium;
- postoperative irrigation.

Adverse Side Effects
None are known.

Warning

Do not use for infusion. Only use the solution if the seal of the container is undamaged and the solution is clear. Opened containers must not be saved; quantities left over must be discarded. Store out of reach of children [3].

18.1.4 Plasma-Lyte148 Injection (Baxter) (Fig. 18.3)

Composition

One liter of Plasma-Lyte 148 contains:

- sodium chloride, USP 526 mg;
- sodium gluconate 502 mg;
- sodium acetate trihydrate, USP 368 mg;
- potassium chloride, USP 37 mg;
- magnesium chloride, USP 30 mg;
  It contains no antimicrobial agents.
  The pH is adjusted with hydrochloric acid. The nominal pH is 5.5 (4.0–8.0).

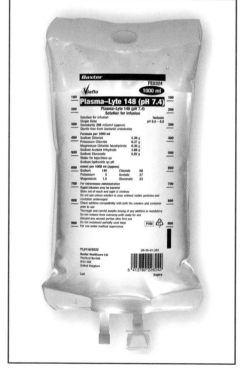

Fig. 18.3 Plasma-Lyte 148 Injection

Indications
Plasma-Lyte 148 injection (multiple electrolytes injection, type 1, USP) is indicated as a source of water and electrolytes or as an alkalinizing agent. It is compatible with blood or blood components and may be administered prior to or following the infusion of blood through the same administration set (i.e., as a priming solution), added to or infused concurrently with blood components, or used as a diluent in the transfusion of packed erythrocytes.

Contraindications
None are known.

Adverse Reactions
Reactions that may occur because of the solution or the administration technique include febrile response, infection at the injection site, venous thrombosis or phlebitis extending from the injection site, extravasation and hypervolemia.

If an adverse reaction does occur, discontinue the infusion, evaluate the patient, institute appropriate therapeutic countermeasures, and save the remainder of the fluid for examination if deemed necessary [4].

18.1.5   Sterofundin (B Braun) (Fig. 18.4)

Composition
One liter of Sterofundin® ISO solution for infusion contains:
- sodium chloride 6.80 g;
- potassium chloride 0.30 g;
- calcium chloride dihydrate 0.37 g;
- magnesium chloride hexahydrate 0.20 g;
- sodium acetate trihydrate 3.27 g;
- L-malic acid 0.67 g;
- excipients;
- water for injection.
  The electrolytes concentration (mmol/L) is:
- sodium 140.0;
- potassium 4.0;
- magnesium 1.0;
- calcium 2.5;
- chloride 127.0;
- acetate 24.0;
- malate 5.0.
  The theoretical osmolarity is 304 mosm/L and the pH is 4.6–5.4.

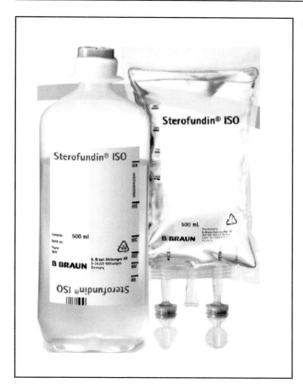

Fig. 18.4 Sterofundin

Indications
Replacement of extracellular fluid losses in the case of isotonic dehydration, in patients in whom acidosis is present or imminent.

Contraindications
Sterofundin ISO must not be administered in the following situations:
- hypervolemia;
- severe congestive cardiac failure;
- renal failure with oliguria or anuria;
- severe general edema;
- hyperkalemia;
- hypercalcemia;
- metabolic alkalosis.

Special Warning
Monitoring of serum electrolytes, fluid balance, and pH is necessary.

Undesirable Effects

Hypersensitivity reactions characterized by urticaria after the intravenous administration of magnesium salts have been occasionally described. Although oral magnesium salts stimulate peristalsis, paralytic ileus has been rarely reported after intravenous infusion of magnesium sulfate. Adverse reactions may be associated with the administration technique and include febrile response, infection at the injection site, local pain or reaction, vein irritation, venous thrombosis or phlebitis extending from the injection site, and extravasation. Adverse reactions also may be associated with the medications added to the solution; the nature of the additive will determine the likelihood of any other undesirable effects [5].

18.2   Colloids on the Market

18.2.1   Dextran$_{70}$

Indication
Shock.

Contraindications
- Known hypersensitivity to dextran or any ingredient in the formulation;
- severe bleeding disorders;
- severe congestive cardiac failure;
- renal failure.

Warnings
Circulatory and/or Volume Overload
May cause circulatory overload; use with caution in patients with impaired renal function, and in those at risk of developing pulmonary edema or cardiac failure.

May cause fluid and/or solute overloading when used as a diluent for serum electrolyte concentrations, overhydration, congested states, or pulmonary edema. The risk of dilutional states is inversely proportional and the risk of solute overloading, resulting in congestion with peripheral and pulmonary edema, directly proportional to the electrolyte concentration of the solution.

Hematologic Effects
Dextran$_{70}$ may interfere with platelet function, especially at doses of approximately 15 mL/kg; use with caution in patients with thrombocytopenia.

Transient prolongation of bleeding time is possible in patients receiving > 1000 mL or approximately 15 mL/kg; a slight increase in bleeding tendency may also occur.

Dextran$_{70}$ causes a marked decrease in factor VIII and an even larger decrease in factors V and IX than expected from the effects of hemodilution alone. These effects usually occur at doses of ~15 mL/kg. Trauma and major surgery patients should be observed for early signs of bleeding complications. The hematocrit should be determined after dextran$_{70}$ administration, avoiding a reduction below 30% by volume.

Increased rouleaux formation is possible; blood samples for typing and cross-matching should be drawn prior to dextran infusion. A sample of the infusion should be reserved for subsequent analysis, if necessary.

Administration of large volumes of dextran solution decreases plasma protein concentrations.

Gastrointestinal Effects
Vomiting and involuntary defecation have occurred in anesthetized patients. Use with caution in patients with pathologic abdominal conditions or in patients undergoing bowel surgery.

Sensitivity Reactions
Hypersensitivity reactions, e.g., urticaria, nasal congestion, wheezing, tightness of chest, and mild hypotension, may occur. These are usually relieved by antihistamines.

Dextran-Induced Anaphylactoid Reactions
Severe dextran-induced anaphylactoid reactions (DIAR), e.g., generalized urticaria, wheezing, hypotension, severe hypotension, shock, cardiac and respiratory arrest, and even death, are rare. They typically occur early in the infusion period in patients with no previous exposure to dextran$_{70}$. Closely monitor these patients, especially during the first minutes of infusion. If severe hypotension occurs, determine whether it is the result of dextran or the initially present shock.

Administration of 20 mL of dextran$_1$ prior to dextran$_{70}$ infusion decreases the likelihood of DIAR; however, serious reactions still may occur.

Discontinue dextran at the first sign of an allergic reaction so long as circulation can be maintained by other means. Immediate medical intervention (e.g., parenteral epinephrine, antihistamines, and other supportive therapy) may relieve symptoms. If circulatory collapse due to anaphylaxis occurs after dextran discontinuation, begin rapid volume substitutions with another agent.

Resuscitative measures should be kept readily available during dextran use.

Local Injection-Site Reactions
Adverse local reactions caused by the IV administration of dextran$_{70}$ include febrile response, infection at the injection site, venous thrombosis or phlebitis extending from the injection site, extravasation, and hypervolemia. If such reactions occur, discontinue the infusion, evaluate the patient, institute appropriate therapeutic countermeasures, and save the remainder of the solution for examination if deemed necessary [6].

18.2.2   Dextran$_{40}$

Indications
* Shock;
* extracorporeal circulation;
* prophylaxis of thromboembolic disorders.

Contraindications
* Known hypersensitivity to dextran or any ingredient in the formulation;
* marked cardiac decompensation;
* renal disease with severe oliguria or anuria;
* marked hemostatic defects of all types (e.g., thrombocytopenia, hypofibrinogenemia), including those caused by drugs (e.g., heparin, warfarin);
* some clinicians consider extreme dehydration a contraindication to dextran 40 therapy.

Warnings
Circulatory and/or Volume Overload

Dextran$_{40}$ is a hypertonic colloidal solution; vascular overload may occur with large doses. Central venous pressure should be closely monitored when the drug is administered by rapid infusion and in patients with poor hydration status needing additional fluid therapy. Immediately discontinue the drug if there is a precipitous rise in central venous pressure or any clinical signs of circulatory overloading. Dextran$_{40}$ may cause fluid and/or solute overloading (especially when large doses are administered), resulting in dilution of serum electrolytes, overhydration, congested states, or pulmonary edema. Do not administer to patients with pulmonary edema; use with caution in those with cardiac decompensation and cardiac failure. The risk of dilutional states is inversely proportional, and the risk of solute overloading, resulting in congestion with peripheral and pulmonary edema, directly proportional to the electrolyte concentration of the solution.

Renal Effects

Increases in the viscosity and specific gravity of urine, especially in patients with decreased urine flow, may occur. Typically, specific gravity increases only slightly in adequately hydrated patients with normal renal function; however, tubular stasis and blocking are reported even in adequately hydrated patients. Low specific gravity of urine during dextran therapy may indicate a failure of renal dextran clearance; in which case dextran should be discontinued. Assess hydration before dextran administration and administer additional fluid if signs of dehydration are present. If the decreased urinary output is secondary to shock, dextran$_{40}$ can still be used so long as urinary output improves after administration of the drug.

Monitor urinary flow rates during administration; discontinue therapy if oliguria or anuria occurs and administer an osmotic diuretic to minimize vascular overloading. Renal failure has been reported, particularly in extremely dehydrated patients. Excessive doses of dextran may precipitate renal failure in patients with advanced renal disease; thus, dosage recommendations should be followed. Tubular vacuolization (osmotic nephrosis) may also occur but is potentially reversible; its clinical importance is not fully known. Abnormal renal function test results are more likely in patients who have undergone surgery or cardiac catheterization. A specific effect of dextran$_{40}$ on renal function has not yet been determined.

Hepatic Effects
Abnormal hepatic function test results (increased AST and ALT) have been reported, generally in patients who have undergone surgery or cardiac catheterization. A specific effect of dextran$_{40}$ on hepatic function has not yet been determined.

Metabolic Effects
Mild to moderate acidosis (usually transient) may develop during perfusion with any priming fluid in pump oxygenators. This condition is not altered by dextran$_{40}$ administration and thus may require an alkalinizing agent.

Hematologic Effects
Dextran$_{40}$ may interfere with platelet function and therefore should be used with caution in patients with thrombocytopenia. A transient prolongation of bleeding time is possible in patients receiving > 1 L of 10% dextran$_{40}$ solution; a slight increase in the bleeding tendency may also occur.

Dextran$_{40}$ causes a marked decrease in factor VIII and an even greater decrease in factors V and IX than expected from the effects of hemodilution alone. Usually, these effects are seen at doses of ~1.5 g/kg (15 mL/kg). Trauma and major surgery patients should be monitored for early signs of bleeding complications. A slightly increased blood loss is possible in postoperative patients. Additional blood loss may occur in patients with active hemorrhage because of the increase in perfusion pressure and improved blood flow. The hematocrit should be determined after the administration of dextran$_{40}$, avoiding reductions below 30% by volume. An increase in rouleaux formation is possible. Blood samples for typing and cross-matching should be drawn prior to dextran infusion. A sample of the administered dextran should be reserved for subsequent use, if necessary. The administration of large volumes of dextran solution reduces plasma protein concentrations.

Sensitivity Reactions
Mild urticarial reactions have been reported.

Dextran-Induced Anaphylactoid Reactions
Severe dextran-induced anaphylactoid reactions, e.g., generalized urticaria, tightness of the chest, wheezing, hypotension, nausea, vomiting, severe

hypotension, shock, cardiac and respiratory arrest, and even death, are rare. They typically occur early in the infusion period in patients with no previous exposure to dextran$_{40}$, even with doses as small as 0.5 g (5 mL). Closely monitor patients with no previous exposure to dextran, especially during the first few minutes of infusion. The administration of 20 mL of dextran$_1$ prior to dextran$_{40}$ infusion decreases the likelihood of anaphylactoid reactions; however, serious reactions may still occur. Discontinue dextran at the first sign of allergic reaction so long as circulation can be maintained by other means. Immediate medical intervention (e.g., parenteral epinephrine, antihistamines, and other supportive therapy) may relieve symptoms. If circulatory collapse due to anaphylaxis occurs after dextran discontinuation, begin rapid volume substitutions with another agent. Resuscitative measures should be kept readily available during dextran use [7].

18.2.3   Gelatin: Gelofusine (B Braun) (Fig. 18.5)

Composition
A 1-L infusion solution contains the following active ingredients:
- succinylated gelatin;

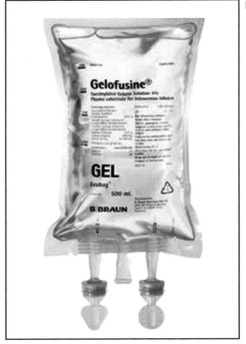

Fig. 18.5 Gelofusine

- water for injections.
  The electrolytes concentrations (mmol/L) are:
- sodium 154;
- chloride 120;
  The relevant physico-chemical characteristics are:
- theoretical osmolarity 274 mOsm/L;
- pH 7.1–7.7;
- gel point ≤ 3 °C.

Indications

Gelofusine can be used as a colloidal volume substitute for:
- prophylaxis and treatment of absolute and relative hypovolemia (e.g., following shock due to hemorrhage or trauma, perioperative blood losses, burns, sepsis);
- prophylaxis of hypotension (e.g., in connection with the induction of epidural or spinal anesthesia);
- hemodilution;
- extra-corporeal circulation (heart-lung machine, hemodialysis);
- increasing the leukocyte yield in leukapheresis.

Contraindications

Gelofusine must not be administered in cases of:
- known hypersensitivity to gelatin;
- hypervolemia;
- hyperhydration;
- severe cardiac insufficiency;
- severe disturbance of blood coagulation.
  Gelofusine may only be administered with great caution in cases of:
- hypernatremia, since additional sodium is administered with Gelofusine;
- dehydration, since in such cases it is primarily the fluid balance that requires correction;
- disturbance of blood coagulation, since administration leads to the dilution of coagulation factors;
- renal insufficiency, since the normal excretion route may be impaired;
- chronic liver disease, since the synthesis of albumin and coagulation factors may be affected and administration brings about a further dilution.

Undesirable Effects

As with all colloidal volume substitutes, allergic (anaphylactic/anaphlactoid) reactions of varying severity can occur after Gelofusine infusion. These can either manifest themselves as skin reactions (urticaria) or result in a flushing of the face and neck. In rare cases, there is a drop in blood pressure, shock, or cardiac and respiratory arrest. The information contained in the standard product information may differ from nationally approved indications, contraindications, etc. [8].

18.2.4   Geloplasma (Fresenius Kabi)

Composition
A 100-ml solution for infusion contains:
- modified liquid gelatin (partially hydrolyzed and succinylated);
- amount expressed as anhydrous gelatin 3.0000 g;
- sodium chloride 0.5382 g;
- magnesium chloride hexahydrated 0.0305 g;
- potassium chloride 0.0373 g;
- sodium (S)-lactate solution;
- amount expressed as sodium lactate 0.3360 g.

   The product contains 0.06% succinic acid as a result of the manufacturing process.

Ionic formula (mmol/l):
- sodium 150;
- potassium 5;
- magnesium 1.5;
- chloride 100;
- lactate 30.

Indications
Emergency treatment of patients in shock:
- hypovolemic shock resulting from: hemorrhage, dehydration, capillary leak, burns;
- vasoplegic shock of traumatic, surgical, septic, or toxic origin.

Treatment of relative hypovolemia associated with hypotension in the context of vasoplegia related to the effects of hypotensive drugs, notably during anesthesia.

Contraindications
Geloplasma must not be used in the following situations:
- known or suspected hypersensitivity to gelatin solutions;
- predominantly extracellular hyperhydration;
- hyperkalemia;
- metabolic alkalosis;
- end of pregnancy.

Adverse Reactions
- Anaphylactic shock;
- allergic skin reaction;
- hypotension;
- slowing of heart rate;

- respiratory difficulties;
- fever, chills [9].

18.2.5 Haemaccel (Piramal Healthcare)

Composition
A 100-mL solution contains:
- polygeline polypeptides of degraded gelatin, cross-linked via urea bridges 3.5 g (equivalent to 0.63g of nitrogen);
- sodium chloride Ph. Eur. 0.85 g;
- potassium chloride Ph. Eur. 0.038 g;
- calcium chloride Ph. Eur. 0.070 g;
- water for injection Ph. Eur.q.s..
  The electrolytes concentration (mmol/L) is:
- sodium 145;
- potassium 5.1;
- calcium 6.25;
- chloride 145.

The mean molecular weight is 30,000.

Indications
Haemaccel is a plasma substitute for volume replacement; it is used to correct or avert circulatory insufficiency due to plasma/blood volume deficiency, either absolute (e.g., resulting from bleeding) or relative (e.g., resulting from a shift in plasma volume between circulatory compartments).

Haemaccel is administered in the following situations:
- hypovolemic shock;
- loss of blood and plasma (e.g. due to trauma, burns, autologous blood or plasma donation prior to surgery);
- heart-lung machine filling.
  In addition Haemaccel can be used as a carrier solution for various drugs.

Contraindications
- Known hypersensitivity to constituents of the preparation;
- existing severe allergic reactions.

The use of Haemaccel is restricted in all conditions in which an increase in intravascular (blood vessel) volume and its consequences (e.g., increased stroke volume, elevated blood pressure) or an increase in interstitial fluid volume or hemodilution could pose a particular risk for the patient. Examples of such conditions are: congestive heart failure, hypertension, esophageal varices, pulmonary edema, hemorrhagic diathesis, renal and postrenal anuria. If the physician considers the infusion necessary, it should be given while taking special precautions:

Caution is also advised in all patients at an increased risk of histamine release, e.g., those with allergic/allergoid reactions or a history of histamine response.

In the above cases, Haemaccel may be given only after taking appropriate prophylactic steps (see Measures of precaution for administration). Use of the preparation in pregnant women and nursing mothers is not contraindicated. Generally, however, particular care is required when fluid or volume replacements are administered during or immediately after pregnancy.

Side Effects
During or after the infusion of plasma substitutes, transient skin reactions (urticaria, wheals), hypotension may occur. Tachycardia, bradycardia, nausea/vomiting, dyspnea, increases in temperature and/or chills are occasionally seen. Rare cases of severe hypersensitivity reactions, even including life-threatening shock, have been observed. Here, the required treatment depends on the nature and severity of the side effect. During the administration of polygeline infusion under pressure, air embolism has been reported albeit very rarely.

If side effects occur, the infusion should be discontinued at once. For mild reactions, administer antihistamines. For severe reactions, if appropriate, immediately inject catecholamines, slowly i.v., plus high doses of corticosteroids, slowly i.v., together with volume replacement and oxygen. Histamine release has been shown to be the cause of anaphylactoid side effects associated with infusions of Haemaccel. Histamine-induced reactions are more likely if the infusion has been rapid.

Furthermore, the above-described reactions may occur as a result of the cumulative effect of several histamine-releasing drugs, e.g., anesthetics, muscle relaxants, analgesics, ganglia blockers, and anticholinergic drugs [10].

18.2.6 Gelaspan (B Braun)

Composition
A 1-L solution contains:
- succinylated gelatin (= modified fluid gelatin) 40.0 g (molecular weight, weight average: 26 500 Daltons);
- sodium chloride 5.55 g;
- sodium acetate trihydrate 3.27 g;
- potassium chloride 0.30 g;
- calcium chloride dihydrate 0.15 g;
- magnesium chloride hexahydrate 0.20 g;
  The electrolytes concentration (mmol/l) is:
- sodium 151;
- chloride 103;

- potassium 4;
- calcium 1;
- magnesium 1;
- acetate 24;
- excipients.

Indications
Gelaspan is a colloidal plasma volume substitute in an isotonic, fully balanced electrolyte solution for the prophylaxis and treatment of imminent or manifest, relative or absolute hypovolemia and shock.

Contraindications
Gelaspan must not be used in the following situations:
- hypersensitivity to gelatin solutions or to any of the other ingredients of Gelaspan;
- hypervolemia;
- hyperhydration;
- hyperkalemia.

Undesirable Effects
- Anaphylactoid reactions;
- tachycardia;
- hypotension;
- respiratory difficulties;
- allergic skin reactions;
- mild transient increase of body temperature, fever, chills [11].

18.2.7 HES 450/0.7/5: HESPAN (B Braun) (Fig. 18.6)

Composition
Hespan (6% hetastarch in 0.9% sodium chloride injection) is a sterile, non-pyrogenic solution for intravenous administration. A 100-mL solution contains:
- hetastarch: 6 g;
- sodium chloride, USP: 0.9 g;
- water for injection, USP: qs;
- pH adjusted with sodium hydroxide, NF if necessary;
  The electrolytes concentration (mEq/L) is:
- sodium 154;
- chloride 154.

The pH is approximately 5.9, with negligible buffering capacity. The calculated osmolarity is approximately 309 mOsM.

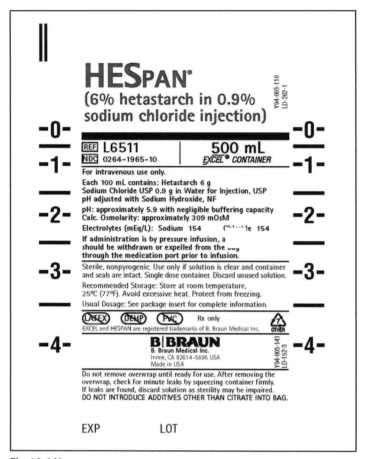

Fig. 18.6 Hespan

Indications

Hespan is indicated in the treatment of hypovolemia, when plasma volume expansion is desired. It is not a substitute for blood or plasma. The adjunctive use of Hespan in leukapheresis has been shown to be safe and efficacious in improving granulocyte harvesting and in increasing the yield of these cells by centrifugal means.

Contraindications

Hespan is contraindicated in patients with known hypersensitivity to hydroxyethyl starch (HES). It is also contraindicated in clinical conditions in which volume overload is a potential problem, such as congestive heart failure or renal disease with anuria or oliguria not related to hypovolemia. Patients with pre-existing coagulation or bleeding disorders should not be given Hespan.

Adverse Reactions
Hypersensitivity
Death, life-threatening anaphylactic/anaphylactoid reactions, cardiac arrest, ventricular fibrillation, severe hypotension, non-cardiac pulmonary edema, laryngeal edema, bronchospasm, angioedema, wheezing, restlessness, tachypnea, stridor, fever, chest pain, bradycardia, tachycardia, shortness of breath, chills, urticaria, pruritus, facial and periorbital edema, coughing, sneezing, flushing, erythema multiforme, and rash.

Cardiovascular
Circulatory overload, congestive heart failure, and pulmonary edema.

Hematologic
Intracranial bleeding, bleeding and/or anemia due to hemodilution and/or factor Vlll deficiency, acquired von Willebrand's-like syndrome, and coagulopathy, including rare cases of disseminated intravascular coagulopathy and hemolysis.

Metabolic
Metabolic acidosis.

Other
Vomiting, peripheral edema of the lower extremities, submaxillary and parotid glandular enlargement, mild influenza-like symptoms, headaches, and muscle pain have all been reported.

HES-associated pruritus has developed in some patients with HES deposits in peripheral nerves [12].

18.2.8 HES 260/0.45: Pentaspan (Bristol-Myers Squibb Canada)

Composition
A 100 mL solution contains the following:
- pentastarch 10.0 g;
- sodium chloride USP 0.9 g;
- water for injection USP qs.

The pH is adjusted with sodium hydroxide. The approximate electrolytes concentration (mEq/L) is:
- sodium 154;
- chloride 154.

The pH is ~5.0 and the calculated osmolality ~326 mOsm/kg.

Indications

Pentaspan is indicated when plasma volume expansion is desired as an adjunct in the management of shock due to hemorrhage, surgery, sepsis, burns, or other trauma. It is not a substitute for red blood cells or coagulation factors in plasma.

Contraindications

Pentaspan is contraindicated in patients with known hypersensitivity to HES, or with bleeding disorders, or with congestive heart failure in which volume overload is a potential problem. Pentaspan should not be used in patients with renal disease and oliguria or anuria not related to hypovolemia.

Adverse Reactions

Coagulation disorders or hemorrhage have been reported in association with the use of Pentaspan as a plasma volume expander. Headache, diarrhea, nausea, weakness, temporary weight gain, insomnia, fatigue, fever, edema, paresthesia, acne, malaise, shakiness, dizziness, chest pain, chills, nasal congestion, anxiety, and increased heart rate have also been reported in clinical studies involving Pentaspan. It is uncertain whether these adverse experiences are attributable to the drug, the medical procedures, concurrent adjunctive medication, or a combination of these factors. Hypersensitivity (wheezing, urticaria, and hypotension) has also been described, as have anaphylactic/anaphylactoid reactions [13].

18.2.9 HES 130/0.4: Voluven (Fresenius Kabi)

Composition

A 100-mL solution contains:
- poly (O-2-hydroxyethyl) starch 6.00 g (molar substitution: 0.4; mean molecular weight: 130,000 Da);
- sodium chloride 0.90 g;
- water for injection qs;
  The pH is adjusted with sodium hydroxide qs or with hydrochloric acid. The approximate electrolytes concentration of (mmol/L) is:
- sodium (Na+) 154;
- chloride (Cl-) 154.
  The theoretical osmolarity is 308 mosmol/L.
  The pH is 4.0–5.5; titratable acidity is < 1.0 mmol NaOH/L.

Indications

Voluven (6% HES 130/0.4) is indicated for the treatment of hypovolemia when plasma volume expansion is required. It is not a substitute for red blood cells or coagulation factors in plasma.

Contraindications

Voluven is contraindicated:
- in patients with fluid overload (hyperhydration) and especially in cases of pulmonary edema and congestive cardiac failure;
- in patients with known hypersensitivity to HES;
- in patients with intracranial bleeding.
  Voluven should not be used:
- in renal failure with oliguria or anuria not related to hypovolemia;
- in patients receiving dialysis treatment;
- in patients with severe hypernatremia or severe hyperchloremia.

Adverse Reactions

Adverse reactions with Voluven, have been reported spontaneously, in clinical trials and in the literature. Anaphylactoid reactions (mild influenza-like symptoms, bradycardia, tachycardia, bronchospasm, non-cardiac pulmonary edema) may occur due to solutions containing HES but are rare. If a hypersensitivity reaction occurs, administration of the drug should be discontinued immediately and the appropriate treatment and supportive measures undertaken until symptoms have resolved.

The concentration of serum amylase commonly rises during HES administration and can interfere with the diagnosis of pancreatitis.

Pruritus is a known complication of HES administration, although it is typically more common with the prolonged use of high doses. In a pivotal study, in which patients were monitored for 28 days postoperatively, pruritus occurred in 10.2% of the patients in the Voluven group and 9.8% of those in the HES group. In both groups, pruritus was mild and self-limiting. However, HES-induced pruritus may be delayed in onset, typically 1–6 weeks after exposure; it may be severe, of protracted (weeks and months) duration, and is generally unresponsive to therapy. The decreased molecular weight of Volvulen, its lower degree of substitution, decreased tissue storage and intravascular persistence in conjunction with a shorter plasma half-life may lower the incidence of pruritus related to its use.

At high doses, dilution effects may commonly result in a corresponding dilution of blood components, such as coagulation factors and other plasma proteins, and in a decrease in the hematocrit. With the administration of HES, blood coagulation disturbances can occur in rare cases, depending on the dosage [14].

18.2.10 HES 130/0.42: Venofundin (B Braun) (Fig. 18.7)

Composition
- Poly(O-2-hydroxyethyl)starch (HES) 60.0 g (molar substitution: 0.42); mean molecular weight: 130,000 Da);
- sodium chloride 9.0 g

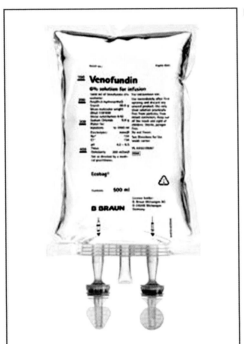

Fig. 18.7 Venofundin

The electrolytes concentration (mmol/L) is:
- sodium 154;
- chloride 154.

The pH is 4.0–6.5; the titration acidity is < 1.0 mmol/L; and the theoretical osmolarity is 309 mOsmol/L.

Indications
Treatment and prophylaxis of hypovolemia and shock.

Contraindications
- Hyperhydration states including pulmonary edema;
- renal failure with oliguria or anuria;
- intracranial bleeding;
- severe hypernatremia or severe hyperchloremia;
- hypersensitivity to HES or to any of the excipients;
- severely impaired hepatic function;
- congestive cardiac failure.

Undesiderable Effects
After HES administration, anaphylactic reactions of varying degrees may

occur. Therefore, all patients given starch infusions must be monitored close-ly for anaphylactic reactions. In case of their occurrence, the Venofundin infu-sion should be stopped immediately, followed by the administration of the usual acute-treatment measures. There may be a drop in the hematocrit and in the concentration of plasma proteins due to blood dilution. Increasing doses of HES infusions lead to the dilution of coagulation factors and may thereby affect blood coagulation. Bleeding time and aPTT may be extended and the level of factor VIII/von Willebrand factor complex reduced after the adminis-tration of large doses. Generally, repeated infusions of HES over several days, especially when high cumulative doses are reached, may lead to pruritus that hardly responds to any form of therapy. Pruritus can appear even several weeks after the termination of HES infusions and may persist for months [15].

18.2.11 HES 130/0.42: Plasma Volume (Baxter)

Composition
A 1-L solution contains:
- poly(O-2-hydroxyethyl) starch (HES) 60.0 g (molar substitution: 0.42); (mean molecular weight: 130 000 Da);
- sodium chloride 6.00 g;
- potassium chloride 0.400 g;
- calcium chloride dihydrate 0.134 g;
- magnesium chloride hexahydrate 0.200 g;
- sodium acetate trihydrate 3.70 g;
  The electrolytes concentration (mmol/L) is:
- sodium 130;
- potassium 5.36;
- calcium 0.912;
- magnesium 0.984;
- chloride 112;
- acetate 27.2.
  The pH is 5.0–7.0; the theoretical osmolarity is ~277 mOsmol/L.

Indications
Treatment of imminent or manifest hypovolemia and hypovolemic shock.

Contraindications
- Hyperhydration states, including pulmonary edema and congestive heart failure;
- renal failure with oliguria or anuria;
- intracranial bleeding;
- known hypersensitivity to HES or any of the excipients;
- severely impaired hepatic function.

Undesirable Effects

Adverse reactions are assessed based on the following frequency rates: very common ($\geq$ 1/10), common ($\geq$ 1/100 to < 1/10), uncommon ($\geq$ 1/1000 to < 1/100), rare ($\geq$ 1/10,000 to < 1/1000), very rare (< 1/10,000), not known (cannot be estimated from the available data). The most commonly reported adverse reactions are directly related to the therapeutic effects of starch solutions and the doses administered, e.g. hemodilution resulting from expansion of the intravascular space without the concurrent administration of blood components. Dilution of coagulation factors may also occur. Very rare hypersensitivity reactions are not dose-dependent.

Disorders of the Blood and Lymphatic System

A very common side effect is a decreased hematocrit and a reduction in the plasma protein concentration as a result of hemodilution. Common (dose-dependent) reactions are associated with higher doses of HES, which cause the dilution of coagulation factors and may thus affect blood clotting. Bleeding time and aPTT may be increased and the concentration of the factor VIII/von Willebrand factor complex may be reduced after the administration of high doses.

Immune System Disorders

Anaphylactic reactions of varying intensity are rare.

General Disorders and Administration-Site Conditions

While uncommon, the repeated infusion of HES for many days, especially if high cumulative doses are reached, usually leads to pruritus that responds very poorly to therapy. It may appear several weeks after the end of the starch infusions and may persist for months. The likelihood of this adverse effect has not been adequately studied for plasma volume Redibag.

Laboratory Tests

Very commonly, HES infusion produces elevated serum concentrations of α-amylase. This effect is the result of the formation of an amylase complex with HES, with delayed renal and extrarenal elimination. It should not be misinterpreted as evidence of a pancreatic disorder. It will disappear 3–5 days after administration.

Anaphylactic Reactions

Anaphylactic reactions of varying intensity may occur after HES administration. All patients receiving starch infusions should therefore be closely monitored. Similarly, the outcome and severity of any such reaction cannot be predicted for any given patient. In the case of an anaphylactic reaction, the infusion must be stopped immediately and suitable emergency measures instituted. There are no specific tests identifying those patients who are likely to suffer an anaphylactic reaction. Equally, the outcome and severity of any such reaction cannot be predicted. Hepatic dysfunction, perhaps due to starch accumulation, has been observed with other HES products. The prophylactic use of corticosteroids has not proved to be effective [16].

18.2.12 HES 130/0.42/6:1: Tetraspan (B Braun) (Fig. 18.8)

Composition
- Poly(O-2-hydroxyethyl) starch (HES) 60.0 g (molar substitution: 0.42); (average molecular weight: 130,000 Da);
- sodium chloride 6.25 g;
- potassium chloride 0.30 g;
- calcium chloride dihydrate 0.37 g;
- magnesium chloride hexahydrate 0.20 g;
- sodium acetate trihydrate 3.27 g;
- L-malic acid 0.67 g; (= mmol/L: Na+ 140, K+ 4.0, Ca2+ 2.5, Mg2+ 1.0;
- Cl- 118, acetate- 24, malate2–5).
  The pH is 5.6–6.4; the theoretical osmolarity is 297 mOsmol/l.

Indications
Treatment of impending or manifest hypovolemia and shock.

Contraindications
- Hyperhydration states, including pulmonary edema;
- renal failure with oliguria or anuria;

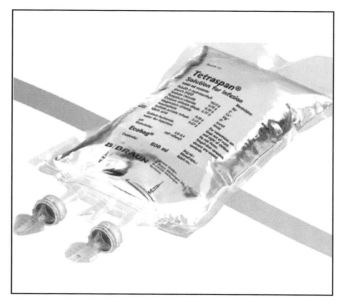

Fig. 18.8 Tetraspan

- intracranial hemorrhage;
- hyperkalemia;
- severe hypernatremia or severe hyperchloremia;
- hypersensitivity to any of the excipients;
- severely impaired hepatic function;
- congestive heart failure.

Undesirable Effects

After HES administration, anaphylactic reactions of varying degrees may occur. Therefore, all patients given starch infusions must be monitored closely. In case of an anaphylactic reaction, the Tetraspan infusion should be stopped immediately, followed by the administration of the usual acute-treatment measures. A drop in the hematocrit and in the concentration of plasma proteins, due to blood dilution, may occur. Increasing doses of HES infusions lead to the dilution of coagulation factors and may thereby affect blood coagulation. Bleeding time and aPTT may be extended and the level of factor VIII/von Willebrand factor complex reduced after the administration of large doses. Generally, repeated infusions of HES over several days, especially when high cumulative doses are reached, can lead to pruritus that hardly responds to therapy. The pruritus can appear even several weeks after the termination of HES infusions and may persist for months [17].

This chapter has highlighted the features, indications, and side effects of the main commercially available products. Here, they have been discussed according to the type of solution, colloid or crystalloid, and in the ascending order of their development, from first-generation to the latest-generation. A feature of the latter is that they are balanced and plasma-adapted.

References

1. http://dailymed.nlm.nih.gov/dailymed/drugInfo.cfm?id=59707. Accessed 03/28/2012
2. http://www.bbraun.com/cps/rde/xchg/bbraun-com/hs.xsl/products.html?prid=PRID00000874. Accessed 03/28/2012
3. http://www.bbraun.com/cps/rde/xchg/bbraun-com/hs.xsl/products.html?prid=PRID00000126. Accessed 03/28/2012
4. http://www.accessdata.fda.gov/drugsatfda_docs/label/2009/017451s060,017378s065lbl.pdf. Accessed 03/28/2012
5. http://www.bbraun.de/cps/rde/xchg/bbraun-de/hs.xsl/products.html?prid=PRID00003097. Accessed 03/28/2012
6. http://www.drugs.com/monograph/dextran-70.html. Accessed 03/28/2012
7. http://www.drugs.com/monograph/dextran-40.html. Accessed 03/28/2012
8. http://www.bbraun.ph/cps/rde/xchg/cw-bbraun-en-ph/hs.xsl/products.html?prid=PRID000 00740. Accessed 03/28/2012
9. http://www.fresenius-kabi.com/6240.htm. Accessed 03/29/2012
10. http://www.piramalcriticalcare.com/products/polygeline/product-info.html#cd. Accessed 03/29/2012
11. http://www.bbraun.com/cps/rde/xchg/bbraun-com/hs.xsl/products.html?id=00020742770000 000152&prid=PRID00007103. Accessed 03/29/2012

12.   http://www.pharmcorpmaine.com/MSDS/Hespan_PI.pdf. Accessed 03/29/2012
13.   http://www.bmscanada.ca/static/products/en/pm_pdf/Pentaspan_EN_PDF.pdf. Accessed 03/29/2012
14.   http://www.fresenius-kabi.ca/pdfs/Voluven%20Product%20Monograph%20Eng%20Oct07.pdf. Accessed 03/29/2012
15.   http://www.bbraun.com/cps/rde/xchg/bbraun-com/hs.xsl/products.html?id=00020742770000000152&prid=PRID00001276. Accessed 03/30/2012
16.   http://www.ecomm.baxter.com/ecatalog/loadResource.do?bid=44366. Accessed 04/02/2012
17.   http://www.bbraun.com/cps/rde/xchg/bbraun-com/hs.xsl/products.html?prid=PRID00003763 04/02/2012

Pharmaco-Economics

19

Felice Eugenio Agrò, Umberto Benedetto and Chiara Candela

When limited economic resources are available, it is necessary to compare the costs and benefits of two (or more) available alternatives. The aim of health economics is to determine the most efficient way to spend limited resources [1].

Pharmaco-economics has been defined as "the description and analysis of the costs of drug therapy to health care systems and society" [1]. In short, pharmaco-economics searches, identifies, measures, and compares the costs and clinical effects of drugs. Spending on drug therapies is one of the main objects of study in pharmaco-economics, mainly because it accounts for a very significant proportion of national budgets, representing about 15% of the health budgets of many nations [1]. This is particularly relevant for patients with multiple chronic conditions, who require several medications [2]. The impressive rise in healthcare system expenditures seen in the last years is largely explained by increased spending on chronic conditions. In the USA, the care of patients with chronic diseases accounts for 78% of that country's health spending [3].

19.1 Costs and Benefits

The key concept in pharmaco-economics is opportunity cost, which does not refer to the costs and benefits of a new treatment but to its added costs and benefits over and above those of the existing treatment.

Costs can be classified as follows:
* *Direct* costs are those spent by the healthcare funder for a specific service or goods, including drug acquisition costs.

U. Benedetto (✉)
Postgraduate School of Anesthesia and Intensive Care, Anesthesia, Intensive Care and Pain Management Department, University School of Medicine, Campus Bio-Medico of Rome, Rome, Italy
e-mail: u2benedetto@libero.it

F. E. Agrò (ed.), *Body Fluid Management*,
DOI: 10.1007/978-88-470-2661-2_19 © Springer-Verlag Italia 2013

- *Indirect* costs are not directly related to a specific item, such as those for administrative staff, equipment rental, and travel to and from the hospital.
- *Intangible* costs are unquantifiable because they cannot be related to a specific service or good; an example is engineering costs. These cannot be measured in terms of money; instead, they only measure quality of life.

  The expected benefits from an intervention can be measured in:
- *Natural* units, which refer to tangible events such as years of life saved and strokes prevented.
- *Utility* units, which refer to the quality-of-health status.

The quality-adjusted life year (QALY) is the most common measure used in health economics. It considers both the quality and the quantity of life and is calculated as Estimated survival × Estimated quality of life (relative to perfect health).

Cost–benefit or outcome analyses are performed using the four common types of economic evaluation discussed below.

19.1.1   Cost Minimization Analysis (CMA)

The CMA is a cost analysis comparing the costs of different, clinically equivalent strategies. As expected, the cheapest therapy is the generally preferred strategy, assuming the same results.

19.1.2   Cost Effectiveness Analysis (CEA)

A CEA evaluation considers health benefits in natural units (e.g., years of life saved, ulcers healed) whereas the costs are considered in terms of money. For instance, in severe reflux esophagitis, it is possible to compare the costs per patient who achieves symptom relief using a proton pump inhibitor compared to those resulting from patients using H2 blockers. The key measure is the incremental cost effectiveness ratio (ICER), expressed as (cost of drug A – cost of drug B)/(benefit of drug A- benefit of drug B).

The four possible results arising in a CEA are the following (Fig. 19.1):
1) If the costs of a new drug are lower and the resulting health benefits higher, this would be the preferred treatment.
2) If the new drug is more expensive but less effective, it is not recommended.
3) Commonly, the new drug is more effective but more expensive than the standard treatment. Based on the ICER, it is necessary to determine whether the extra benefits justify the additional costs, i.e., if the new drug is "cost-effective." This can be evaluated using a threshold value, previously established.

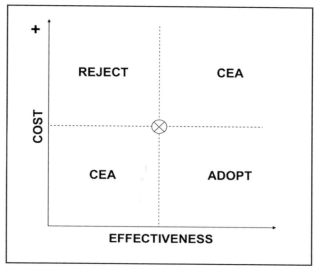

Fig. 19.1 Four possible results arising in a cost effectiveness analysis

4) Finally, the new drug is more expensive but more effective than the standard treatment. This case is similar to the previous one. The extra benefits are assessed to determine whether they justify the additional costs if the new drug becomes the preferred treatment.

19.1.3   Cost Utility Analysis (CUA)

The CUA considers a specific outcome, evaluating the costs to reach a goal measured in money. However, in this analysis, the outcome is measured in terms of survival and quality of life. Thus, the outcome may not be directly related to health status. A CUA can compare strategies in different areas of medicine.

19.1.4   Cost Benefit Analysis (CBA)

The benefit is assessed as the economic benefit of a strategy, and costs and benefits are expressed as money. A CBA will not account for intangible costs, as they cannot be measured in terms of money (e.g., relief of anxiety). This approach is rarely used in health economics.

19.2   Pharmaco-Economics in Fluid Management

Cost is a main concern in decision-making for fluid therapy. Only a few reports have compared the total costs of care adopting different fluid therapies. Those studies were carried out in specific clinical settings [4].

In addition, there are no data on the costs associated with late outcomes after fluid therapy, including those incurred after intensive care unit (ICU) or hospital discharge. These aspects need to be evaluated to correctly assess the cost–benefit ratios in fluid therapy [5], based on well-designed health economics studies.

In addition, recent data on the different effects of fluid therapy strategies and the biological properties of the various available crystalloid and colloid solutions must be taken into account. All of these elements may help physicians in choosing the best fluid type in different clinical situations.

For example, the widespread use of balanced instead of unbalanced solutions has raised concerns due to their increased costs. The clinical benefits related to their use, however, are expected to overcome the greater expense. Thus, the cost-effectiveness of balanced solutions should be rigorously addressed, taking into account potential advantages in outcomes, such as morbidity, mortality, and length of ICU or hospital stay when compared to unbalanced solutions.

In fact, the administration of large volumes of 0.9% saline or colloids dissolved in isotonic saline (unbalanced) is associated with the development of dilutional-hyperchloremic acidosis. Although moderate, this transient side-effect (24–48 h) may increase the ICU stay [6]. Balanced or physiological fluids are not associated with the same disturbance of acid/base physiology [6]. Moreover, several reports indicated that the use of unbalanced solutions and the consequences may have detrimental effects on the clinical course of the patient. Improved gastric and renal perfusion, thus reducing the incidence of renal impairment, has been shown in patients receiving balanced solutions. In addition, these solutions are better than unbalanced solutions in preserving hemostasis [7].

Balanced crystalloid solutions have been available for many years. Colloid solutions (hydroxyethyl starch, HES 130/0.42) presented in a "balanced" form are now becoming widely available. On the base of accumulated observations, the extra benefits provided by balanced solutions justify the additional costs over the cheaper but less effective unbalanced solutions. Their cost-effectiveness is expected to be relevant on the ward as well as in the ICU.

Example 1 (see also Table 19.1). Assuming:

- hospital stay (HS) cost of 480€/day;
- unbalanced and non-plasma-adapted colloid or crystalloid cost: 7€/L;
- balanced and plasma-adapted colloid or crystalloid: 10€/L;
- WARD stay length of 8 days with fluid therapy (FT) consisting of 2 L per day, as typically required by patients with multiple chronic diseases.

Table 19.1 Total cost comparison adopting or not a balanced plasma-adapted solution

	Unbalanced and non-plasma-adapted solutions	Balanced and plasma-adapted solutions
Cost of HS/day	480 €	480 €
Cost of FT/day	14 €	20 €
Cost of HS for 8 days	(480 x 8) = 3,840 €	(480 x 8) = 3,840 €
Cost of FT for 8 days	(14 x 8) = 112 €	(20 x 8) = 160 €
Total cost	(3,840 + 112) = 3,952€	(3,840 + 160) = 4,000€

FT, fluid therapy; *HS*, hospital stay.

As previously mentioned, the recent introduction of balanced and plasma-adapted solutions has allowed many of the side effects of older-generation solutions to be avoided, especially regarding acid-base and metabolic disorders [6]. This advantage is due to their electrolytic composition, which is very close to that of plasma.

In particular, balanced and plasma-adapted solutions avoid the dilutional acidosis caused by the older-generation solutions. The replacement of HCO3- with metabolizable anions reduces the risk of dilutional acidosis.

According to these observations, it can be expected that patients receiving the older solutions will develop dilutional acidosis and/or hyperchloremic acidosis and/or metabolic disorder, thus requiring an additional day of hospitalization to treat these side effects.

In patients receiving unbalanced non-plasma adapted solution, one additional day will increase overall costs by (3,952+480+14)= 4,446 €

SAVING: (4,446 - 4,000) = 446 € using balanced and plasma-adapted solutions.

This benefit becomes much more relevant if the total number of patients treated per year is considered.

Assuming:
- patient-volume of 1,000 patients hospitalized per year;
- mean hospital stay of 5 days;
- fluid therapy of 2 L/day.

A crude analysis of the cost of adopting new balanced solutions vs. the old unbalanced non-plasma-adapted solutions yields the result shown in Table 19.2.

Assuming that 15% of patients treated with unbalanced and non-plasma-adapted solutions develop metabolic and acid-base balance alterations, thus requiring one additional day of hospital stay, the overall costs in the group using the unbalanced non-plasma-adapted solution have to be corrected as shown in Table 19.3.

Table 19.2 Total cost comparison adopting or not a balanced plasma-adapted solution

	Unbalanced and non-plasma-adapted solutions	Balanced and plasma-adapted solutions
Cost of HS/day	480 €	480 €
Cost of FT/day	14 €	20 €
Mean HS	5 days	5 days
No. patients/year	1,000	1,000
Total cost in 1 year	(480 + 14) x 5 x 1,000 = 2,470,000 €	(480 + 20) x 5 x 1,000 = 2,500,000 €

FT, fluid therapy; *HS*, hospital stay.

Table 19.3 Total cost comparison adopting or not a balanced plasma-adapted solution taking into account the side effects related to the use of unbalanced solutions

	Unbalanced and non-plasma-adapted solutions		Balanced and plasma-adapted solutions
	Without side effects 850 patients	With side effects 150 patients	Without side effects 1000 patients
Cost of HS/day	480 €	480 €	480 €
Cost of FT/day	14 €	14 €	20 €
Mean HS	5 days	6 days	5 days
Total cost in 1 year	(480 + 14) x 5 x 850 = 2,099,000 €	(480 + 14) x 5 x 150 = 444,600 €	(480 + 20) x 5 x 1,000 = 2,500,000 €
Total cost	2,544,100 €	2,500,000 €	

FT, fluid therapy; *HS*, hospital stay.

SAVING: (2,544,100-2,500,000)= 44,100,000 € by using balanced and plasma-adapted solutions.

Therefore, balanced and plasma-adapted fluid therapy results in a remarkable cost saving compared to unbalanced and plasma-adapted fluid therapy.
Example 2. Assuming:
- ICU stay cost of € 1,000/day;
- unbalanced plasma-adapted colloid or crystalloid cost of € 7;
- balanced plasma-adapted colloid or crystalloid cost of € 10;
- mean hospital stay length of 3 days and fluid therapy of 3 L/day in patients with multiple chronic diseases.

The use of unbalanced and non-plasma-adapted solutions commonly leads to the onset of metabolic and acid-base balance disorders, requiring an additional day of hospital stay (Table 19.4).

The overall cost assuming the use of unbalanced solution as fluid therapy corresponds to:

$$(3,063 + 1,000 + 21) = 4,084 \text{ €}$$

Table 19.4 Total cost comparison adopting or not a balanced plasma-adapted solution

	Unbalanced and non-plasma-adapted solutions	Balanced and plasma-adapted solutions
Cost of HS/day	1,000 €	1,000 €
Cost of FT/day	21 €	30 €
Cost HS for 3 days	(1,000 x 3) = 3,000 €	(1,000 x 3) = 3,000 €
Cost FT for 3 days	(21 x 3) = 63 €	(30 x 3) = 90 €
Total cost	(3,000 + 63) = 3,063 €	(3,000 + 90) = 3,090 €

FT, fluid therapy; *HS*, hospital stay.

Table 19.5 Total cost comparison adopting or not a balanced plasma-adapted solution

	Unbalanced and non-plasma-adapted solutions	Balanced and plasma-adapted solutions
Cost of HS/day	1,000 €	1,000 €
Cost of FT/day	21 €	30 €
Mean HS	3 days	3 days
No. patients/year	500	500
Total cost in 1 year	(1,000 + 21) x 3 x 500 = 1,531,500 €	(1,000 + 30) x 3 x 500 = 1,545,000 €

FT, fluid therapy; *HS*, hospital stay.

SAVING: 4,084 – 3,090 = 994 € by using balanced and plasma-adapted solution.

Assuming:
- ICU patient-volume of 500 patients per year;
- mean hospital stay length of 3 days and fluid therapy of 3 L/day.

Crude analysis of the costs incurred by adopting the new balanced solutions vs. the old, unbalanced non-plasma-adapted solutions yields the results shown in Table 19.5.

Assuming that 15% of patients treated with unbalanced and non-plasma-adapted solutions develop metabolic and acid-base balance alterations, thus requiring one additional day of hospital stay, the overall costs in the group using the unbalanced non-plasma-adapted solution have to be corrected as shown in Table 19.6.

SAVING: (2,067,825 - 1545,000) = 522,825 € by using balanced and plasma-adapted solutions.

Thus, the use of balanced and plasma-adapted fluid therapy could produce a savings compared to unbalanced and plasma-adapted fluid therapy.

Table 19.6 Total cost comparison adopting or not a balanced plasma-adapted solution taking into account the side effects related to the use of unbalanced solutions

	Unbalanced and non-plasma-adapted solutions		Balanced and plasma-adapted solutions
	Without side effects 425 patients	With side effects 75 patients	Without side effects 500 patients
Cost of HS/day	1,000 €	1,000 €	1,000 €
Cost of FT/day	21 €	21 €	30 €
Mean HS	3 days	4 days	3 days
Total cost in 1 year	(1,000 + 21) x 3 x 425 = 1,301,775 €	(1,000 + 21) x 4 x 75 = 766,050 €	(1,000 + 30) x 3 x 500 = 1,545,000 €
Total cost	2,067,825 €	1,545,000 €	

FT, fluid therapy; *HS*, hospital stay.

This cost/benefit of plasma-adapted and balanced fluid therapy can vary from country to country according to the cost of the fluids on the market and the clinical condition of the patients.

Considering site-specific costs, the result of a CBA on fluid therapy can be summarized by the following formulas, which can be used by individual institutions to evaluate the cost saving related to the use of balanced plasma-adapted solutions.

Assuming that:

- EXC is the extra cost of 1 L of balanced plasma-adapted solution;
- L is the overall amount of fluid therapy per day, expressed in liters;
- CSD is the cost of a hospital stay per day;
- n is the number of patients/year;
- d is the average hospital stay length.

COST SAVING per year [€/$]: n 0.15*CDS [€/$] - d*L* EXC [€/$]*

As an example, for a mean hospital stay of 5 days and fluid therapy of 2 L/day, the cost-saving will correspond to: n (0.15*CDS-10*EXC). Thus, the extra cost should be < 1.5% (0.15/10) of the hospital stay cost per day to obtain a cost savings.

Therefore, for a mean cost of hospital stay of 400 [€/$] per day, we can accept an extra cost for the use of balanced plasma-adapted solution of up to 6 [€/$] (1.5% of 400) per liter of fluid therapy per day.

The graph in Figure 19.2 allows a quick assessment of whether the additional cost of using balanced plasma-adopted solutions translates into cost saving. If the intercept between extra-cost for 1 L of balanced plasma-adapted solution and hospital stay cost per day lies in the green area, a cost saving should be expected.

In addition, we can use Table 19.7, which shows the maximum ratio (μ) between the extra cost and the hospital stay cost for each combination of hos-

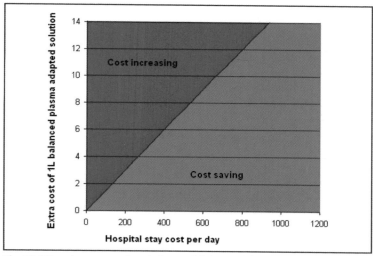

Fig. 19.2 Based on a mean hospital stay of 5 days and fluid therapy of 2 L/day

Table 19.7 Maximum ratio (μ) between the extra cost and the hospital stay cost for each combination of hospital stay length and average amount of fluid therapy per day

Length of stay (days)	Amount of fluid (L/day)			
	1 L/day	2 L/day	3 L/day	4 L/day
1 day	0.15	0.075	0.05	0.0375
2 days	0.075	0.0375	0.025	0.01875
3 days	0.05	0.025	0.016667	0.0125
4 days	0.0375	0.01875	0.0125	0.009375
5 days	0.03	0.015	0.01	0.0075
6 days	0.025	0.0125	0.008333	0.00625
7 days	0.021428571	0.010714	0.007143	0.005357

pital stay length and average amount of fluid therapy per day. Taking into account site specific average hospital stay length (day) and average amount of fluid therapy per day (liter), we can obtain the site-specific μ. Multiplying μ * site-specific hospital stay cost per day, we obtain the cut-off value of the extra cost to obtain a cost saving.

In case of an average ICU stay length of 4 days and an average amount of fluid therapy of 3 L, the maximum ratio is 0.0125. Assuming a hypothetical cost of € 600 for 1 day in the ICU, the extra cost for 1 L of balanced plasma-adapted solution should not exceed € 7.5 (0.0125*600) to obtain a cost saving. Therefore if 1 L of balanced plasma-adapted solution costs € 8 and 1 L of unbalanced solution costs € 3, the extra cost will be € 5 (8-3), and the use of a balanced solution will translate into a cost saving.

These examples underline the importance of a cost/benefit analysis in assessing fluid therapy based on the available, balanced plasma-adapted solutions.

However, it should be noted that the main objective in fluid management is not to achieve a saving in terms of money, but rather to guarantee the best quality of care.

Key Concepts
- Expenditures on drug therapy as a target for health economics
- Relevance of multiple chronic conditions, which are associated with the consumption, on average, of more medications
- Evaluation of the costs and benefits of different therapeutic choices
- Costs as a key concern in fluid management

Key Words
- Health economics
- Pharmaco-economics
- Costs and benefits
- Cost effectiveness analysis

Focus on...
- Vogeli C, Shields AE, Lee TA (2007) Multiple chronic conditions: prevalence, health consequences, and implications for quality, care management, and costs. J Gen Intern Med 22 Suppl 3:391-395
- Vincent JL (2000) Fluid management: the pharmacoeconomic dimension. Crit Care 4 (suppl 2):S33–S35

References

1. Chunningham S (2001) An introduction to economic evaluation of health care. JO 3:246
2. Wood Johnson R (2002) Foundation partnership for solutions. Chronic conditions: making the case for ongoing care
3. Vogeli C (2007) Multiple chronic conditions: prevalence, health consequences, and implications for quality, care management, and costs. J Gen Intern Med 22 Suppl 3:391-5
4. Vincent JL (2000) Fluid management: the pharmacoeconomic dimension. Crit Care 4 (suppl 2):S33–S35
5. Burchardi H, Schneider H (2004) Economic aspects of severe sepsis: a review of intensive care unit costs, cost of illness and cost effectiveness of therapy. Pharmacoeconomics 22:793-813
6. Guidet B (2010) A balanced view of balanced solutions. Crit Care 14:325
7. Grocott MPW (2005) Perioperative Fluid Management and Clinical Outcomes in Adults. Anesth Analg 100:1093–106
8. Boldt J (2009) Cardiopulmonary bypass priming using a high dose of a balanced hydroxyethyl starch versus an albumin-based priming strategy. Anesth Analg 109:1752

Fluid Management: Questions and Answers

20

Maria Benedetto, Chiara Candela and Felice Eugenio Agrò

20.1 How Is Water Distributed in Body Compartments?

Body water accounts for approximately 60% of body weight; it is mainly distributed in the extracellular and intracellular spaces (ECS and ICS, respectively). The ICS contains nearly 55% of the water, and the ECS 45% (about 15 L in a normal adult). The ECS is further divided into the intravascular space (IVS), the interstitial space (ISS), and the transcellular space (TCS), containing about 15%, 45%, and 40% of ECS water, respectively. The TCS is a functional compartment represented by the amount of fluid and electrolytes continually exchanged (in and out) by cells with the ISS and by the IVS with the ISS.

20.2 What Is the Physiological Role of Electrolytes Contained in the Plasma?

Sodium is the main cation in the ECS and the main determinant of ECS volume. It has an important hemodynamic role as it is involved in the renin-angiotensin system. It is necessary for the regulation of blood and body fluids, for the transmission of nerve impulses, and for cardiac activity.

Potassium is the major cation in the ICS. It is important in allowing cardiac muscle contraction and conduction and participates in sending nerve impulses. It also plays a key role in kidney function.

Calcium is involved in exocrine, endocrine, and neuro-endocrine secretions, the coagulation system, muscle contraction, cell growth, and enzymatic regulation.

C. Candela (✉)

Postgraduate School of Anesthesia and Intensive Care, Anesthesia, Intensive Care and Pain Management Department, University School of Medicine Campus Bio-Medico of Rome, Rome, Italy
e-mail: chiaracandela@yahoo.it

F. E. Agrò (ed.), *Body Fluid Management*,
DOI: 10.1007/978-88-470-2661-2_20 © Springer-Verlag Italia 2013

Magnesium is the physiological antagonist of calcium. It is crucial in neuromuscular stimulation. In addition, it acts as a cofactor of several enzymes involved in the energy metabolism contributed by three major categories of nutrients: carbohydrates, lipids, and proteins.

Chloride is the most important anion of the ECS. Together with sodium, it determines the ECS volume. It is also responsible for membrane potential, acid-base balance, and plasma osmotic pressure.

Bicarbonate is the main buffer-system of the blood and thus has a crucial role in maintaining acid-base balance.

20.3   What Is Acid-Base Balance?

Acid-base balance represents a complex mechanism through which the body maintains a neutral pH (7.38–7.42) in order to prevent protein degradation and pathologic alterations in biochemical reactions. The control of pH includes an inorganic (bicarbonate) and an organic (hemoglobin) buffer system. The kidneys and lungs are involved in the elimination of overproduced and accumulated acids or and that are overproduced or accumulated.

20.4   What Is the Difference Between Osmolarity, Osmolality, and Tonicity?

Osmolarity is determined by the number of particles per one *liter* of a solution.

Osmolality is determined by the number of particles per one *kilogram* of a solution.

Tonicity is represented by the *sum of all small particles* contained in a solution.

20.5   What Is the Role of Osmotic and Oncotic Pressures in Water Movement Through a Semipermeable Membrane?

Osmotic pressure (μ) is exerted by osmotically active particles (electrolytes) that do not freely pass through semi-permeable biological membranes. It is one of the forces that regulate fluid movement across biological membranes. According to the osmotic pressure, water will pass from a solution of low to one of high electrolytic concentration to re-equilibrate the amounts of electrolytes on either side of the membranes [1, 2].

Oncotic pressure, or colloid-osmotic pressure (π), is a form of osmotic pressure exerted by macro-molecules (proteins, particularly albumin) that cannot easily cross a semi-permeable membrane [1]. Thus, water passes from a solution of low to one of high protein concentration [1, 2].

20.6 What Are the Effects of a Hypotonic vs. a Hypertonic Solution?

A hypotonic solution reduces plasma osmotic pressure, leading to water movement from the ECS to the ICS [3]. Consequently, cellular edema and cell lysis (e.g., hemolysis) may occur. Larger volumes of hypotonic solutions have been known to produce a transient increase in intracranial pressure (ICP) [4], because of cerebral edema. The magnitude of this increase can be predicted by the reduction in plasma osmolarity [5]. Patients whose osmolality is < 240 mOsmol/kg will fall into a coma, with a mortality rate of 50% [6].

Hypertonic solutions increase plasma osmotic pressure, leading to water movement from the ICS to the ECS and cellular dehydration.

In hyperosmolar hyperglycemic non-ketotic syndrome and in diabetic keto-acidosis, mortality is clearly correlated with plasma osmolality [7]. Hypovolemic shock also triggers hyperglycemia with hyperosmolarity [8], through the release of epinephrine [9] or through an increase in blood lactate levels [10].

20.7 What Are the Advantages of Balanced Plasma-Adapted Solutions?

A balanced, plasma-adapted solution is a solution qualitatively and quantitatively similar to plasma. Its use avoids the development of hyperchloremic acidosis, while assuring the same volume effect as unbalanced solutions and potentially reducing morbidity and mortality.

Balanced, plasma-adapted solutions also reduce the effects on acid-base balance. Specifically, they avoid the dilutional acidosis caused by older-generation solutions, because they contain adequate concentration of metabolizable anions, which may be converted into HCO3- in the tissues. Replacing HCO3- with metabolizable anions reduces the risk of dilutional acidosis.

20.8 What Are the Main Crystalloids on the Market and What Are Their Properties?

Normal or physiologic saline solution, i.e., 0.9% NaCl solution, contains only sodium and chloride, at high concentrations (154 mmol/L). The osmolarity of a 0.9% NaCl solution is 308 mmol/l. Despite its name, it is not physiologic because it is neither isotonic, nor balanced, nor plasma-adapted.

Ringer solutions are second-generation crystalloids. Compared to saline solutions, they have lower sodium (130 mmol/L) and chloride (112 mmol/L) contents. They contain potassium, calcium and magnesium (Ringer acetate) as well as metabolizable ions: lactate (Ringer lactate) and acetate (Ringer acetate). Both Ringer solutions are more plasma-adapted than normal saline, while remaining unbalanced.

0.9% saline is indicated in patients with hypochloremia, while avoiding hypernatremia. Fluid losses from ileostomy, diarrhea, and small-bowel fistula should be replaced with balanced solutions [21].

In case of acute blood loss, absolute hypovolemia should first be treated-with balanced crystalloids and colloids, until blood is available. Patients with sepsis, peritonitis, pancreatitis, and relative hypovolemia should receive balanced crystalloids and colloids.

Intravenous fluids are administered in order to achieve an optimal stroke volume during surgery and up to 8 h thereafter [21].

20.14 In Major Abdominal Surgery, What Are the Advantages of Total Balanced GDT?

A total balanced GDT has been demonstrated to reduce the incidence of peri-operative complications [22], such as gut disorders, while improving healing of the wound and anastomosis and reducing the length of hospital stay [23].

20.15 How Should Fluid Administration Be Managed in Thoracic Surgery?

First of all, blood losses should be appropriately replaced. It is advisable that the total positive fluid balance in the first 24 h of the peri-operative period does not exceed 20 mL/kg.

For an average adult patient, crystalloid administration should be limited to < 3 L in the first 24 h. Urine output > 0.5mL/kg/h is unnecessary.

If increased tissue perfusion is needed postoperatively, it is preferable to use invasive monitoring and inotropes to avoid fluid overload.

Central venous pressure monitoring is beneficial particularly in the presence of a thoracic epidural.

Intravascular colloid retention during the treatment of hypovolemia may approach 90% vs. 40% during normovolemia.

20.16 How Should Lung Transplantation Patients Be Managed?

The interruption of lymphatic drainage in the graft may predispose the patient to peri-operative pulmonary interstitial fluid overload.

If large quantities of crystalloids/colloids are needed, potential interstitial pulmonary edema may be prevented by intra-operative ventilation with moderate-to-high PEEP. However, excessive fluid replacement becomes harmful after tracheal extubation because the increase in venous return, following the withdrawal of mechanical ventilation, may determine pulmonary congestion.

If the PiCCO system has been used for hemodynamic monitoring, it will probably show an increased intra-thoracic blood volume, with a significant expansion of extravascular lung water [24]. Quite often, the presence of renal dysfunction associated with lung transplantation complicates peri-operative fluid management, rendering these patients more vulnerable to fluid retention.

20.17 Which Fluid Is the Best Choice in Thoracic Surgery?

The most recent data are in favor of the use of colloids for the replacement of volume losses due to fluid shifting and/or bleeding. It is likely that the greater effectiveness of colloids in this context is due to a better effect on volume expansion [25] and minimized shifting of fluid through a potentially damaged capillary membrane [26, 27].

In patients undergoing esophagectomy, the choice of crystalloids vs. colloids as intraoperative fluid therapy and the effects on intestinal anastomotic healing are debatable.

20.18 Why Does Regional Anesthesia Cause Hypotension?

Regional anesthesia blocks the fibers of the sympathetic nervous system that innervates the smooth muscle of arteries and veins, causing vasodilatation, blood pooling, and a decreased venous return to the heart. There may be significant changes in systemic blood pressure, especially in patients who are already intravascularly depleted.

In this setting, vasodilatation induced by regional anesthesia produces hypotension due to relative hypovolemia, rather than a reduction of blood volume.

20.19 How Can Hypotension Following Spinal Anesthesia for a Cesarean Section Be Prevented?

For many years, crystalloids were used to prevent hypotension related to spinal anesthesia in women undergoing cesarean section, but recent evidence does not support this practice. In fact, several studies have shown that HES is better than crystalloid solutions in preventing hypotension [28, 29].

Among the various possible colloids, HES are certainly among those to be preferred, despite its higher cost compared to other colloids because it offers prophylaxis for venous thrombosis and is associated with fewer allergic reactions. In addition, HES guarantee central volume expansion by preventing the onset of hypotension. This effect is due to the increase in preload and the fact that HES are quickly removed from the circulation [30, 31].

20.20   How Much Fluid Is Needed in Orthopedic Surgery?

In patients undergoing minor surgery, the preoperative administration of 1–2 L of fluids (mainly crystalloids) appears rational to correct dehydration. This approach has been shown to reduce postoperative complications, such as drowsiness, dizziness, nausea, and vomiting, as well as post-surgical pain [32-34].

In major surgery, there are strategies for fluid administration: liberal, restricted, or goal-directed therapy. While studies on liberal-restricted strategies do not provide unanimous results, many studies have shown that GDT is a valid approach for managing patients undergoing major surgery, due to the reduction in hospital stay and postsurgical complications [35-37].

The purpose of GDT is to optimize perfusion and tissue oxygenation under the guidance of hemodynamic variables that suggest the need for fluids or other therapies (such as vasoactive inotropic drugs).

20.21   Which Fluid Is the Best Choice in Orthopedic Surgery?

Hypovolemia is the most important condition that may occur during major orthopedic surgery and it must be prevented during the entire peri-operative period. Patients with hypovolemia due to bleeding must be promptly treated with balanced crystalloid associated with a colloid rather than crystalloids alone.

While many studies comparing the effects of colloids and crystalloids on clotting have shown that colloids interfere with clotting to a greater extent than crystalloids [38, 39], this is not the case with the latest-generation HES. In fact, comparisons of Voluven with older-generation HES showed a much less pronounced effect on coagulation for the former [40-43].

More recent studies have focused on HES diluted in balanced solutions, suggesting that they could be used throughout the peri-operative period. In fact, in a recent study, patients undergoing orthopedic surgery who received balanced and plasma-adapted solutions had fewer side effects than those receiving non-balanced HES [44].

20.22   What Is the Best Fluid Management Strategy in Cardiac Patients?

In cardiac surgery, the use of colloids rather than crystalloids seems to be more appropriate for volume replacement. A considerable amount of crystalloids, with interstitial distribution, is needed in order to achieve the same IVS volume replacement as a comparatively minute amount of colloids [45].

Indeed, the administration of a large volume may facilitate fluid overload and hemodilution. The use of crystalloids is suggested for continuous loss (total water body loss such as due to perspiration and urinary output) and the use of colloids for temporary losses (IVS loss such as due to hemorrhage).

20.23   Which Fluid Should Be Used in Cardiopulmonary Bypass Priming?

The central role of CPBP in cardiac surgery is well-recognized. In fact, the choice of the solution is one of the major factors that influence patient outcome. Nevertheless, the ideal priming protocol has not yet been identified, and there are no specific guidelines on this topic.

During cardiopulmonary bypass, the colloid-osmotic pressure decreases because of hemodilution. The main goal of CPBP is to avoid this drop.

Several lines of evidence suggest that the use of crystalloids alone is not indicated for priming. In fact, crystalloids have been shown to reduce the oncotic pressure and to increase the risk of postoperative organ dysfunctions as well as pulmonary edema [46, 47].

According to many studies, colloids are preferable to crystalloids, in particular HES in balanced solutions, given that the latest-generation HES seem to be related to fewer post-operative clinical alterations [48-51].

However, it is important to note that there is not enough evidence to advocate the "default" use of HES for CPBP. Moreover, it should be borne in mind that HES are true drugs, with potential benefits and side effects, and thus should be used with caution.

20.24   What Is the Best Choice for Fluid Therapy in Septic Patients?

The choice of a specific fluid for the management of septic patients is controversial, but it seems rational that fluid resuscitation in patients with severe sepsis/septic shock should be mainly based on the use of crystalloids. This conclusion is in agreement with many recently published reviews on this topic [52, 53]. The use of HES should be limited to patients whose hemodynamic status is particularly compromised. Low-molecular-weight HES, such as HES 130/0.4, have been associated with less nephrotoxicity and coagulopathy than medium-molecular-weight forms. As already recommended by the guidelines on sepsis therapy, crystalloids and colloids in balanced solution are preferred. Current studies on the safety of HES 130/0.4 in balanced solutions will clarify whether this colloid can be considered the first-choice fluid for patients with severe sepsis or septic shock.

The Surviving Sepsis Campaign guidelines recommend a goal-directed fluid management with an initial target CVP ≥ 8 mm Hg and the continuation of fluid therapy until the achievement of hemodynamic stability [54].

20.25   How Is Fluid Resuscitation Managed in Trauma Patients?

According to the eighth edition of Advanced Trauma Life Support, fluid resuscitation in trauma starts with warm isotonic crystalloids (Ringer lactate or saline). Hypertonic solutions are alternative fluids in the early stages of trauma, especially in patients with brain injury, based on their ability to decrease the ICP [55] with a greater efficacy than mannitol.

Another possible benefit of hypertonic solutions is a rapid increase in the mean arterial pressure by using small volumes, and a consequent reduction of lung edema in the days following resuscitation [56].

Trauma patients in whom hemodynamic instability or cognitive deterioration occurs, should be administered an intravenous bolus of 500 mL HES [57]. If the patient remains in shock, a new bolus should be repeated after 30 min, but the total volume of intravenous HES should not exceed 1000 mL

20.26   Can GDT Be Useful in Non-Surgical Patients?

We carried out a systematic review and meta-analysis of randomized controlled trials comparing GDT with the standard of care. The primary aim was to evaluate the effects of hemodynamic GDT on mortality and morbidity in non-surgical critically ill patients.

The review showed that hemodynamic optimization could reduce mortality in these patients. However, as determined in the subgroup analysis, the benefit was relevant only for septic or trauma patients but was not observed in a mixed population of critically ill patients. In these cases, there was no reduction in hospital mortality.

20.27   What Are the Guidelines for Fluid Therapy in Burn Patients?

According to the American Burn Association guidelines, patients with burns > 20 % of total body surface area (TBSA) must receive fluid replacement based on the total burned area estimation. A need for crystalloids of 2–4 mL/kg/% TBSA has been estimated in the first 24 h (Parkland formula according to Baxter). A half-volume should be administered during the first 8 h and the remaining volume in the following 16 h [58]. The guidelines also support the use of colloids between 12 and 24 h from the injury, when the integrity of capillary membranes has been restored. The use of colloids may result in a reduction of tissue edema and of the overall fluid requirement [58, 59].

Fluid administration should be carried out in order to obtain, in the first phase, a mean arterial pressure > 65 mmHg, urine output > 0.5 mL/kg/h, CVP 10–15 mmHg (if necessary 20 mmHg), and no increase in the hemoglobin-concentration or hematocrit.

20.28 How Should Fluid Administration Be Managed in Children?

Recommendations for infusion therapy in children indicate the use of crystalloids with an osmolality and electrolyte concentration similar to plasma (plasma-adapted solutions) and a glucose concentration of 1–2.5% [60].

Gelatins are used in children between the ages of 1 and 12 years, while HES should not be administered to children younger than 2 years because of the immaturity of the kidneys [61].

Fourth-generation HES have the advantage of being diluted in balanced, plasma-adapted solutions. Thus, both alterations of acid-base balance and electrolyte imbalances are significantly reduced compared to the use of third-generation HES, which are diluted in simple saline solution [62]. Since the composition of the ECS or IVS in children and adults is comparable, the concept of balanced fluid resuscitation should benefit both, especially when high volumes of colloids are provided [11].

Recently, HES 130/0.42 was shown to be safe and effective for volume replacement and well tolerated when used in pediatric surgery [63].

20.29 What Are the Advantages of Balanced Plasma-Adapted Solutions in Children?

The literature supports the use of isotonic, balanced, plasma-adapted solutions in children to avoid dilutional and hyperchloremic acidosis (caused by normal saline solution) and to reduce the risk of peri-operative hyponatremia, especially when a large amount of fluid is needed [63-65]. These properties may decrease the negative effects on acid-base balance and the electrolytic alterations involving renal and cardiac function, particularly in children with kidney disease or those who have undergone cardiac surgery [66, 67]. As a consequence, even if outcome studies examining balance solutions in pediatric patients are still lacking, clinical experience suggests that these solutions should be used in the peri-operative period also in children, as in adults, for their obvious positive effects [63, 68].

20.30 Why Is Hemodilution Associated with Fluid Administration?

Fluid administration can lead to hemodilution, resulting in a decrease in hemoglobin/hematocrit. [69, 70]. This is a compensatory mechanism to increase cerebral blood flow despite a reduction of arterial oxygen content. It is absent or reduced when there is brain damage; thus, excessive hemodilution resulting from inadequate fluid management may further aggravate brain injury [71-73].

20.31   What Is the Best Approach to Patients Undergoing Neurosurgery?

The main goal of peri-operative fluid management is to ensure adequate tissue oxygenation and prevent oxygen debt following an increase in the cerebral metabolic rate of oxygen ($CMRO_2$) during surgery.

One of the most important complications, which must be avoided and prevented, is iatrogenic cerebral edema due to a decrease in plasma osmolality. Tommasino emphasized that iatrogenic cerebral edema will not occur when the normal values of osmolality and oncotic pressure are maintained, regardless of whether colloids or crystalloids are used [74]. However, fluid therapy should be adjusted also to prevent/counteract the increase in ICP.

Therefore, in neurosurgical patients, an isovolemic state is acquired by the infusion of iso-osmolar crystalloid (~300 mOsm; 0.9% saline solution), in order to avoid affecting plasma osmolality, the main determinant of fluid balance in the brain, and water accumulation in the brain parenchyma.

Hyperosmotic solutions should be used in cases of intracranial hypertension, reserving the use of hypertonic saline to those cases refractory to conventional therapy (hyperventilation, mannitol, diuretics).

It is worth noting that it is always advisable to monitor postoperative osmolality [75].

20.32   What Is the Major Complication in Childbirth?

Bleeding is a major cause of maternal mortality and complications of childbirth [76]. In fact, the transfusion of blood is required in 1–2% of pregnancies. [77, 78] The main causes of bleeding are: uterine atony, retained placenta, trauma, placenta previa, and abruption placenta [77].

Maintenance of perfusion pressure and blood volume is provided initially with crystalloids or colloids while waiting for blood products. The optimal fluid type for use in hypovolemic patients has been the subject of much debate. According to Van der Linden, there is no advantage in using albumin rather than saline solution in terms of morbidity and mortality [79]. However, other studies suggested that saline solution 0.9% causes hyperchloremic acidosis and therefore cannot be recommended. There is an argument supporting balanced fluid resuscitation using fluids (crystalloids and colloids) containing a physiological balance of electrolytes [80]. Hypertonic saline has been advocated in patients with hemorrhagic shock, but studies demonstrating the effectiveness of this solution are lacking [81]. The presence of relative anemia requires that the administration of clear fluids be limited and, to ensure perfusion, adapted to the intravascular volume [82].

20.33 What Is the Optimal Management Approach to Pregnancy-Induced Hypertension with Oliguria?

In the treatment of pregnancy-induced hypertension the infusion of 500–1000 mL of crystalloids has been recommended [83]. If the hypertension persists, it is important to consider the state of fluid balance because excess fluid can lead to pulmonary or cerebral edema. The lack of response to the infusion of crystalloids in patients with oliguria may require alternative treatments depending on the cause [83]. In the case of intravascular volume depletion, a further infusion of crystalloids is needed. If, instead, oliguria is due to renal artery vasospasm then dopamine is required, without the infusion of fluids. In patients requiring volume expansion, due to the decrease in postpartum colloid osmotic pressure, colloids are the first choice [84].

20.34 What Is Palliative Sedation?

Palliative sedation is a medical procedure that consists of reduction/abolishment of consciousness as the only therapeutic resource to relieve refractory symptoms, which are intolerable for the patient. It is carried out through the gradual titration of a sedative with periodic monitoring of the patient's vital signs, level of sedation, and degree of symptom relief.

20.35 What Is the Role of Hydration in Terminally Ill Patients?

Hydration aims to prevent or correct the symptoms that may occur with dehydration, especially delirium and the neurotoxicity of opioids. Numerous studies have shown that the hydration of terminally ill cancer patients can prevent the onset of delirium [85-87]; in Canada, vigorous hydration resulted in a decrease in the incidence of delirium in patients in a palliative care unit [86].

Some authors have reported side effects associated with hydration, including vomiting, nausea, increased secretions, edema, ascites, urinary tract infections, and the presence of secretions in the airways [88]. However, according to Dalal and Bruera [89], there is no concrete evidence for an association; instead, they claimed, the side effects are due to excessive fluid administration.

In terminally ill patients hypoalbuminemia may occur [90], which can lead to pulmonary or peripheral edema and ascites, if crystalloids are administered. If serum albumin is < 26 g/L, then Dunlop et al. [91] advise against the administration of fluids either intravenously or subcutaneously to avoid adverse effects. Instead, the administration of intravenous colloids is preferred.

Hydration of a terminally ill patient should not be seen an act of "charity" but as a medical gesture. Indeed, to ensure proper hydration does not mean extending the life of the patient but simply to prevent complications that arise due to sedation, such as electrolyte disorders.

20.36 What Are the Local Complications Related to Infusion Therapy?

Infusion therapy, as all medical procedures, is not free from complications, which may differ in their gravity. Complications may arise due to incorrect positioning of the catheter or to the side effects of the infused fluid.

Phlebitis is a local complication due to an inflammation of the vessel intima, characterized by erythema, swelling, and pain.

Infiltration is defined as a loss of fluid into the surrounding tissue, mainly following displacement of the catheter.

Extravasation is the administration of medications or fluids into the tissues surrounding the point of infusion. It can be prevented selecting a well fitting vein. It is advisable to avoid hand and wrist veins because of richness of nerves and tendons.

Hematoma is another common complication during fluid infusion. It occurs due to vessel wall damage. In order to prevent hematomas, a compressive dressing at the site where the needle entered the vein is suggested.

20.37 What Are the Systemic Complications Related to Infusion Therapy?

Infusion therapy may be associated with clotting disorders, ranging from the onset of bleeding to the formation of intravascular thrombi. Bleeding disorders can arise due to the dilution of coagulation factors in the blood or the interference of colloids molecules with platelet adhesion or clot formation.

Blood stream infections are severe infections that can increase patient morbidity and mortality. They are frequently related to the use of intravenous devices and can result in serious complications.

Venous air embolism is a potential complication of infusion therapy, with effects on morbidity and mortality. It occurs when there is a communication between the venous system and a source of air while a pressure gradient allows the passage of air into the vessel [92]. In severe cases, venous air embolism may cause arrhythmias. Severe inflammatory alterations in the pulmonary vessels may also occur, such as direct endothelial damage and the accumulation of platelets, fibrin, neutrophils, and lipid droplets.

20.38   Is It Possible To Quantify the Third Space?

Third-space fluid losses have never been directly determined and the actual location of the lost fluid remains unclear. Instead, these losses have only been quantified indirectly by continually measuring peri-operative changes in the ECV via tracer-dilutional techniques, assuming that the total ECV (functional plus non-functional) remains constant. These techniques are based on the administration of a known quantity of a proper tracer into a definite body fluid space.

However, different studies using these techniques have demonstrated that a classic third space quantitatively does not exist. It is a pathologic compartment that reflects the peri-operative fluid shift. Therefore, we suggest abolishing this vague notion and dealing with the given facts: fluid is peri-operatively shifted inside the functional ECV, from the IVS toward the ISS.

20.39   What Are the Main Indications for Balanced and Plasma-Adapted Solutions?

- In major orthopedic surgery, in which there is a high risk to develop bleeding and coagulation disorders.
- In major abdominal surgery, due to the bleeding risk and possible "third space" syndrome.
- In polytrauma and head trauma, with a risk of an increase in ICP and cerebral edema.
- In cardiac surgery, especially cardiopulmonary by-pass priming.
- In patients with reduced kidney function who are at risk of hyperkalemia .
- In patients with reduced colloid-oncotic pressure and possible interstitial edema.
- In pediatric patients with acid-base imbalance and electrolyte alterations.
- In patients with capillary leak syndrome, adult lung injury, adult respiratory distress syndrome, or pulmonary edema.
- In patients with hyperchloremic acidosis and a possible reduction in renal blood flow.

20.40   What Are the Cost/Benefit Advantages of Balanced and Plasma-Adapted Solutions?

Balanced and plasma-adapted solutions cause fewer side effects than either older-generation colloids or crystalloids, thus shortening the hospital stay. For example, the large-volume administration of 0.9% saline or colloids dissolved in isotonic saline (unbalanced) is associated with the development of dilutional-hyperchloremic acidosis. Although moderate, this transient side effect (24–48 h) may increase the length of the ICU stay. Furthermore, balanced and plasma-adapted solutions are not associated with disturbances of acid-base physiology [90].

Patients randomized to balanced solutions, when compared with those randomized to saline-based fluids, were less likely to have impaired hemostasis while gastric perfusion improved [93]. Renal function may also be better preserved [94].

Based on these observations, the extra benefits provided by balanced solutions justify the additional costs over cheaper but less effective unbalanced ones. Their cost-effectiveness is expected to be relevant in both the ICU and on the ward, suggesting that the use of balanced plasma-adapted solutions will improve patient outcome while conserving economic resources at the same time.

References

1. Voet D, Voet JG, Pratt CW (2001) Fundamentals of Biochemistry (Rev. ed.). New York, Wiley
2. Amiji MM, Sandmann BJ (2002) Applied Physical Pharmacy. McGraw-Hill Professional
3. Williams EL, Hildebrand KL, McCormick SA et al (1999) The effect of intravenous lactated Ringer's solution versus 0.9 % sodium chloride solution on serum osmolality in human volunteers. Anesth Analg 88:999-1003
4. Tommasino C, Moore S, Todd MM (1988) Cerebral effects of isovolemic hemodilution with crystalloid or colloid solutions. Crit Care Med 16:862-868
5. Schell RM, Applegate RL, Cole DJ (1996) Salt, starch, and water on the brain. J Neurosurg Anesth 8:179-182
6. Arieff AI, Llach F, Massry SG (1976) Neurological manifestations and morbidity of hyponatremia: Correlation with brain water and electrolytes. Medicine 55:121-129
7. Jayashree M, Singhi S (2004) Diabetic ketoacidosis: Predictors of outcome in a pediatric intensive care unit of a developing country. Pediatr Crit Care Med 5:427-433
8. Boyd DR, Mansberger AR Jr (1968) Serum water and osmolal changes in hemorrhagic shock: An experimental and clinical study. Amer Surg 34:744-749
9. Järhult J (1973) Osmotic fluid transfer from tissue to blood during hemorrhagic hypotension. Acta Physiol Scand 89:213-226
10. Kenney PR, Allen-Rowlands CF, Gann DS (1983) Glucose and osmolality as predictors of injury severity. J Trauma 23:712-71
11. Sukanya Mitra and Purva Khandelwal (2009) Are All Colloids Same? How to Select the Right Colloid? Indian Journal of Anaesthesia 53:592
12. Dubois MJ, Vincent JL (2007) Colloid Fluids. In: Hahn RG, Prough DS, Svensen CH (eds.) Perioperative Fluid Therapy, 1 edn. New York, Wiley, pp 153-611
13. Kaminski MV, Williams SD (1990) Review of the rapid normalization of serum albumin with modified total parenteral nutrition solutions. Crit Care Med 18:327-35
14. Rajnish KJ et al (2004) Albumin: an overview of its place in current clinical practice. J Indian An
15. Schnitzer JE, Carley WW, Palade GE (1988) Specific albumin binding to microvascular endothelium in culture. Am J Physiol 254:H425-27
16. Moran M, Kapsner C (1987) Acute renal failure associated with elevated plasma oncotic pressure. N Engl J Med 317:150-3
17. Levi M, Jonge E (2007) Clinical relevance of the effects of plasma expanders on coagulation. Semin Thromb Haemost 33:810–815

18. Solanke TF, Khwaja MS, Kadomemu EL (1971) Plasma volume studies with four different plasma volume expanders. J Surg Res 11:140-43
19. Mitral S, Khandelwal P (2009) Are All Colloids Same? How to Select the Right Colloid? Indian J Anaesth 53:592–607
20. Ramani Moonesinghe S, Mythen MG, Grocott MPW (2011) High risk surgery: epidemiology and Outcomes. Anesth Analg 112:891-901
21. Soni N (2009) British Consensus Guidelines on Intravenous Fluid Therapy for Adult Surgical Patients (GIFTASUP): Cassandra's view. Anaesthesia 64:235-8
22. Brandstrup B, Tonnesen H, Beier-Holgersen R et al (2003) Effects of intravenous fluid restriction on postoperative complications: Comparison of two perioperative fluid regimens - a randomized assessor-blinded multicenter trial. Ann Surg 238:641-8
23. Lobo DN, Bostock KA, Neal KR et al (2002) Effect of salt and water balance on recovery of gastrointestinal function after elective colonic resection: A randomised controlled trial. Lancet 359:1812-8
24. Della Rocca G, Costa MG (2005) Volumetric monitoring: principles of application. Minerva Anestesiol 71:303–306
25. McIlroy DR, Kharasch ED (2003) Acute intravascular volume expansion with rapidly administered crystalloid or colloid in the setting of moderate hypovolemia. Anesth Analg 96:1572–7
26. Matharu NM, Butler LM, Rainger GE et al (2008) Mechanisms of the anti-inflammatory effects of hydroxyethyl starch demonstrated in a flow-based model of neutrophil recruitment by endothelial cells. Crit Care Med. May 36:1536-42
27. Jacob M, Bruegger D, Rehm M et al (2006) Contrasting effects of colloid and crystalloid resuscitation fluids on cardiac vascular permeability. Anesthesiology 104:1223-31
28. Vercauteren HP, Hoffman V, Coppejans HC (1996) Hydroxyethyl starch compared with modified gelatin as volume preload before spinal anaesthesia for caesarean section. Br J Anaesth 76:731–3
29. Riley ET, Cohen SE, Rubenstein AJ, Flanagan B (1995) Prevention of hypotension after spinal anesthesia for cesarean section: Six percent hetastarch versus lactated Ringer's solution. Anesth Analg 81:838–42
30. Laxenaire M, Charpentier C, Feldman L (1994) Réactions anaphylactoïdes aux substituts colloïdaux du plasma: incidence, facteurs de risque, mécanismes. Enquête prospective, multicentrique française. Annales Françaises d'Anesthésie et Reanimation 13:301–310
31. Svensen C, Hahn RG (1997) Volume kinetics of Ringer solution, dextran 70, and hypertonic saline in male volunteers. Anesthesiology 87:204–12
32. Connolly CM, Kramer GC, Hahn RG et al (2003) Isoflurane but not mechanical ventilation-promotes extravascular fluid accumulation during crystalloid volume loading. Anesthesiology 98:670–81
33. Holte K, Kehlet H (2002) Compensatory fluid administration for preoperative dehydration – does it improve outcome? Acta Anaesthesiol Scand 46:1089–93
34. Maharaj CH, Kallam SR, Malik A et al (2005) Preoperative intravenous fluid therapy decreases postoperative nausea and pain in high risk patients. Anesth Analg 100:675–8
35. Ali SZ, Taguchi A, Holtmann B, Kurz A (2003) Effect of supplemental pre-operative fluid on postoperative nausea and vomiting. Anaesthesia 58:780–4
36. Gan TJ, Soppitt A, Maroof M et al (2002) Goal-directed intraoperative fluid administration reduces length of hospital stay after major surgery. Anesthesiology 97:820–6
37. Wakeling HG, McFall MR, Jenkins CS et al (2005) Intraoperative oesophageal Doppler guided fluid management shortens postoperative hospital stay after major bowel surgery. Br J Anaesth 95:634–42
38. Fries D, Innerhofer P, Klingler A et al (2002) The effect of the combined administration of colloids and lactated Ringer's solution on the coagulation system: an in vitro study using thrombelastograph coagulation analysis (ROTEG. Anesth Analg 94:1280–7
39. VG (2005) Colloids decrease clot propagation and strength: role of factor XIII-fibrin polymer and thrombin-fibrinogen interactions. Acta Anaesthesiol Scand 49:1163–71

40. Langeron O, Doelberg M, Ang ET et al (2001) Voluven®, a lower substituted novel hydrox-yethyl starch (HES 130/0.4) causes fewer effects on coagulation in major orthopedic surgery than HES 200/0.5 Anesth Analg 92:855-62

41. Oeveren W, Hagenaars A, Tigchelaar I et al (1998) Increased von Willebrand factor after low molecular weight hydroxyethyl starch priming solution in cardiopulmonary bypass. Br J Anaesth 80 (Suppl 1):A267

42. Huet R, Siemons W, Hagenaars A, van Oeveren W (1998) Is hydroxyethyl starch 130/0.4 the optimal starch plasma substitute in adult cardiac surgery? Anesth Analg 86(Suppl 4):SCA80

43. Konrad CJ, Markl TJ, Schuepfer GK et al (2000) In vitro effects of different medium molec-ular hydroxyethyl starch solutions and lactated ringer's solution on coagulation using sono-clot for analysis. Anesth Analg 90:274–9

44. Papakitsos G, Papakitsou T, Kapsali A (2010) A total balanced volume replacement strategy using a new balanced 6% hydroxyethyl starch preparation Tetraspan (HES 130/0.42) in pa-tients undergoing major orthopaedic surgery: 6AP3-1. European Journal of Anaesthesiology 27:106

45. Rackow EC, Falk JL, Fein IA et al (1983) Fluid resuscitation in circulatory shock: a compar-ison of the cardio-respiratory effects of albumin, hetastarch, and saline solutions in patients with hypovolemic and septic shock. Crit Care Med 11:839-850

46. Foglia RP, Lazar HL, Steed DL et al (1978) Iatrogenic myocardial edema with crystalloid primes: effects on left ventricular compliance, performance and perfusion. Surg Forum 29:312-315

47. Hoeft A et al (1991) Priming of cardiopulmonary bypass with human albumin or Ringer's Lac-tate: effect on colloiosmotic pressure and extravascular lung water. Br J Anesth 66:73-80

48. Sade RM, Stroud MR, Crawford FA Jr et al (1985) A prospective randomized study of hy-droxyethyl starch, albumin, and lactated Ringer's solution as priming fluid for cardiopulmonary bypass. The Journal of Thoracic and Cardiovascular Surgery 89:713-722

49. Gallandat Huet RC, Siemons AW, Baus D et al (2000) A novel hydroxyethyl starch (Voluven) for effective perioperative plasma volume substitution in cardiac surgery. Can J Anaesth 47:1207–1215

50. Haisch G, Boldt J, Krebs C et al (2001) Influence of a new hydroxyethylstarch preparation (HES 130/0.4) on coagulation in cardiac surgical patients. J Cardiothorac Vasc Anesth 15:316–321

51. American Thoracic Society Consensus Statement (2004) Evidence-based colloid use in the critically ill. Am J Respir Crit Care Med1247–1259

52. Groeneveld ABJ, Navickis RJ, Wilkes MM (2011) Update on the comparative safety of col-loids: a systematic review of clinical studies. Ann Surg 253:470–483

53. Hartog CS, Bauer M, Reinhart K (2011) The efficacy and safety of colloid resuscitation in the critically Ill. Anesth Analg 112:156 –64

54. Dellinger RP et al (2008) Surviving Sepsis Campaign: international guidelines for manage-ment of severe sepsis and septic shock: 2008. Crit Care Med 36:296-327

55. Bratton SL et al (2007) Guidelines for the management of severe traumatic brain injury. II. Hyperosmolar therapy. J Neurotrauma 24(suppl1):S14-20

56. Patanwala AE et al (2010) Use of hypertonic saline injection in trauma. Am J Health Syst Pharm 67:1920-8

57. Cotton BA et al (2009) Guidelines for prehospital fluid resuscitation in the injured patient. J Trauma 67:389-402

58. Tam N et al. American Burn Association (2008) American Burn Association practice guide-lines burn shock resuscitation. J Burn Care Res 29:257-66

59. Vlachou E et al (2010 Nov) Hydroxyethylstarch supplementation in burn resuscitation—a prospective randomised controlled trial. Burns 36:984-91

60. Su¨mpelmann R, Becke K, Crean P et al (2011) European consensus statement for intraoper-ative fluid therapy in children. Eur J Anaesthesiol 28:637–639

61. Haas T, Preinreich A, Oswald E et al (2007) Innerhofer Effects of albumin 5% and artificial colloids on clot formation in small infants) Anaesthesia 62:1000-7

62. Suempelmann R, Witt L, Brütt M et al (2010) Changes in acid-base, electrolyte and hemoglobin concentrations during infusion of hydroxyethyl starch 130/0.42/6:1 in normal saline or in balanced electrolyte solution in children. Paediatr Anaesth 20:100-4. Epub

63. Bailey AG, McNaull PP, Jooste E, Tuchman JB (2010) Perioperative crystalloid and colloid fluid management in children: where are we and how did we get here? Anesth Analg 110:375-390

64. Moritz M, Ayus JC (2010) Water water everywhere: standardizing postoperative fluid therapy with 0.9% normal saline. Anesth Analg 110:293–5

65. Montañana PA, Modesto i Alapont V, Ocón AP et al (2008) The use of isotonic fluid as maintenance therapy prevents iatrogenic hyponatremia in pediatrics: a randomized, controlled open study. Pediatr Crit Care Med 9:589–97

66. Neville KA, Sandeman DJ, Rubinstein A et al (2010) Prevention of hyponatremia during maintenance intravenous fluid administration: a prospective randomized study of fluid type versus fluid rate. J Pediatr 156:313–9

67. Waters J, Gottlieb A, Schoenwald P (2001) Normal saline versus lactated Ringer's solution for intra-operative fluid management in patients undergoing abdominal aortic aneurysm repair: an outcome study. Anesth Analg 93:817–22

68. Houghton J, Wilton N (2011) Choice of isotonic perioperative fluid in children. Anesth Analg 112:246–7; Roth JV. Pediatric postoperative fluid therapy: avoiding hyponatremia

69. Harrison MJG (1989) Influence of haematocrit in the cerebral circulation. Cerebrovasc Brain Metabol Rev 1:55-67

70. Hudak ML, Koehler RC, Rosenberg AA et al (1986) Effect of hematocrit on cerebral blood flow. Am J Physiol 251:H63-70

71. Todd MM, Wu B, Warner DS (1994) The hemispheric cerebrovascular response to hemodilution is attenuated by a focal cryogenic brain injury. JNeurotrauma 11:149-60

72. Tommasino C, Ravussin P (1994) Oncotic pressure and hemodilution. Ann Fran Anesth Reanim 13:62-7

73. DK, Ryu KH, Hindman BJ et al (1996) Marked hemodilution increases neurologic injury after focal cerebral ischemia in rabbits. Anesth Analg 82:61-7

74. Tommasino C (2002) Fluids and the neurosurgical patient. Anesthesiology Clin N Am 20:329-346

75. Shenkin HA, Benzier HO, Bouzarth W (1976) Restricted fluid intake: rational management of the neurosurgical patient. J Neurosurg 45:432- 6

76. Atrash HK, Koonin LM, Lawson HW et al (1990) Maternal mortality in the United States, 1979 - 1986. Obstet Gynecol 76:1055

77. Kamani AA, McMorland GH, Wadsworth LD (1988) Utilization of red blood cell transfusion in an obstetric setting. Am J Obstet Gynecol 159:1177

78. Kapholz H (1990) Blood transfusion in contemporary obstetric practice. Obstet Gynecol 75:940

79. Van der Linden P, Ickx BE (2006) The effects of colloid solutions on hemostasis. Can J Anaesth 53(6 Suppl):S30–S39

80. Finfer S, Bellomo R, Boyce N et al (2004) A comparison of albumin and saline for fluid resuscitation in the intensive care unit. N Engl J Med 350:2247–2256

81. Boldt J (2007) The balanced concept of fluid resuscitation. Br J Anaesth 99:312-315

82. Mion G, Rüttimann M (1997) Loading with hypertonic saline solution during pregnancy toxemia. Ann Fr Anesth Reanim 16:1046-1047

83. Clark SL, Greenspoon JS, Aldahl D et al (1986) Severe preeclampsia with persistent oliguria: Management of hemodynamic subsets. Am J Obstet Gynecol 154:490

84. Kapholz H (1990) Blood transfusion in contemporary obstetric practice. Obstet Gynecol 75:940

85. Seymour DG, Henschke PJ, Cape RD, Campbell AJ (1980) Acute confusional states and dementia in the elderly: the roles of dehydration/volume depletion, physical illness and age. Age Ageing 9:137–146

86. Bruera E, Franco JJ, Maltoni M, Watanabe S, Suarez-Almazor M (1995) Changing patterns of agitated impaired mental status in patients with advanced cancer: association with cognitive monitoring, hydration, and opioid rotation. J Pain Symptom Manage 10:287–291

87. Inouye SK, Bogardus ST Jr, Charpentier PA et al (1999) A multicomponent intervention to prevent delirium in hospitalized older patients. N Engl J Med 340:669–676
88. Wildiers H, Menten J (2002) Death rattle: prevalence, prevention and treatment. J Pain Symptom Manage 23:310–7
89. Dalal S, Bruera E (2004) Dehydration in cancer patients: to treat or not to treat. J Support Oncol 2:467–487
90. Ellershaw JE, Sutcliffe JM, Saunders CM (1995) Dehydration and the dying patient. Journal of pain and symptom management 10:192–197
91. Dunlop RJ, Ellershaw JE, Baines MJ, Sykes N, Saunders CM (1995) On withholding nutrition and hydration in the terminally ill: has palliative medicine gone too far? A reply Journal of medical ethics 21:141-143
92. Van Hulst RA, Klein J, Lachmann B (2003) Gas embolism: pathophysiology and treatment. Clin Physiol Funct Imaging 23:237-46
93. Guidet B (2010) A balanced view of balanced solutions. Crit Care 14:325
94. Grocott MPW (2005) Perioperative fluid management and clinical outcomes in adults. Anesth Analg 100:1093-106

Printed in August 2012